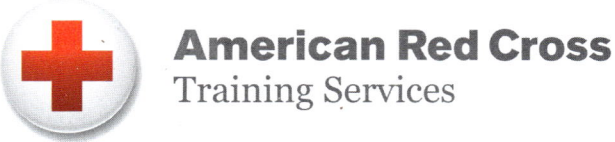

American Red Cross
First Aid
CPR
AED

Participant's Manual

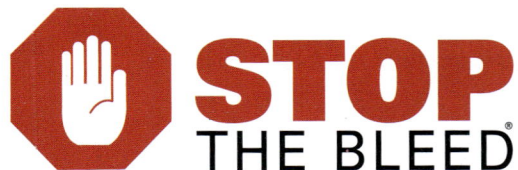

DoD recommends the use of CoTCCC approved tourniquets.

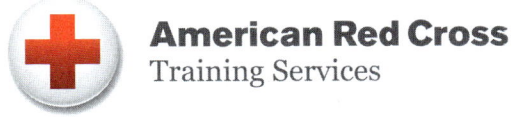

This Participant's Manual is part of the American Red Cross First Aid/CPR/AED program. The emergency care procedures outlined in the program materials reflect the standard of knowledge and accepted emergency practices in the United States at the time this manual was published. It is the reader's responsibility to stay informed of changes in emergency care procedures.

PLEASE READ THE FOLLOWING TERMS AND CONDITIONS (the "Terms and Conditions") BEFORE AGREEING TO ACCESS, USE OR DOWNLOAD THE FOLLOWING AMERICAN NATIONAL RED CROSS MATERIALS. BY PURCHASING, DOWNLOADING, OR OTHERWISE USING OR ACCESSING THE MATERIALS, YOU ACKNOWLEDGE AND HEREBY AGREE TO BE LEGALLY BOUND BY BOTH THESE TERMS AND CONDITIONS AND THE AMERICAN NATIONAL RED CROSS TERMS OF USE (AVAILABLE AT redcross.org/terms-of-use). YOU AGREE THAT THE INCLUDED COURSE MATERIALS ARE PROVIDED "AS IS" AND WITHOUT WARRANTIES OF ANY KIND, AND THAT **ANY ACCESS TO OR USE OF THESE COURSE MATERIALS IS AT YOUR OWN RISK.**

The following materials (including downloadable electronic materials, as applicable) including all content, graphics, images and logos, are copyrighted by, and the exclusive property of, The American National Red Cross ("Red Cross"). Unless otherwise indicated in writing by the Red Cross, the Red Cross grants you ("Recipient") the limited right to download, print, photocopy and use the electronic materials only for use in conjunction with teaching or preparing to teach a Red Cross course by individuals or entities expressly authorized by the Red Cross, subject to the following restrictions:

- The Recipient is prohibited from creating new electronic versions of the materials.
- The Recipient is prohibited from revising, altering, adapting or modifying the materials, which includes removing, altering or covering any copyright notices, Red Cross marks, logos or other proprietary notices placed or embedded in the materials.
- The Recipient is prohibited from creating any derivative works incorporating, in part or in whole, the content of the materials.
- The Recipient is prohibited from downloading the materials, or any part of the materials, and putting them on Recipient's own website or any other third-party website without advance written permission of the Red Cross.
- The Recipient is prohibited from removing these Terms and Conditions in otherwise-permitted copies, and is likewise prohibited from making any additional representations or warranties relating to the materials.

Any rights not expressly granted herein are reserved by the Red Cross. The Red Cross does not permit its materials to be reproduced or published without advance written permission from the Red Cross. To request permission to reproduce or publish Red Cross materials, please submit your written request to The American National Red Cross by going to the Contact Us page on redcross.org and filling out the General Inquiry Form.

Copyright © 2011, 2016, 2021 by The American National Red Cross. ALL RIGHTS RESERVED.

The Red Cross emblem and the American Red Cross® name and logos are trademarks of The American National Red Cross and protected by various national statutes.

Printed in the United States of America
ISBN: 978-1-7367447-8-9

Science and Technical Content

The scientific content and evidence within the American Red Cross First Aid/CPR/AED course is consistent with the *American Red Cross Focused Updates and Guidelines 2020* and the most current science and treatment recommendations from:

- The International Liaison Committee on Resuscitation (ILCOR)
- The International Federation of Red Cross and Red Crescent Societies
- The Policy Statements, Evidence Reviews and Guidelines of:
  - American Academy of Pediatrics (AAP)
  - American College of Emergency Physicians (ACEP)
  - American College of Obstetrics and Gynecology (ACOG)
  - American College of Surgeons (ACS)
  - Committee on Tactical Combat Casualty Care (CoTCCC)
  - Obstetric Life Support™ (OBLS)
  - Society of Critical Care Medicine (SCCM) and the American College of Critical Care Medicine (ACCM)
  - Surviving Sepsis Campaign (SSC)

Guidance for this course was provided by the American Red Cross Scientific Advisory Council, a panel of 60+ nationally and internationally recognized experts from a variety of medical, nursing, EMS, advanced practice, allied health, scientific, educational and academic disciplines. Members of the Scientific Advisory Council have a broad range of professional specialties including resuscitation, emergency medicine, critical care, obstetrics, pediatrics, anesthesia, cardiology, surgery, trauma, toxicology, pharmacology, education, sports medicine, occupational health, public health and emergency preparedness. This gives the Scientific Advisory Council the important advantage of broad, multidisciplinary expertise in evaluating existing and new assessment methodologies, technologies, therapies and procedures—and the educational methods to teach them.

More information on the science of the course content can be found at the following websites:

- ilcor.org
- redcross.org/science

Dedication

This program is dedicated to the thousands of employees and volunteers of the American Red Cross who contribute their time and talent to supporting and teaching lifesaving skills worldwide and to the thousands of course participants who have decided to be prepared to take action when an emergency strikes.

Acknowledgments

Many individuals shared in the development of the American Red Cross Basic Life Support program in various technical, editorial, creative and supportive ways. Their commitment to excellence made this manual possible.

American Red Cross Scientific Advisory Council

We would like to extend our gratitude to the following members of the American Red Cross Scientific Advisory Council for their guidance and review of this program:

David Markenson, MD, MBA, FCCM, FAAP, FACEP, FACHE
Scientific Advisory Council Co-Chair
Chief Medical Officer, American Red Cross

E. M. "Nici" Singletary, MD, FACEP
Scientific Advisory Council Co-Chair
Professor, Department of Emergency Medicine
University of Virginia

Aquatics Subcouncil

Peter G. Wernicki, MD, FAAOS
Aquatics Subcouncil Chair
Orthopedic Surgeon, Pro Sports
Vero Beach, Florida
Assistant Clinical Professor of Orthopedic Surgery
Florida State University College of Medicine

William Dominic Ramos, MS, PhD
Aquatics Subcouncil Vice Chair
Indiana University
Bloomington, Indiana

Angela K. Beale-Tawfeeq, PhD
Chair Associate Professor
Department of STEAM Education
College of Education, Rowan University
Glassboro, New Jersey

Jodi Jensen, PhD
Assistant Professor and Director of Aquatics
Hampton University
Hampton, Virginia

Stephen J. Langendorfer, PhD
Bowling Green, Ohio

Bridget L. McKinney, PhD(h), MS, BS
District Supervisor, Miami Dade PSS
PSWAP-Mentoring and Swim Organization, Inc.

Linda Quan, MD
Bellevue, Washington

Kevin M. Ryan, MD
Assistant Professor of Emergency Medicine
Boston University School of Medicine
Associate Medical Director, Boston EMS
Boston, Massachusetts

Andrew Schmidt, DO, MPH
Assistant Professor
Department of Emergency Medicine
University of Florida College
of Medicine—Jacksonville
Jacksonville, Florida

Leslie K. White, BRec
Supervisor—Citizen Services (Access 311)
Department of Community Services
City of St. John's
Newfoundland and Labrador, Canada

Education Subcouncil

Jeffrey L. Pellegrino, PhD, MPH, EMT-B/FF, EMS-I
Education Subcouncil Chair
Assistant Professor of Emergency Management and Homeland Security
University of Akron
Akron, Ohio

Nicholas Asselin, DO, MS
Education Subcouncil Vice Chair
Department of Emergency Medicine Division of EMS
Alpert Medical School of Brown University
LifePACT Critical Care Transport
Providence, Rhode Island

Rita V. Burke, PhD, MPH
Department of Preventive Medicine
University of Southern California
Los Angeles, California

Brian Miller, MS, MSEd, MEd, CHES
Program Director, Health Sciences
Murphy Deming College of Health Sciences
Chair, Institutional Review Board
Mary Baldwin University
Fishersville, Virginia

Gamze Ozogul, PhD
Instructional Systems and Technology Department
School of Education, Indiana University
Bloomington, Indiana

Thomas E. Sather, Ed.D, MS, MSS, CAsP, CDR, MSC, USN
Branch Chief, Training Operations
Defense Health Agency Life Support Training Manager
Assistant Professor, Uniformed Services University of the Health Sciences
Education and Training, Military Medical Treatment Facility Operations Division
J-7 Education and Training Directorate
Defense Health Agency (DHA)
Falls Church, Virginia

First Aid Subcouncil

Nathan P. Charlton, MD
First Aid Subcouncil Chair
Associate Professor
Department of Emergency Medicine
University of Virginia Health System
Charlottesville, Virginia

S. Robert Seitz, MEd, RN, NRP
First Aid Subcouncil Vice Chair
Center of Emergency Medicine
University of Pittsburgh
Pittsburgh, Pennsylvania

David C. Berry, PhD, MHA, AT, ATC, ATRIC, CKTP
Professor/Professional Athletic Training Program Director
Department of Kinesiology
College of Health and Human Services Saginaw Valley State University
University Center, Michigan

Adelita G. Cantu, PhD, RN
Associate Professor, UT Health San Antonio School of Nursing
San Antonio, Texas

Jestin Carlson, MD, MS, FACEP
St. Vincent Hospital
Erie, Pennsylvania

Sarita A. Chung, MD, FAAP
Department of Medicine
Division of Emergency Medicine
Children's Hospital
Boston, Massachusetts

Theodore John Gaensbauer, MD, FAPA, FAACAP
Clinical Professor, Department of Psychiatry
University of Colorado Health Sciences Center
Denver, Colorado

Craig Goolsby, MD, MEd, FACEP
Professor and Vice Chair, Department of Military and Emergency Medicine
Science Director, National Center for Disaster Medicine and Public Health
Uniformed Services University
Bethesda, Maryland

Elizabeth Kennedy Hewett, MD
Assistant Professor of Pediatrics
University of Pittsburgh School of Medicine Faculty Physician
UPMC Children's Hospital of Pittsburgh
Pittsburgh, Pennsylvania

Morgan Hillier, MD, BSc, BKin, FRCPC, MSc
Staff Emergency Physician
Sunnybrook Health Sciences Centre Toronto
Medical Director
Toronto Fire Services
Toronto, Ontario, Canada

Angela Holian, PharmD, BCPS
Clinical Pharmacy Specialist, Emergency Medicine, Department of Pharmacy
UVA Health System
Charlottesville, Virginia

Deanna Colburn Hostler, DPT, PhD, CCS
Clinical Assistant Professor
Department of Rehabilitation Sciences
University at Buffalo
Buffalo, New York

Robin M. Ikeda, MD, MPH, RADM, USPHS
Associate Director for Policy and Strategy Office of the Director
Centers for Disease Control and Prevention
Atlanta, Georgia

Amy Kule, MD, FACEP
Loyola University Medical Center
Maywood, Illinois

Matthew J. Levy, DO, MSc, FACEP, FAEMS, NRP
Johns Hopkins University School of Medicine
Department of Emergency Medicine
Baltimore, Maryland
Howard County Government
Department of Fire and Rescue Services
Columbia, Maryland

Edward J. McManus, MD
I.D. Care, Inc./I.D. Associates, P.A.
Hillsborough, New Jersey

Nathaniel McQuay, Jr, MD
Chief, Acute Care Surgery
University Hospitals Cleveland Medical Center
Cleveland, Ohio

Aaron M. Orkin, MD, MSc, MPH, PhD(c), CCFP(EM), FRCPC
Assistant Professor
Department of Family and Community Medicine
University of Toronto
Emergency Physician
St. Joseph's Health Centre and Humber River Hospital
Toronto, Ontario, Canada

Amita Sudhir, MD
Associate Professor
University of Virginia
Department of Emergency Medicine

Jeffrey S. Upperman, MD
Professor of Surgery and Surgeon-in-Chief
Vanderbilt Children's Hospital
Nashville, Tennessee

Preparedness and Health Subcouncil

Dr. Steven J. Jensen, DPPD
Preparedness and Health Subcouncil Chair
Advisor, Emergency Management
Lecturer
California State University at Long Beach
Long Beach, California

James A. Judge II, BPA, CEM, FPEM EMT-P
Preparedness and Health Subcouncil Vice Chair
Emergency Management Director
Volusia County Department of Public Protection
Daytona Beach, Florida

Lauren M. Sauer, MS
Assistant Professor of Emergency Medicine
Department of Emergency Medicine
Johns Hopkins Medical Institutions
Baltimore, Maryland

Samir K. Sinha, MD, DPhil, FRCPC, AGSF
Mount Sinai Hospital
Toronto, Ontario, Canada

Jacqueline Snelling, MS
Arlington, Virginia

Resuscitation Subcouncil

Joseph W. Rossano, MD
Resuscitation Subcouncil Chair
Chief, Division of Cardiology
Co-Executive Director of the Cardiac Center
Jennifer Terker Endowed Chair in Pediatric Cardiology
Associate Professor of Pediatrics at the Children's Hospital of Philadelphia
and the Perelman School of Medicine at the University of Pennsylvania
Philadelphia, Pennsylvania

Michael G. Millin, MD, MPH, FACEP, FAEMS
Resuscitation Subcouncil Vice Chair
Department of Emergency Medicine
Johns Hopkins University School of Medicine
Baltimore, Maryland
Medical Director
Maryland and Mid-Atlantic Wilderness Rescue Squad/Austere Medical Professionals

Bruce J. Barnhart, MSN, RN, CEP
Senior Program Manager
Arizona Emergency Medicine Research Center
The University of Arizona College of Medicine-Phoenix
Phoenix, Arizona

Lynn Boyle, MSN, RN, CCRN
Nurse Manager-PICU
The Children's Hospital of Philadelphia
Philadelphia, Pennsylvania

Richard N. Bradley, MD
147th Medical Group
Houston, Texas

Meredith Gibbons, MSN, CPNP
Pediatric Nurse Practitioner
Columbia University Medical Center
New York, New York

Wendell E. Jones, MD, MBA, CPE, FACP
Chief Medical Officer
Veteran's Integrated Service, Network 17
Arlington, Texas

Andrew MacPherson, MD, CCFP-EM, FCFP
Clinical Professor
Department of Emergency Medicine
University of British Columbia
Royal Jubilee Hospital
Victoria, British Columbia, Canada

Bryan F. McNally, MD, MPH
Professor, Emergency Medicine
Department of Emergency Medicine
Emory University School of Medicine
Atlanta, Georgia

Ira Nemeth, MD
Medical Director
Ben Taub Emergency Department
Senior Faculty, Baylor College of Medicine
Houston, Texas

Joshua M. Tobin, MD
Adjunct Clinical Associate Professor
Stanford University Medical Center
Stanford, California

Bryan M. White, Lt Col, USAF, MC MD, FACC, FASE, RPVI
Las Vegas, Nevada

Lynn White, MS, FAEMS
National Director of Clinical Practice, Global Medical Response

Content Direction

The development of this program would not have been possible without the leadership, valuable insights and dedication of the subject matter experts, who generously shared their time to ensure the highest quality program:

David Markenson, MD, MBA, FCCM, FAAP, FACEP, FACHE
Scientific Advisory Council Co-Chair
Chief Medical Officer, American Red Cross

Edward J. McManus, MD
I.D. Care, Inc./I.D. Associates, P.A.
Hillsborough, New Jersey

E. M. "Nici" Singletary, MD, FACEP
Scientific Advisory Council Co-Chair
Professor, Department of Emergency Medicine
University of Virginia

Joseph W. Rossano, MD
Resuscitation Subcouncil Chair
Chief, Division of Cardiology
Co-Executive Director of the Cardiac Center
Jennifer Terker Endowed Chair in Pediatric Cardiology
Associate Professor of Pediatrics at the Children's Hospital of Philadelphia and the Perelman School of Medicine at the University of Pennsylvania
Philadelphia, Pennsylvania

Nathan P. Charlton, MD
First Aid Subcouncil Chair
Associate Professor
Department of Emergency Medicine
University of Virginia Health System
Charlottesville, Virginia

S. Robert Seitz, MEd, RN, NRP
First Aid Subcouncil Vice Chair
Center of Emergency Medicine
University of Pittsburgh
Pittsburgh, Pennsylvania

David C. Berry, PhD, MHA, AT, ATC, ATRIC, CKTP
Professor/Professional Athletic Training Program Director
Department of Kinesiology
College of Health and Human Services Saginaw Valley State University
University Center, Michigan

Matthew J. Levy, DO, MSc, FACEP, FAEMS, NRP
Johns Hopkins University School of Medicine
Department of Emergency Medicine
Baltimore, Maryland
Howard County Government
Department of Fire and Rescue Services
Columbia, Maryland

Michael G. Millin, MD, MPH, FACEP, FAEMS
Resuscitation Subcouncil Vice Chair
Department of Emergency Medicine
Johns Hopkins University School of Medicine
Baltimore, Maryland
Medical Director
Maryland and Mid-Atlantic Wilderness Rescue Squad/Austere Medical Professionals

Wendell E. Jones, MD, MBA, CPE, FACP
Chief Medical Officer
Veteran's Integrated Service, Network 17
Arlington, Texas

Lynn White, MS, FAEMS
National Director of Clinical Practice, Global Medical Response

Program Development

Special thanks to the program development team for their expertise and mix of patience and persistence to bring this program through to completion: Dominick Tolli, Danielle DiPalma, Laura Scott, Sarah Kyle, Nichole Steffens, Alyssa Dreikorn, Stephanie Shook, Whitney Wilson, Katie Loizou, Jennifer Surich, Maureen Pancza, Maureen Schultz, Anna Pruett, Sealworks, FreshFly, Surround Mix Group and The StayWell Company.

Supporting Organizations

Special thanks to Clifton Salas, Deb Gress, Nancy Tobin and the staff of the Philadelphia American Red Cross for accommodating the Red Cross and coordinating resources for this program's video production.

Table of Contents

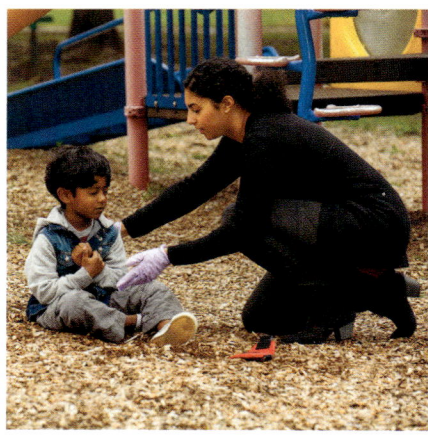
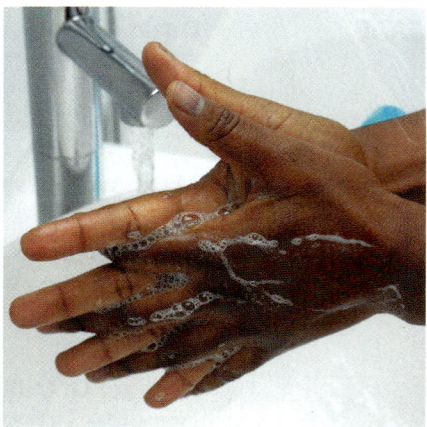
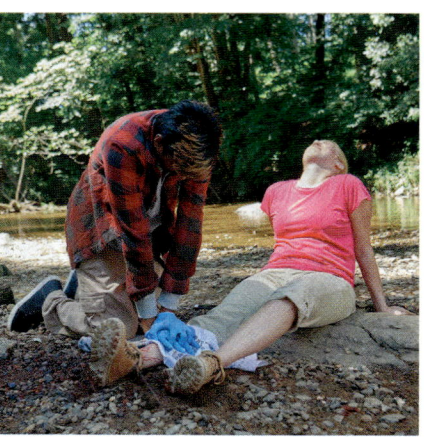

Part 1
First Aid Basics | 1

CHAPTER 1: FIRST AID, CPR, AED FOUNDATIONS

Lowering the Risk for Infection	**4**
Preparing for Emergencies	**8**
Your Role in the EMS System	**10**
Recognizing That an Emergency Exists and Gaining Confidence to Take Action	**11**
Emergency Action Steps	**12**

PUTTING IT ALL TOGETHER 1-1

Checking an Injured or Ill Person **25**

Part 2
First Aid for Cardiac Arrest and Choking | 27

CHAPTER 2: ADULT CPR AND AED

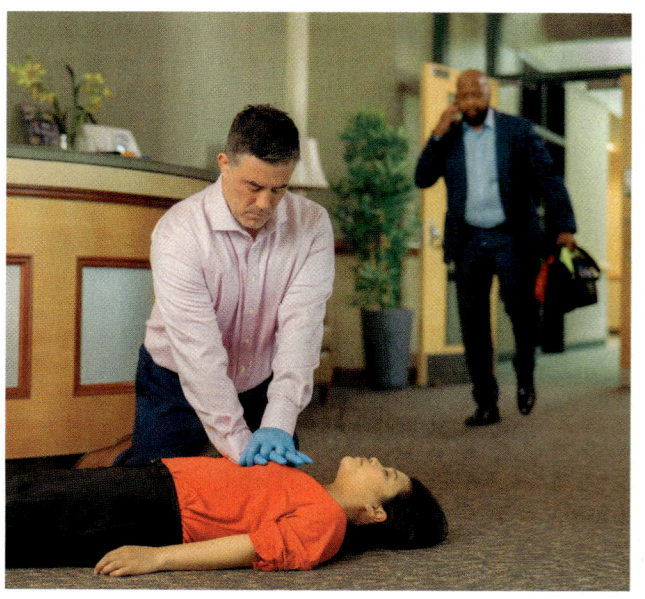

Recognizing Cardiac Arrest	**30**
Components of High-Quality CPR	**31**
Giving CPR	**32**
CPR Special Considerations	**38**
Using an AED	**38**

PUTTING IT ALL TOGETHER 2-1

Giving CPR and Using an AED for an Adult **44**

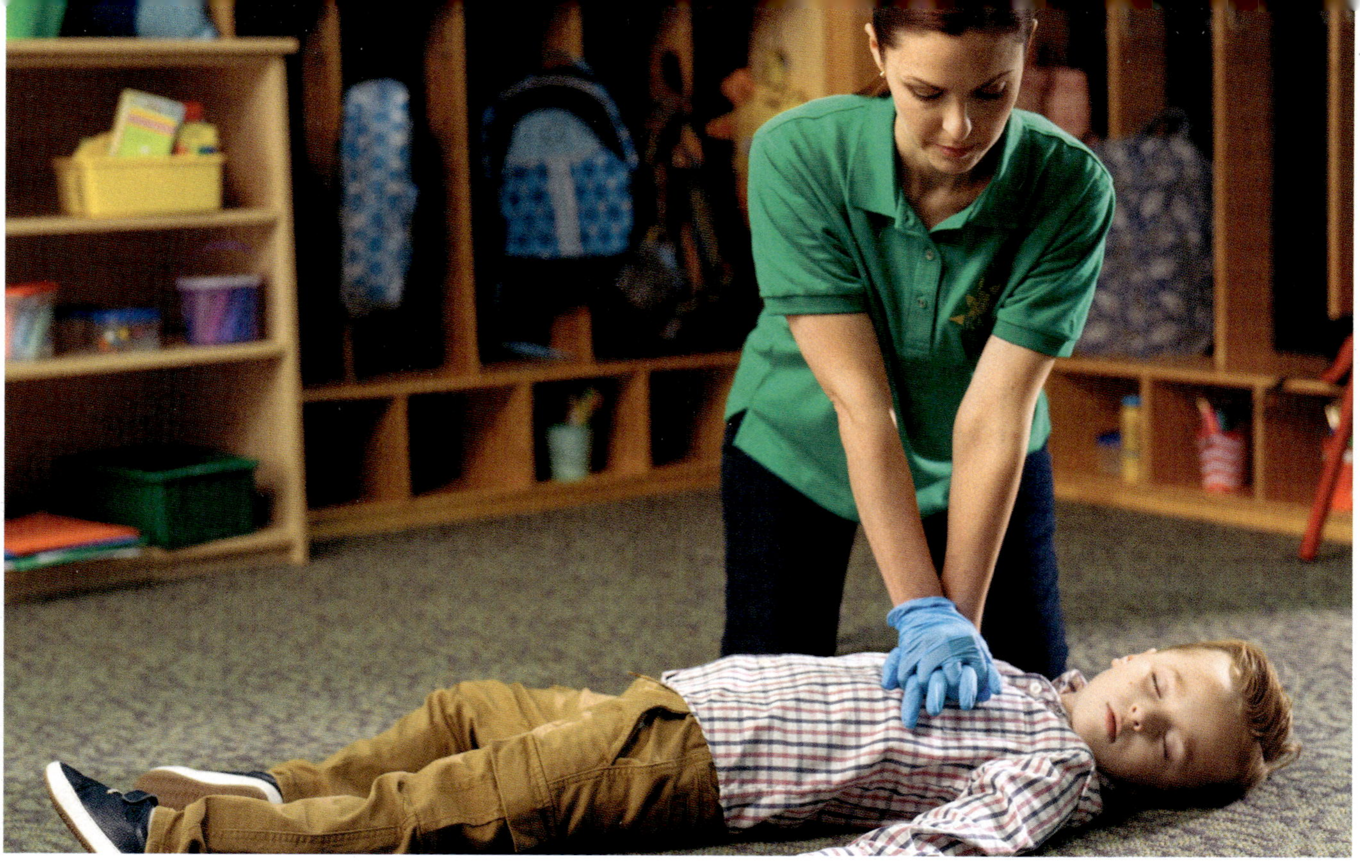

CHAPTER 3: PEDIATRIC CPR AND AED

Defining Children and Infants **50**
Pediatric Cardiac Chain of Survival **50**
Components of High-Quality CPR. **51**
CPR and AED Differences Among Adults,
    Children and Infants **51**

PUTTING IT ALL TOGETHER 3-1

Giving CPR and Using an AED for a Child **57**

PUTTING IT ALL TOGETHER 3-2

Giving CPR and Using an AED for an Infant. **61**

CHAPTER 4: CHOKING

Risk Factors for Choking. **66**
Recognizing Choking **66**
Giving First Aid Care for an Adult or Child
    Who Is Choking **67**
Giving First Aid Care for an Infant Who Is Choking . . . **70**

PUTTING IT ALL TOGETHER 4-1

Caring for an Adult or Child Who Is Choking. **72**

PUTTING IT ALL TOGETHER 4-2

Caring for an Infant Who Is Choking **74**

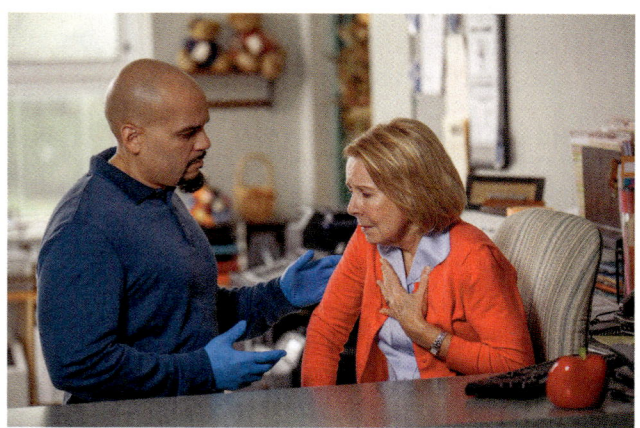

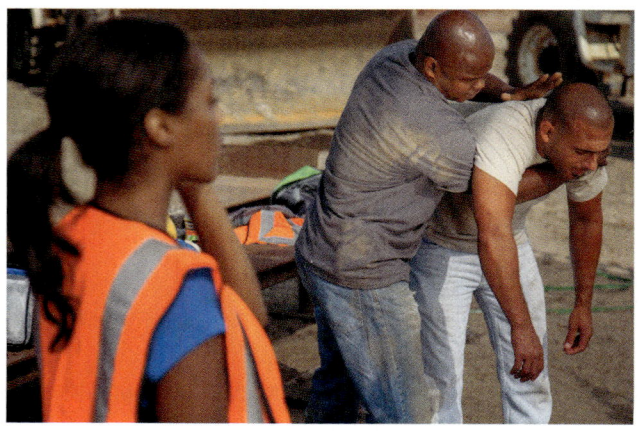

American Red Cross | Table of Contents   **ix**

Part 3
First Aid for Sudden Illnesses and Injuries | 77

CHAPTER 5: SUDDEN ILLNESS

General Approach to Sudden Illness	80
Heart Attack	82
Respiratory Distress	84
Asthma and Asthma Attack	86
Allergic Reactions and Anaphylaxis	88
Opioid Overdose	90
Diabetic Emergencies	92
Seizures	94
Shock	95
Stroke	96
Fainting	97
Sickle Cell Crisis and Acute Chest Syndrome	98
Fever in Young Children and Infants	99
Vomiting, Diarrhea and Dehydration in Young Children and Infants	100

PUTTING IT ALL TOGETHER 5-1

Assisting with an Asthma Inhaler for a Person Experiencing an Asthma Attack ... 101

PUTTING IT ALL TOGETHER 5-2

Assisting with an Epinephrine Auto-Injector for a Person Experiencing Anaphylaxis ... 103

CHAPTER 6: WOUNDS AND BLEEDING

Open Wounds and External Bleeding	106
Life-Threatening Internal Bleeding	114
Minor Closed Wounds	114

PUTTING IT ALL TOGETHER 6-1

Using Direct Pressure to Control Life-Threatening Bleeding ... 116

PUTTING IT ALL TOGETHER 6-2

Using Direct Pressure and a Windlass Rod Tourniquet to Control Life-Threatening Bleeding ... 119

CHAPTER 7: INJURIES AND ENVIRONMENTAL EMERGENCIES

General Approach to Injuries and Environmental Emergencies	124
Injuries	124
Burns	124
Head, Neck and Spinal Injuries	127
Muscle, Bone and Joint Injuries	130
Nose and Mouth Injuries	132
Chest Injuries	133
Abdominal Injuries	135
Pelvic Injuries	135
Environmental Emergencies	136
Heat-Related Illnesses	136
Cold-Related Illnesses and Injuries	138
Poison Exposure	141
Bites and Stings	144
Exposure to Rash-Causing Plants	151
Lightning-Strike Injuries	152

Appendices | 155

APPENDIX A: EMERGENCY MOVES

Emergency Moves ... 157

APPENDIX B: INJURY PREVENTION

Injury Prevention	159
General Strategies for Reducing the Risk for Injury	159
Vehicle Safety	159
Fire Safety	160
Safety at Home	161
Safety at Work	163
Safety at Play	163

APPENDIX C: SKILL PRACTICE SHEETS FOR CORE COURSE

Skill Practice Sheets for Core Course	165
Skill Practice Sheet: Checking a Person Who Appears Unresponsive	166
Skill Practice Sheet: Giving Chest Compressions to Adults	168

Skill Practice Sheet: Giving Breaths to Adults with a Face Shield **169**

Skill Practice Sheet: Giving Breaths to Adults with a Pocket Mask. **170**

Skill Practice Sheet: Giving CPR Cycles to Adults. . . **171**

Skill Practice Sheet: Using an AED for Adults **172**

Skill Practice Sheet: Giving Chest Compressions to Children. **174**

Skill Practice Sheet: Giving Breaths to Children with a Face Shield **176**

Skill Practice Sheet: Giving Breaths to Children with a Pocket Mask. **177**

Skill Practice Sheet: Giving CPR Cycles to Children. **178**

Skill Practice Sheet: Giving CPR Cycles to Infants . . **179**

Skill Practice Sheet: Using an AED for Children and Infants. **180**

Skill Practice Sheet: Giving Back Blows and Abdominal Thrusts to Adults and Children **182**

Skill Practice Sheet: Giving Back Blows and Chest Thrusts to Infants **184**

Skill Practice Sheet: Using Direct Pressure to Control Life-Threatening Bleeding. **186**

APPENDIX D: SKILL PRACTICE SHEETS FOR SKILL BOOSTS

Skill Practice Sheets for Skill Boosts **189**

Skill Practice Sheet: Administering Quick-Relief Medication Using an Inhaler **190**

Skill Practice Sheet: Administering Quick-Relief Medication Using a Nebulizer **191**

Skill Practice Sheet: Administering Using an Auto-Injector . . . .

Skill Practice Sheet: Administering Using a Nasal Spray . . . .

Skill Practice Sheet: Administering Nalo Using a Nasal Atomizer. . . . .

Skill Practice Sheet: Using Direct Pressure Control Life-Threatening Bleeding. **197**

Skill Practice Sheet: Using Direct Pressure and a Windlass Rod Tourniquet to Control Life-Threatening Bleeding. **199**

Skill Practice Sheet: Using Direct Pressure and a Ratcheting Tourniquet to Control Life-Threatening Bleeding. **201**

Skill Practice Sheet: Using Direct Pressure and an Elastic Tourniquet to Control Life-Threatening Bleeding. **203**

Skill Practice Sheet: Wound Packing **205**

Skill Practice Sheet: Applying a Rigid Splint to a Leg. **206**

Skill Practice Sheet: Applying a Sling and Binder . . . **208**

Skill Practice Sheet: Applying a Vacuum Splint to a Leg **210**

Glossary **213**

Sources. **219**

Photography Credits. **221**

Index **225**

PART 1
First Aid Basics

CHAPTER 1: First Aid, CPR, AED Foundations

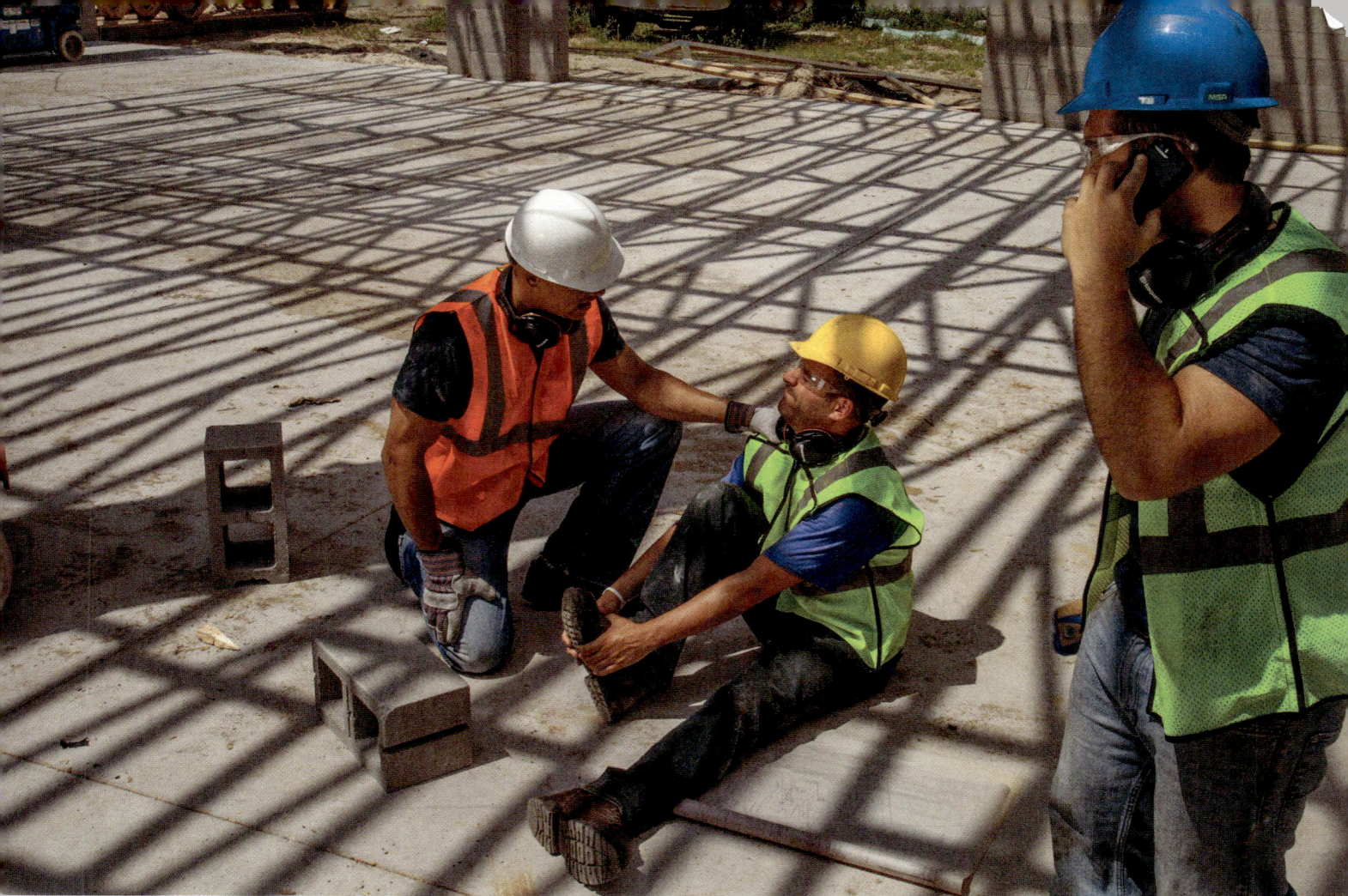

CHAPTER 1
First Aid, CPR, AED Foundations

Being knowledgeable and skilled in providing first aid can help you to make your workplace, home and community a safer place to be. When a person is injured or becomes suddenly ill, your quick action can prevent the injury or illness from worsening, and it may even save the person's life. Although every emergency situation is unique, understanding basic principles of giving first aid care will always serve you well.

Lowering the Risk for Infection

Giving first aid care is a hands-on activity. Though the risk of getting infected when giving first aid care is very low, providing this care can put you in close contact with another person's body fluids (such as saliva, mucus, vomit or blood), which may contain **pathogens** (harmful microorganisms that can cause disease). Pathogens can be spread from person to person through direct or indirect contact. With direct contact, the pathogen is passed through close physical contact between two people (or with droplets). With indirect contact, the pathogen is spread by way of a contaminated surface or object.

Some pathogens that you could be exposed to when providing first aid care pose particular risk because of their long-term effects on your health (Box 1-1).

- **Bloodborne pathogens** are spread when blood or other potentially infectious material from an infected person enters the bloodstream of a person who is not infected. Bloodborne illnesses that are of particular concern include human immunodeficiency virus (HIV) infection and hepatitis B and C. Fortunately, although bloodborne pathogens can cause serious illnesses, they are *not* easily transmitted and are not spread by casual contact. Remember, for infection to occur, an infected person's blood must enter your bloodstream. This could happen through direct or indirect contact with an infected person's blood if it comes in contact with your eyes, the mucous membranes that line your mouth and nose, or an area of broken skin on your body. You could also become infected if you stick yourself with a contaminated needle (a "needlestick injury") or cut yourself with broken glass that has been contaminated with blood.
- **Pathogens transmitted via air:**
  - **Airborne transmission** is infection spread through exposure to infectious respiratory droplets comprised of smaller droplets (usually less than 5 micrometers) that can remain suspended in the air for longer periods of time and can travel greater distances (usually greater than 6 feet). Small particles, like a fine spray or mist, stay suspended in the air longer and travel farther. Examples of illnesses spread by airborne transmission include measles, tuberculosis and chicken pox.
  - **Droplet transmission** is infection spread through exposure to infectious respiratory droplets (i.e., larger particles) that are propelled through the air for short distances due to coughing, sneezing, talking or being

---

Box 1-1 Bloodborne Illnesses and Illnesses Transmitted via Air

Although the risk of catching a disease when giving first aid care is very low, whenever you give care, there is the potential to be exposed to an infectious disease. Of particular concern are diseases that are not easily treated and can have long-term effects on your health, should you become infected. Using personal protective equipment (PPE) significantly reduces your risk for catching an infectious disease.

Bloodborne Illnesses

- **HIV** is a virus that invades and destroys the cells that help us to fight off infections. A person who is infected with HIV may look and feel healthy for many years. However, during this time, the virus is breaking down the person's immune system. Eventually, a person who is infected with HIV may develop acquired immunodeficiency syndrome (AIDS). A person with AIDS is unable to fight off infections that a healthy person would be able to resist or control. The person can die from one of these infections. Although medications have been developed to help slow the progression of HIV infection, currently there is no cure.
- **Hepatitis** is inflammation of the liver, an organ that performs many vital functions for the body. There are many different types and causes of hepatitis. Hepatitis B and hepatitis C are caused by infection with bloodborne viruses. Chronic infection with the viruses that cause hepatitis B or C can lead to liver failure, liver cancer and other serious conditions.

Illnesses Transmitted via Air (Airborne and Droplet Transmission)

- **Tuberculosis** is a bacterial infection of the lungs that is spread through airborne transmission from one person to another. Although tuberculosis primarily affects the lungs, it can also affect the bones, brain, kidneys and other organs. If not treated, tuberculosis can be fatal. Treatment is complex and involves taking many different medications over an extended period of time.
- **Influenza** is a viral illness that is spread when virus-containing droplets are released into the air when an infected person coughs or sneezes. These droplets land on other people's mouths or noses or other surfaces or are inhaled. Symptoms of infection include sudden onset of fever, aches, chills, fatigue, cough and headache. Complications from the flu are common and can lead to serious infections, such as pneumonia. Every year, thousands of people in the United States die from complications of influenza. There is no cure for influenza, and treatment, including antiviral medication, is focused on lessening the severity of symptoms. However, there is an annual vaccine available that is effective in preventing infection and/or reducing the severity of infection if infected.

in close contact with an infected person. Larger particles are heavier and quickly fall to the ground where they can no longer be inhaled and cause infection. Transmission is most likely to occur when someone is close to the infectious person, generally within about 6 feet. An example of illness spread by droplet transmission is influenza.

Limiting Your Exposure to Pathogens

There are two main steps you can take to limit your exposure to pathogens that have the potential to infect you while giving first aid care: wash your hands after giving care (and before, if possible) and use personal protective equipment (PPE). In addition to limiting your own risk for infection, washing your hands and using PPE also can provide protection for the person you are caring for.

Handwashing

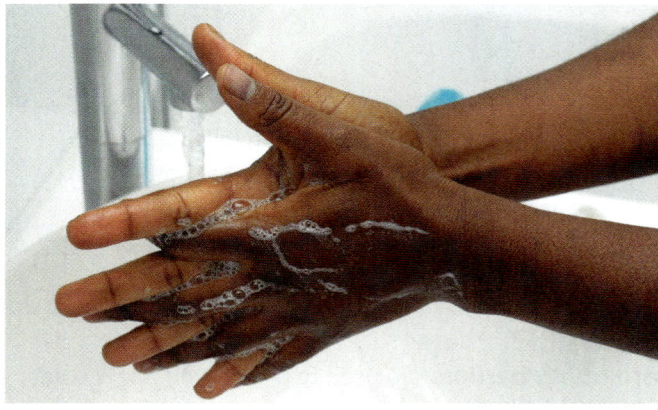

The best approach to lowering the risk for infection is handwashing. Always wash your hands after giving care, and if time allows, wash your hands before giving care. At minimum, hands should be washed:

- Before providing care (if possible).
- After providing care, even if gloves were worn.
- After touching blood or other potentially infectious materials.
- After touching objects or surfaces that could be contaminated with blood or other potentially infectious materials.
- Before putting on and after removing gloves or other PPE.
- Before and after eating and drinking.
- After using the restroom.

Wash your hands thoroughly with soap and warm or cold running water when you have finished giving care, even if you wore disposable gloves. Wash for at least 20 seconds and make sure to cover all surfaces of both hands: the palms and backs of your hands, in between your fingers including the sides of your thumbs and under your fingernails.

If soap and water are not available, you may use an alcohol-based hand sanitizer to decontaminate your hands. When using an alcohol-based hand sanitizer, dispense the recommended amount of product into the palm of one hand. Read the label to determine the correct amount. Rub the gel over all surfaces of your hands and fingers. Continue rubbing your hands until they are dry. This should take about 20 seconds.

Even if you use alcohol-based hand sanitizer, wash your hands with soap and water as soon as you have access to handwashing facilities.

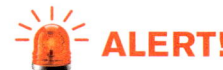 **ALERT!**

Alcohol-based hand sanitizers may not be as effective if your hands are visibly soiled with dirt or body fluids. In addition, although using an alcohol-based hand sanitizer properly will reduce the number of pathogens on your hands, it may not eliminate all pathogens. For these reasons, always wash your hands with soap and water as soon as you can, even if you used an alcohol-based hand sanitizer!

Personal Protective Equipment

Personal protective equipment (PPE) includes barrier devices used to prevent pathogens from contaminating your skin, mucous membranes or clothing. This equipment includes latex-free disposable gloves, gowns, protective eyewear, masks, CPR breathing barriers and shoe covers. PPE can help lower your risk for getting or transmitting an infectious disease when giving care, and you should use PPE whenever possible.

ALERT!

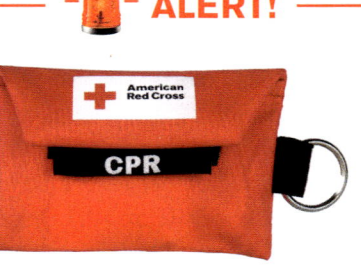

Be prepared by having a first aid and bleeding control kit handy and adequately stocked with PPE. You can also carry a keychain kit containing a pair of latex-free disposable gloves and a breathing barrier so that you always have this equipment readily available.

American Red Cross | First Aid Basics

Latex-Free Disposable Gloves

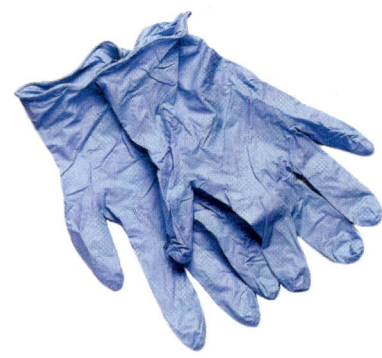

Not all latex-free gloves are impermeable to blood and other potentially infectious materials. It is important to check that the latex-free gloves you are using will not allow blood and other potentially infectious materials to seep through. Nitrile gloves meet this requirement.

Latex-free disposable gloves are meant to be worn once and then discarded. Never clean or reuse disposable gloves. Disposable gloves should fit properly and be free of rips or tears. You should wear latex-free disposable gloves:

- When providing care, especially whenever there is a possibility that you will come in contact with a person's blood or other potentially infectious materials.
- When there is a break in the skin on your own hands. (Cover any cuts, scrapes or sores before putting on the gloves.)
- When you must handle items or surfaces soiled with blood or other potentially infectious materials.

When you are wearing gloves, try to limit how much you touch other surfaces with your gloved hands. Pathogens from your soiled gloves can transfer to other items or surfaces that you touch, putting the next person who handles the item or touches the surface at risk for infection. If possible, remove soiled gloves and replace them with a clean pair before touching other surfaces or equipment in your first aid kit. When you are finished providing care, remove your gloves using proper technique to avoid contaminating your own skin (Box 1-2). Dispose of the gloves properly and wash your hands. Follow facility policies for when gloves need to be disposed in a red biohazard waste bag. When multiple people are in need of care, remove your gloves, wash your hands and replace your gloves with a clean pair before assisting the next person.

If you have gloves, put them on. If available, using gloves is always best. However, sometimes gloves won't be available when a person has a life-threatening injury or illness. In these cases, don't wait until you have gloves to begin providing care. If gloves are not available, you should wash your hands as soon as possible after giving care, and especially after handling blood, and avoid contact with your mouth and eyes. Your risk of infection from HIV and other bloodborne illnesses is very low. In fact, the risk of contracting HIV from infected blood coming into contact with non-intact skin (such as scrapes and lacerations) is less than 0.1 percent. There is no risk of contracting HIV if infected blood comes into contact with intact skin. (Source: CDC https://www.cdc.gov/hai/pdfs/bbp/exp _to_blood.pdf.) Still, if you are exposed to blood, report the exposure incident to EMS personnel or your healthcare provider. (See Handling an Exposure Incident.) Know and follow your employer's guidelines for what PPE to wear and when.

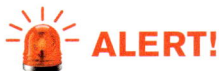 **ALERT!**

Because many people are allergic to latex, the American Red Cross recommends the use of latex-free disposable gloves.

Breathing Barriers

Breathing barriers are used to protect you from contact with saliva and other body fluids, such as blood, as you give breaths. Breathing barriers also protect you from breathing the air that the person exhales. The most basic and portable type of breathing barrier is a **face shield**, a flat piece of thin plastic that you place over the person's face, with the

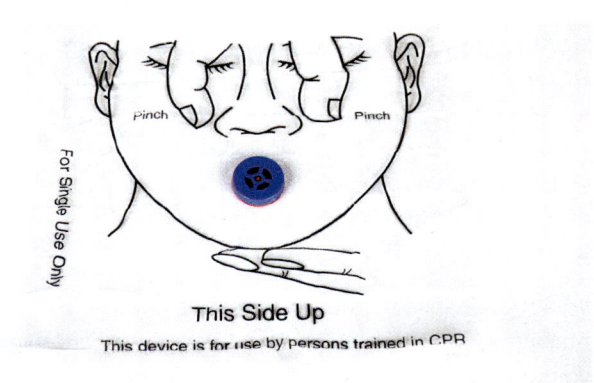

opening over the person's mouth. The opening contains a one-way valve that protects you from coming into contact with the person's body fluids and exhaled air.

A **pocket mask** is a transparent, flexible device that creates a tight seal over the person's nose and mouth to allow you to give breaths without making mouth-to-mouth contact or inhaling exhaled air. A pocket mask is the most common device that can be found with AEDs and first aid kits in public locations. Pocket masks sized specifically for children and infants are available. Always use equipment that is sized appropriately for the injured or ill person.

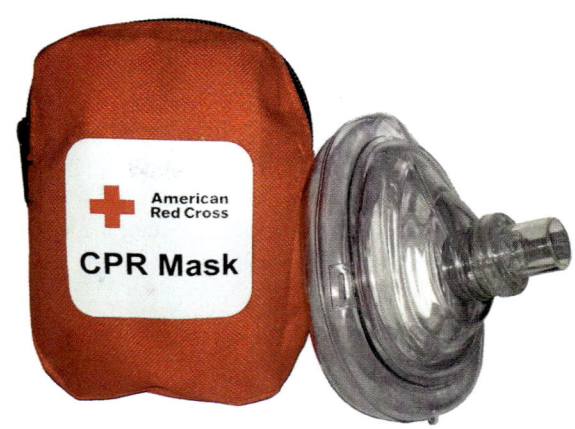

Box 1-2 Removing Latex-Free Disposable Gloves

1. Pinch the palm side of one glove on the outside near your wrist.

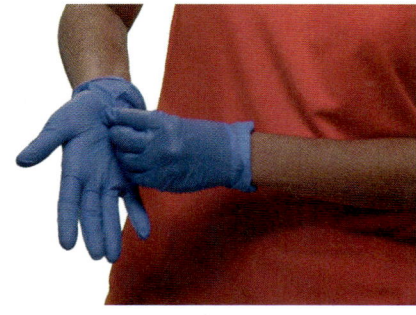

2. Pull the glove toward your fingertips, turning it inside out as you pull it off your hand.

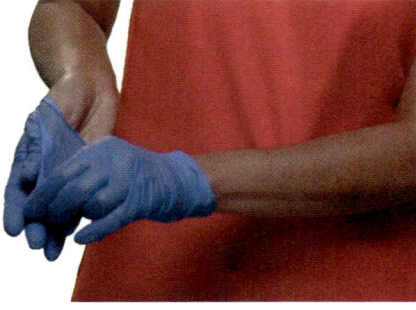

3. Hold the glove in the palm of your other (still-gloved) hand.

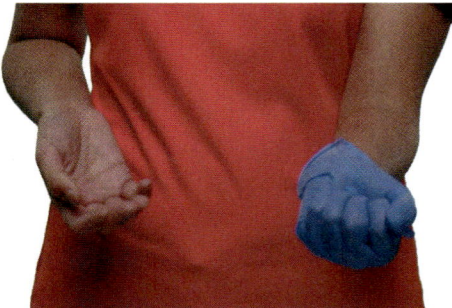

4. Carefully slip two fingers under the wrist of the other glove. Avoid touching the outside of the glove.

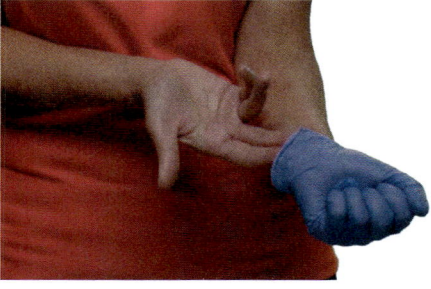

5. Pull the glove toward your fingertips, turning it inside out as you pull it off your hand. The other glove is now contained inside.

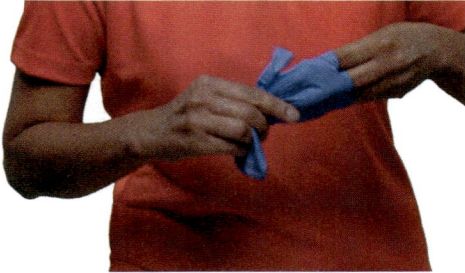

6. Dispose of the gloves properly and wash your hands. (Follow facility policies for when gloves need to be disposed in red biohazard waste bag.)

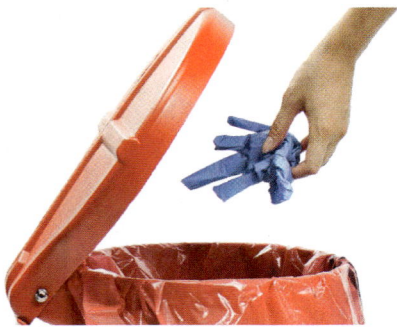

American Red Cross | First Aid Basics 7

Cleaning and Disinfecting Surfaces and Equipment

Reusable equipment and surfaces that have been contaminated by blood or other potentially infectious materials need to be properly cleaned and disinfected before the equipment is put back into service or the area is reopened. Clean and disinfect surfaces and equipment as soon as possible after the incident occurs. Remember to wear appropriate PPE.

If blood or other potentially infectious materials have spilled on the floor or another surface, prevent others from accessing the area. If the spill contains a sharp object (e.g., shards of broken glass), do not pick the object up with your hands. Instead, use tongs or a disposable scoop and scraper to remove and dispose of the object. Clean as per the protocol of the area or facility. If there is not a specific protocol or policy, follow the general approach of wiping up or absorbing the spill using absorbent wipes or a solidifier (a fluid-absorbing powder). After wiping up the spill, you'll need to disinfect the area. Before taking this step, you should first remove the disposable latex-free gloves worn while cleaning the spill, dispose of them and clean your hands. You should then put on a new pair of gloves to protect yourself while using the disinfectant. Flood the area with a freshly mixed disinfectant solution of approximately 1½ cups of bleach to 1 gallon of water (1 part bleach to 9 parts water, or about a 10 percent solution), or use another approved disinfectant product. When using a bleach solution, always ensure good ventilation and wear gloves and eye protection. Let the bleach solution stand on the surface for at least 10 minutes. Then use clean absorbent materials (such as paper towels) to wipe up the disinfectant solution and dry the area. Dispose of all materials used to clean up the blood spill in a labeled biohazard container. If a biohazard container is not available, place the soiled materials in a sealable plastic bag or a plastic container with a lid, seal the plastic bag or container, and dispose of it properly.

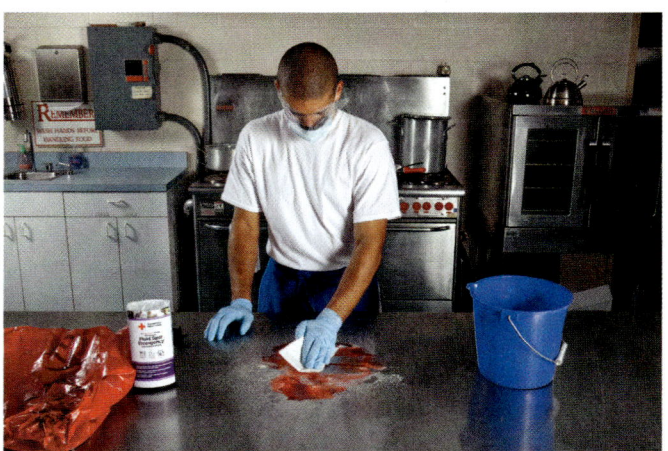

Handling an Exposure Incident

If another person's blood or other potentially infectious material comes into contact (or if you are unsure if it came into contact) with your eyes, the mucous membranes of your mouth or nose, or an opening or break in your skin, or if you experience a needlestick injury, then you have been involved in an exposure incident.

If the exposure incident occurred in a workplace setting, follow your company's exposure control plan for reporting the incident and receiving post-exposure follow-up care.

If the exposure incident occurs outside a workplace setting and no policy is in place, follow these steps. Decontaminate the exposed area. If your skin was exposed, wash the contaminated area with soap and water. For splashes into your mouth or nose, flush the area with water. For splashes into the eyes, irrigate the eyes with water, saline or a sterile irrigant for 15 to 20 minutes. Seek medical care immediately.

Preparing for Emergencies

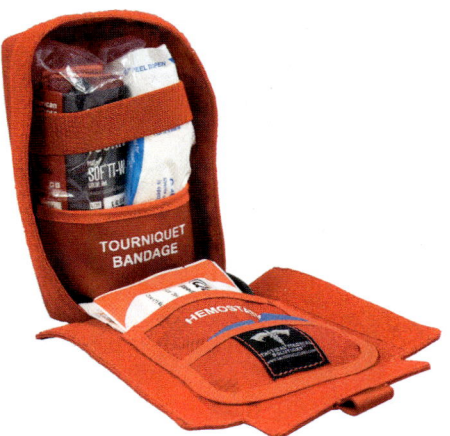

By definition, emergencies are unexpected situations that require immediate action. But by expecting the unexpected and taking general steps to prepare, you can increase the likelihood of a positive outcome should an emergency situation arise.

By reading this manual and participating in an American Red Cross First Aid/CPR/AED course, you have taken an important first step in preparing for emergencies. You will learn the concepts and skills you need to recognize emergency situations and respond appropriately until emergency medical services (EMS) arrives and begins their care of the person. Once you have learned these concepts and skills, review and practice them regularly so that if you ever have to use them, you will be well prepared and have the confidence to act.

Make sure you have ready access to items that will make it easier to respond to an emergency, should one occur. Keep a first aid kit in your home and vehicle (Box 1-3) and know the location of the first aid kit, automated external defibrillator (AED) and bleeding control kit in your workplace. Download the American Red Cross First Aid app to your mobile device so that you always have a first aid reference at your fingertips.

Keep a current list of emergency telephone numbers in your mobile phone, by the telephones in your home and workplace, and in your first aid kit. Most communities are served by the emergency telephone number 9-1-1. If your community does not operate on a 9-1-1 system, look up the numbers for the police department, fire department and emergency medical services (EMS) system. Also include the number for the national Poison Help hotline (1-800-222-1222) on your list. Teach everyone in your home how and when to use these numbers.

Take steps to make it easier for EMS personnel and others to help you should an emergency occur.

- Make sure your house or apartment number is large, easy to read and well-lit at night. Numerals are easier to read than spelled-out numbers.
- Keep relevant medical information, such as a list of the medications that each family member takes, in an accessible place (e.g., on the refrigerator door and in your wallet or mobile phone).
- If you have a chronic medical condition such as diabetes, epilepsy or allergies, it is a good idea to wear a medical identification tag (Figure 1-1, A) to alert responders to the presence of the condition in case you are not able to tell them. You can also create a digital medical identification tag in your mobile phone that can be accessed without unlocking the phone (Figure 1-1, B). In addition to information about chronic medical conditions, blood type and so on, you can enter contact information for the person you would want contacted on your behalf in case of an emergency.

In a life-threatening emergency, every second counts. By preparing for emergencies, you can help ensure that care begins as soon as possible—for yourself, a family member, a friend, a co-worker or a member of your community.

Box 1-3 First Aid Kits

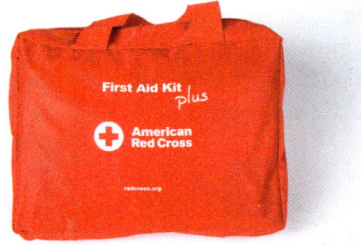

You can purchase first aid kits and supplies from the Red Cross store (redcross.org) or a local store. Whether you buy a first aid kit or assemble one yourself, make sure it has all of the items you may need. Check the kit regularly and replace any used or expired supplies. The Red Cross recommends that first aid kits include the following at a minimum:

- 2 pairs latex-free (nitrile) disposable gloves
- Supplies to control bleeding (8 sterile pads; 4 x 4 inches)
- Supplies to secure dressing (4 roller bandages; 2, 3 or 4 inches x 4 yards)
- 1 roll of adhesive tape (⅜ inch x 2.5 yards)
- 2 triangular bandages (40 x 40 x 56 inches)
- Latex-free adhesive bandages (3 each of the following sizes):
  - 1 x 3 inches
  - ¾ x 3 inches
  - large fingertip
  - knuckle

- Topical wound gel or ointment (10 packets, 0.03 ounce/0.9 gram each)
- 1 compact, moldable splinting device with securing mechanism (e.g., roller bandage, triangular bandage, tape)
- 4 plastic bags (1 quart or 1 gallon) for application of ice water and/or 2 instant cold packs
- 4 low-dose aspirin (81 mg each) or 1 adult aspirin (325 mg), chewable
- Oral glucose tablet, minimum of 20 grams
- Saline solution
- 1 pair of 7-inch utility shears/scissors
- Alcohol-based hand sanitizer
- Splinter forceps/tweezers
- 1 latex-free face shield
- First aid guide book

Optional items:
Antiseptic towelettes (10 packets; 0.14 ounce/0.5 gram each)
2 trauma pads (5 x 9 inches)
Topical antibiotic (10 packets; 0.14 ounce/0.5 gram each)
1 manufactured windlass rod tourniquet
1 eye covering with means of attachment (2 x 9 inches)
1 burn dressing (4 x 4 inches)

For a list of the recommended contents for a workplace first aid kit, see ANSI Z308.1-2015 Minimum Class A First Aid Kit Supplies and ANSI Z308.1-2015 Minimum Class B First Aid Kit Supplies in the ARC SAC Scientific Review: First Aid Kit.

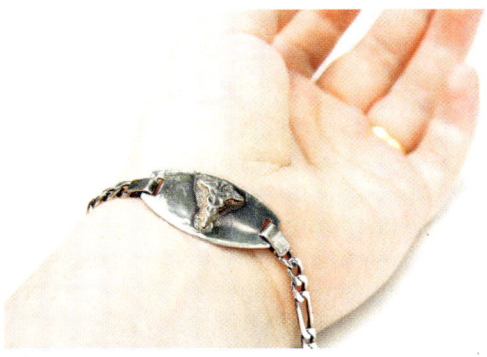
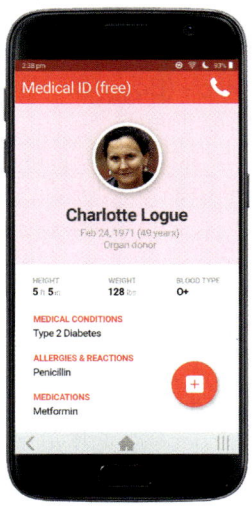

Figure 1-1. A medical identification tag (A) or an application on your phone (B) can give responders important information about you in case you are not able to do so.

Your Role in the EMS System

The **emergency medical services (EMS) system** is a network of professionals linked together to provide the best care for people in all types of emergencies (Box 1-4). As a member of the community, you play a major role in helping the EMS system to work effectively. Your role in the EMS system includes:

Box 1-4 The Emergency Medical Services System

The EMS system is a network of professionals linked together to provide the best care for people in all emergencies.

The system begins when someone sees an emergency and decides to take action by calling 9-1-1 or the designated emergency number.

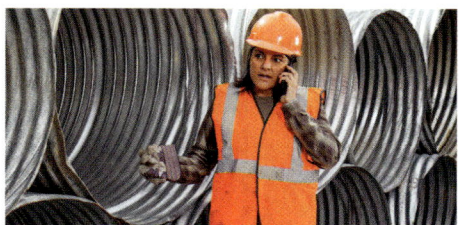

This action allows the EMS dispatcher to take down information about the emergency and provide it to the trained EMS professionals who will respond to the scene. Many EMS dispatchers are also trained to provide first aid and CPR instructions over the phone to assist the lay responder until the professional responders arrive.

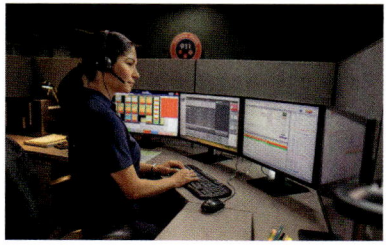

EMS professionals have advanced training that allows them to provide medical care outside of the hospital setting. Once on the scene, these professionals will begin the care of the person, including transportation to a hospital or other facility for the best medical care if needed.

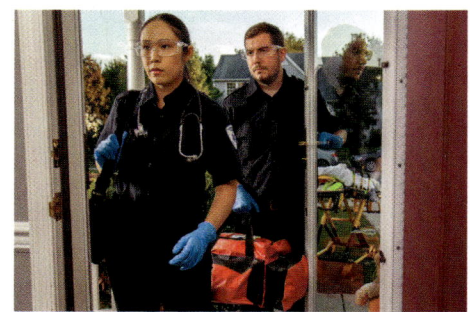

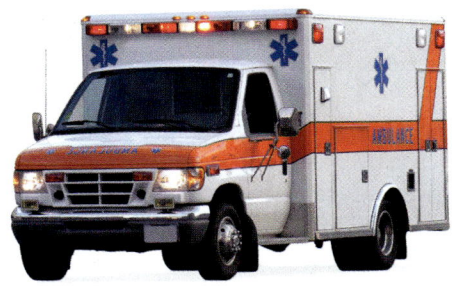

---

10   Chapter 1 | First Aid, CPR, AED Foundations

- Recognizing that an emergency exists and gaining confidence to take action.
- Performing the emergency action steps:
  - **Check** the scene and the person.
  - **Call** 9-1-1 and get equipment.
  - Give **care** until EMS personnel arrive and begin their care of the person.

Recognizing That an Emergency Exists and Gaining Confidence to Take Action

Sometimes it will be obvious that an emergency exists—for example, unusual noises, unusual odors, or unusual appearances or behaviors. But other times, the signs of an emergency may be less obvious, such as a slight change in a person's normal appearance or behavior or an unusual silence. In order to determine if an emergency exists, you will use all of your senses. Your eyes, ears, nose and even your gut instincts can alert you that an emergency situation exists (Box 1-5).

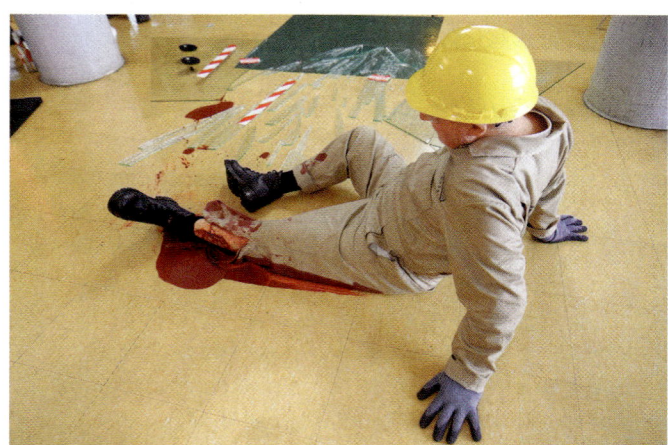

Box 1-5 Signs of an Emergency

Unusual Noises
- Screaming, moaning, yelling, crying or calls for help
- Sudden, loud noises such as breaking glass, crashing metal, a thud or screeching tires
- A change in the sound made by machinery or equipment
- Unusual silence

Unusual Odors
- A foul or unusually strong chemical odor
- The smell of smoke
- The smell of gas
- An unrecognizable odor
- An inappropriate odor (e.g., a sickly-sweet odor on a person's breath)

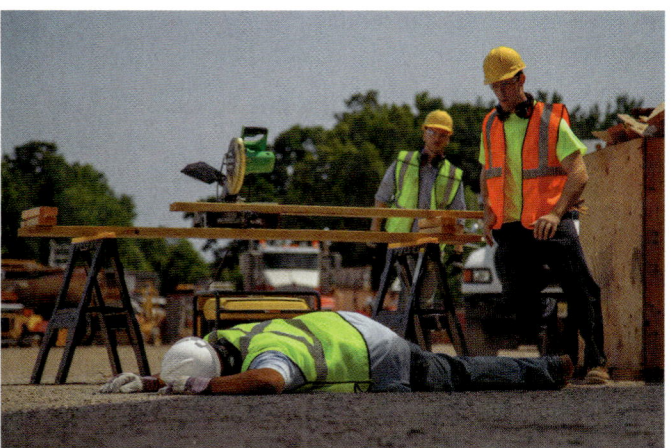

Unusual Appearances or Behaviors
- A stopped vehicle on the roadside or a car that has run off the road
- Downed electrical wires
- Sparks, smoke or fire
- A person who suddenly collapses or is lying motionless
- Signs or symptoms of illness or injury, such as a person clutching their throat or heart, a person having a seizure, a person with swollen lips, difficulty breathing, sudden weakness on one side of the body, profuse sweating for no apparent reason or an uncharacteristic skin color, pool of blood or blood pulsating or person's limb at an unusual angle or bent in the middle
- Confusion in a person who is normally alert
- Unusual drowsiness
- A person moaning, staggering or slurring their speech or unable to speak
- Personality or mood changes (e.g., agitation in a person who is normally calm, irritability in a person who is normally pleasant)

Once you recognize an emergency situation, you must decide to take action. In an emergency, deciding to act is not always as simple as it sounds. Some people are slow to act in an emergency because they panic, are not exactly sure what to do or think someone else will take action. But in an emergency situation, your decision to take action could make the difference between life and death for the person who needs help.

The training you receive from taking an American Red Cross First Aid/CPR/AED course will give you the confidence to take action when an emergency occurs. The goal is for you to gain knowledge and skills and build confidence so that you know how to respond appropriately to an emergency.

Your decision to act in an emergency can save a life. However, even if you decide not to give care, you should at least call or instruct someone to call 9-1-1 or the designated emergency number to get emergency medical help to the scene.

Several tips to give you the confidence to take action and respond in an emergency are presented below.

- **Always call 9-1-1 or tell someone to do so if you think the situation is an emergency.** If you are not sure if the situation is an emergency, err on the side of caution and call 9-1-1 or the designated emergency number or tell someone to do so.
- **Be confident in your ability to give care based on your first aid training.** Getting trained in first aid will give you the knowledge, skills and confidence you need to respond appropriately to an emergency. If you are not sure what to do, call 9-1-1, or tell someone to do so, and follow the EMS dispatcher's instructions. The worst thing to do is nothing.
- **Don't assume that the situation is already under control.** Although there may be a crowd of people around the injured or ill person, it is possible that no one has taken action. If no one is giving care or directing the actions of bystanders, you can take the lead. If someone else is already giving care, confirm that someone has called 9-1-1 and ask how you can help.
- **Be confident in your ability to handle unpleasant sights, sounds or smells.** You may have to turn away for a moment and take a few deep breaths to regain your composure before you can give care if faced with upsetting sights, sounds or smells, such as blood, vomit or a traumatic injury. Knowing that you are trained to give care in these situations will often help you to push through these unpleasant

situations. In the rare case that you are unable to give care due to feeling faint or nauseated, you can volunteer to help in other ways, such as by calling 9-1-1 and bringing necessary equipment and supplies to the scene.
- **Lower your risk for infection.** The risk of getting infected with a communicable disease while giving care to another person is low. Although it is possible for diseases to be transmitted in a first aid situation, it is extremely unlikely that you will get infected this way. Taking additional precautions as you have been trained, such as putting on latex-free disposable gloves and using a CPR breathing barrier, can reduce your risk even further.
- **Know your legal protections.** It is important for you to know that the majority of states and the District of Columbia have Good Samaritan laws in place to help protect people who voluntarily give care in good faith without accepting or expecting anything in return. If you have questions regarding whether or not you are protected when providing first aid, refer to your state's Good Samaritan laws.

Emergency Action Steps

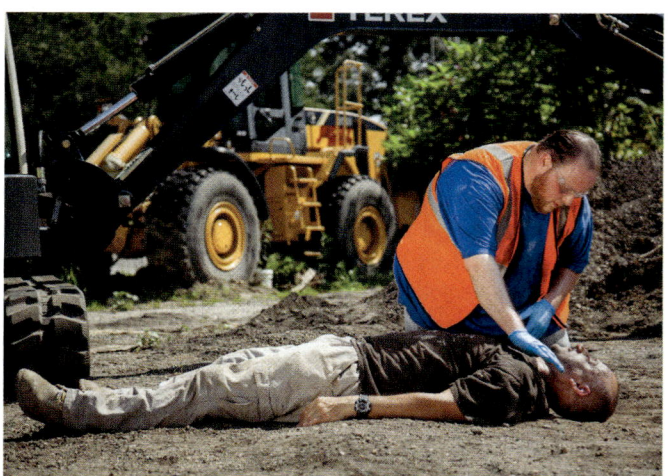

An emergency can be stressful, but you can take steps to help a person in any emergency situation, from cardiac arrest to choking to life-threatening bleeding.

In any emergency situation, there are three simple steps to take to guide your actions. If you remember these three emergency action steps you will be calm and confident in all emergencies:

1. **CHECK** the scene, check the person by forming an initial impression, obtain consent and continue checking the person.
2. **CALL** 9-1-1 and get equipment.
3. **CARE** for the person.

> **THE PROS KNOW.** The **CHECK-CALL-CARE** emergency actions steps are taught as a linear sequence. However, in an emergency these steps may be completed simultaneously or repeated depending on the situation.
>
>
>
> For example, if during your initial **CHECK** you determine that a person is experiencing a life-threatening emergency (e.g., trouble breathing), immediately move to the **CALL** step. Next, give general **CARE** (e.g., have the person rest in a comfortable position). As you give **CARE**, continue to **CHECK** them to find out more information and determine whether additional **CARE** is needed (e.g., if you find they are having an asthma attack, assist them with their medication).

number, or tell someone to do so. Once professional responders make the scene safe, you can offer your assistance as appropriate.

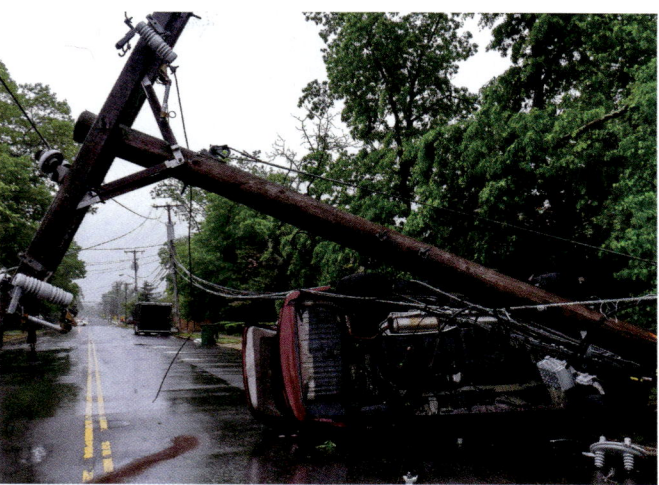

Check the Scene and the Person

In an emergency situation, it is very important that you first check the scene for safety before rushing to help an injured or ill person. Then, before touching the person, you need to form an initial impression and obtain consent. Once you have determined that the scene is safe, and you have an initial idea of what is happening, and you have obtained consent, you then conduct a more thorough check of the person to determine what is wrong and what care is needed.

Check the Scene for Safety

Checking the scene includes checking for safety risks. When doing so, try to answer the following questions.

- **Is the scene safe to enter?** Check for hazards that could jeopardize your safety or the safety of bystanders, such as fire, downed electrical wires, spilled chemicals, an unstable building or traffic. Do not enter bodies of water unless you are specifically trained to perform in-water rescues (Box 1-6). Avoid entering confined areas with poor ventilation and places where natural gas, propane or other substances could explode. Do not enter the scene if there is evidence of criminal activity or the person is hostile or threatening suicide. If these or other dangers threaten, stay at a safe distance and immediately call 9-1-1 or the designated emergency

- **What happened?** Take note of anything that might tell you the cause of the emergency. If the person is unresponsive and there are no witnesses, your check of the scene may offer the only clues as to what happened. Use your senses to detect anything out of the ordinary, such as broken glass, a spilled bottle of medication or an unusual smell or sound. Keep in mind that the injured or ill person may not be exactly where they were when the injury or illness occurred—someone may have moved the person, or the person may have moved in an attempt to get help.

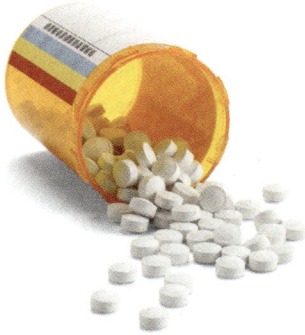

- **How many people are involved?** Look carefully for more than one injured or ill person. A person who is moving or making noise or who has very visible injuries will likely attract your attention right away, but there may be a person who is silent and not moving or a person obscured by debris or wreckage that you do not notice at first. It also is easy to overlook a small child or an infant. In an emergency with more than one injured or ill person, 9-1-1 needs this information to determine the needed resources, and you may need to prioritize care (in other words, decide who needs help first).

American Red Cross | First Aid Basics

- **Is anyone else available to help?** Take note of bystanders who can be of assistance. A bystander who was there when the emergency occurred or who knows the injured or ill person may be able to provide valuable information about the situation or the person. Bystanders can also assist in other ways, such as by calling 9-1-1 or the designated emergency number, getting needed items (such as an AED and first aid kit), waiting for EMS personnel and leading them to the site of the emergency, controlling crowds and reassuring the injured or ill person.

Box 1-6 Reach or Throw, Don't Go!

Do not enter water in an attempt to rescue a person who is in trouble unless you are specifically trained to perform in-water rescues. Instead, get help from a trained responder, such as a lifeguard, to get the person out of the water as quickly and safely as possible or call 9-1-1 or the local emergency number and wait for help. Never go out onto the ice in an attempt to rescue a person who has fallen through the ice. Because a person has just fallen through it, the ice is unsafe. A responder who rushes out onto the ice is likely to become a victim as well. Instead call or send someone to call 9-1-1 immediately and then attempt a reaching or throwing assist.

Reaching and throwing assists allow you to help a conscious person who is in trouble without entering the water yourself. These types of assists are the safest assists for responders who are not professionally trained lifeguards to perform during an aquatic emergency. They are also the best type of assist to use when someone has fallen through ice. To keep yourself safe, always remember "Reach or throw, don't go!"

When doing a reaching or throwing assist:

- Start the rescue by talking to the person, if possible. Let the person know help is coming.
- Use gestures to communicate with the person if it is too noisy or if the person is too far away to hear.
- Tell the person what he or she can do to help with the rescue, such as grasping a line, rescue buoy or other floating device.
- Encourage the person to move toward safety by kicking or stroking. Some people are able to reach safety by themselves with calm encouragement from a person on the deck or shore.

Reaching Assist

If the person is close enough, use a reaching assist to help him or her out of the water. To do a reaching assist, use any available object that will extend your reach and give something for the person to grab so you can pull the person in. Items that work well for reaching assists include a pole, an oar or paddle, a tree branch, a shirt, a belt or a towel. Community or hotel pools and recreational areas often have reaching equipment, such as a shepherd's *crook* (an aluminum or fiberglass pole with a large *hook* on one end) located close to the water.

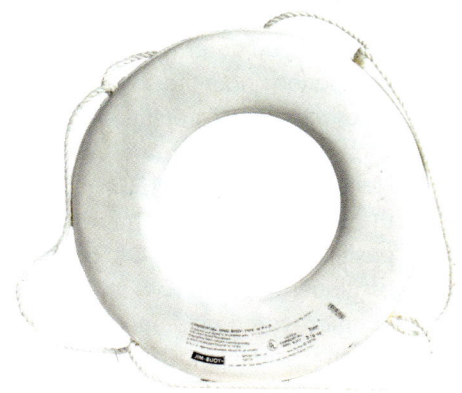

You can perform a reaching assist from the pool deck, pier surface or shoreline. If no equipment is available and you are close enough, you may be able to perform a reaching assist by extending your arm to the person.

You can also perform a reaching assist from a position within the water by extending an arm or a leg to the person, if you are already in the water and you have something secure to hold on to.

Throwing Assist

A throwing assist involves throwing an object to the person so that they can grasp it and be pulled to safety. A floating object with a line attached (such as a ring buoy) is ideal for a throwing assist; however, an object that floats (such as a life jacket or cooler) can also be used. In some situations, you may have to improvise with an object that floats but is not specifically meant for throwing assists. If possible, keep a throwing object with a coiled line in a prominent location that is accessible to the water, so that anyone can quickly access it to throw to someone in trouble. All boats should have rescue equipment onboard for throwing assists.

Wading Assist

A wading assist involves wading into the water and using a reaching assist to help pull the person to safety. Only use a wading assist in water that is less than chest deep. If a current or soft bottom makes wading dangerous, do not enter the water. For your own safety, wear a life jacket if one is available and take something to extend to the person, such as a ring buoy, branch, pole, air mattress or paddle.

Check the Person

After checking the scene for safety, check the person and obtain consent. Checking the person includes forming an initial impression, then conducting a more thorough check. You should obtain consent after you have formed an initial impression but before you touch the person to complete your check.

Before you can give first aid care, you need to gather information to determine what is wrong with the person, which will guide your next actions. Remember that before you touch the person you must obtain consent. Your first goal is to identify and care for any life-threatening conditions. If the person does not appear to have any life-threatening conditions, you can check the person for other types of injuries or conditions that may require care. The observations you make and the information you gather will help you to better understand the nature of the emergency and give appropriate, effective care.

Form an Initial Impression

First, form an initial impression about the nature of the person's illness or injury. You can usually get an idea of what's going on with the person as you approach them. Before you touch the person, try to form an initial impression about the person's condition and what is wrong. For example, does the person seem alert, or confused or sleepy? Look at the person's skin—does it appear to be its normal color, or does it seem pale, ashen (gray) or flushed? Is the person moving or motionless? Does the person have any immediately identifiable injuries?

Look for signs of a life-threatening illness or injury, such as:

- Does the person appear unresponsive?
- Does the person seem to be breathing or are they having trouble breathing?
- Does the person appear to have life-threatening bleeding or another life-threatening condition?

If the person appears unresponsive, check for responsiveness (see Check the Person Who Appears Unresponsive).

If the person is responsive and appears to have life-threatening bleeding or another life-threatening condition, move immediately to the call step. Then, give care for the condition found according to your level of training. At the same time, you may need to continue checking the person to obtain more information and determine whether additional care is needed (see Continue Checking the Person).

If the person is responsive and appears to have a non-life-threatening condition, continue checking them to see if they have conditions that may require EMS and first aid care (see Continue Checking the Person).

Obtain Consent

After checking the scene for safety and forming an initial impression, you need to obtain consent.

Before touching the person or giving first aid care, you need to obtain **consent** (permission) from the injured or ill person (or the person's parent or guardian if the person is a minor). To obtain consent tell the person:

- Your name.
- The type and level of training that you have (such as training in first aid or CPR).
- What you plan to do.

With this information, an ill or injured person can grant their consent for care or state that they do not wish you to do anything.

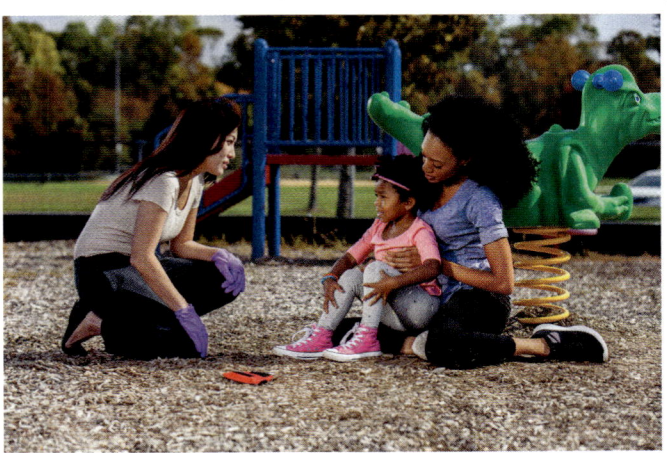

Someone who appears unresponsive or mentally altered, for example, they're confused or disoriented, may not be able to grant consent. In these cases, consent is implied under the law (**implied consent**). Basically, the law assumes the person would give consent if they could. Implied consent also applies when a minor needs emergency medical assistance and the minor's parent or guardian is not present.

An injured or ill person may refuse care, even if they desperately need it. A parent or guardian also may refuse care for a minor in their care. You must honor the person's wishes. Explain to the person why you believe care is necessary, but do not touch or give care to the person if care was refused. If you believe the person's condition needs emergency care, call EMS personnel to evaluate the situation. If the person gives consent initially but then withdraws it, stop giving care and call for EMS personnel if you have not already done so.

If you do not speak the same language as the injured or ill person, obtaining consent may be challenging. Find out if someone else at the scene can serve as a translator. If a translator is not available, do your best to communicate with the person by using gestures and facial expressions. When you call 9-1-1 or the designated emergency number, explain that you are having difficulty communicating with the person, and tell the dispatcher which language you believe the person speaks. The dispatcher may have someone available who can help with communication.

Check the Person Who Appears Unresponsive

If the person appears to be unresponsive based on your initial impression, check for responsiveness by using the **shout-tap-shout sequence**. Shout, using the person's name if you know it. If there is no response, tap the person's shoulder (if the person is an adult or child) or the bottom of the foot (for an infant) and shout again. If the person does not respond to you in any way—such as by moving, opening their eyes, or moaning—they're unresponsive.

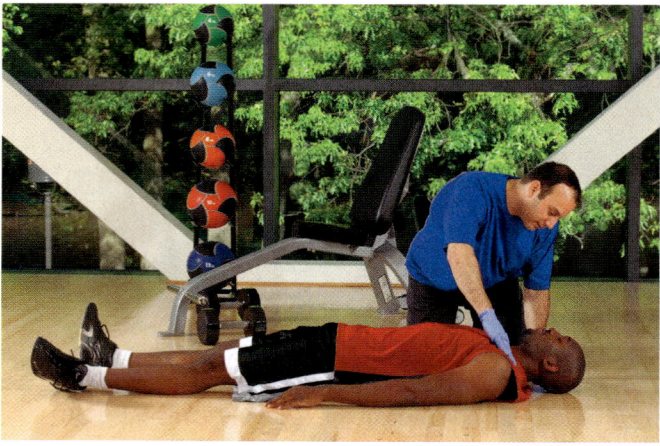

During this shout, tap, shout check, you are also going to check to see if the person is breathing and you are going to check again for life-threatening bleeding or another obvious life-threatening illness or injury that you might not have seen during the initial impression.

When checking for breathing, make sure the person is face-up. If they are face-down, roll them onto their back, taking care not to create or worsen a suspected injury. Look to see if the person's chest is rising and falling.

Normal breathing is quiet, regular and effortless. Agonal breaths, or isolated or infrequent gasps, are not considered breathing. To check for life-threatening bleeding or another life-threatening condition, quickly scan down the person's body looking for blood or other signs and symptoms.

Checking for responsiveness, breathing, life-threatening bleeding or another life-threatening condition should take no more than 10 seconds.

If you determine the person is **unresponsive**, responsive but **not fully awake**, **not breathing**, has **life-threatening bleeding**, or another **life-threatening condition**:

- Immediately go to the call step.
- Give care immediately for the condition found and continue your check (as appropriate) to obtain more information and determine whether additional care is needed (see Continue Checking the Person).
  Note: *For a person who is unresponsive and not breathing, start CPR and use an AED immediately (see Chapters 2 and 3).*

If you determine the person is **responsive** and experiencing a non-life-threatening emergency, continue checking them (see Continue Checking the Person).

Continue Checking the Person

To gather additional information about the nature of the person's illness or injury, ask them questions using the mnemonic SAM (Figure 1-2) and do a focused check.

The reason you as a first aid responder should ask questions and do a focused check is because as time goes on, the person may be less able to say things. You may be able to gather information that others will not be able to. Also, this information will help you provide care. So again, if the person is responsive and does not appear to have a life-threatening illness or injury (or, as needed, for a life-threatening emergency, after calling 9-1-1, getting equipment and giving immediate care according to your level of training), ask questions using the mnemonic SAM, and then do a focused check.

Interview the Person Begin by asking the person's name and use it when you speak to the person. Position yourself at eye level with the person and speak clearly, calmly and in a friendly manner, using age-appropriate language. Try to provide as much privacy as possible for the person while

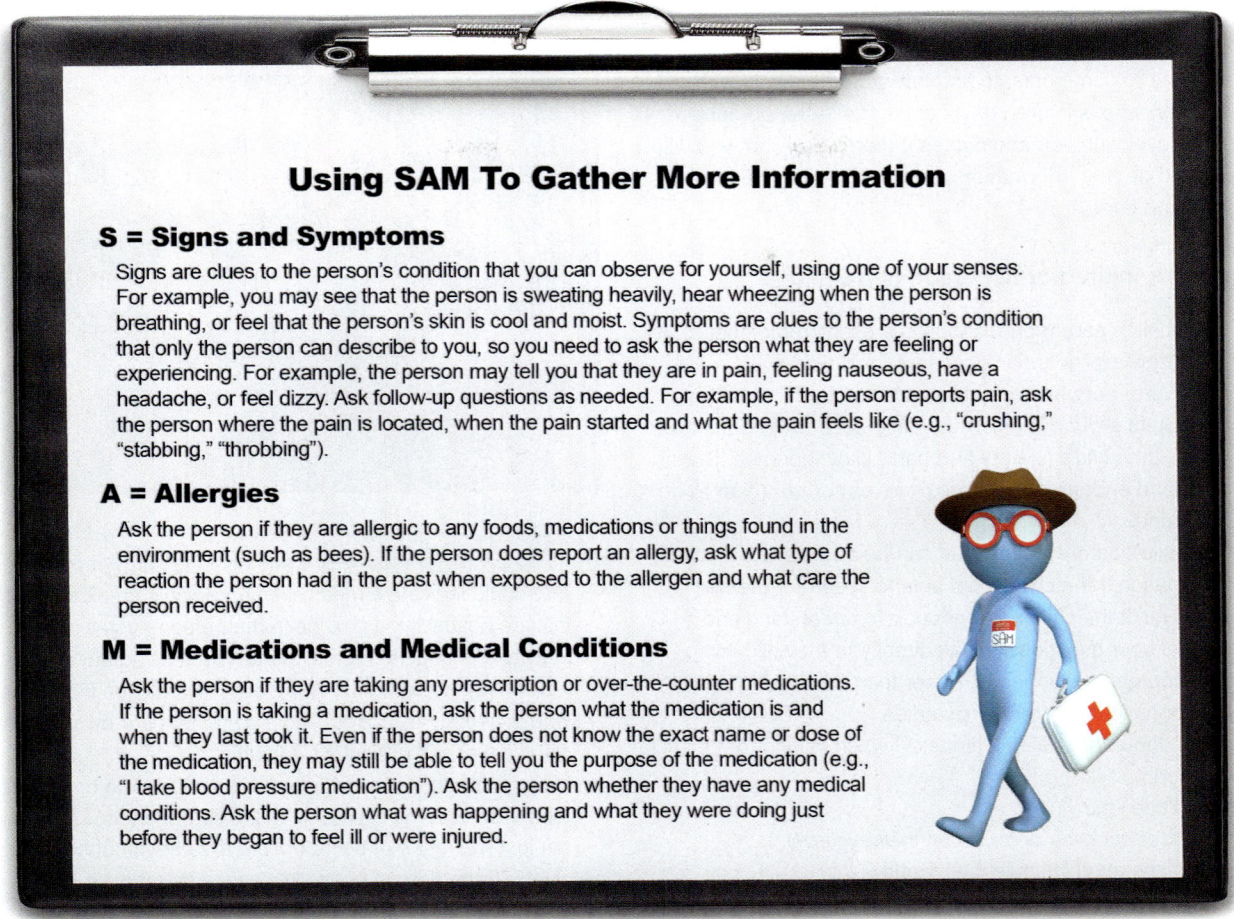

Figure 1-2. The mnemonic SAM can help you remember what to ask the injured or ill person.

you are conducting the interview and keep the interview brief. Tailor your approach to the age of the person, as well as to any special circumstances (Box 1-7). The mnemonic SAM can help you remember what you should ask about. If possible, write down the information you learn during the interview or, preferably, have someone else write it down for you. Be sure to give the information to emergency medical services (EMS) personnel when they arrive. It may help them to determine the type of medical care that the person should receive.

For children and infants, you will interview the parents or guardians. If the child is at an age where they talk, it is also important to ask them what is bothering them because all children, especially older children, wish to be part of the process.

Other people at the scene may be able to provide useful information as well. They may have witnessed what happened. If there are people at the scene who know the injured or ill person well (such as family members or friends), they may also be able to provide information about the person's medical history if the person is not able to do so, for example, because of the effects of the injury or illness.

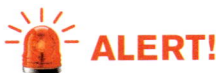 **ALERT!**

Sometimes people who have been injured or become suddenly ill may act strangely; be uncooperative; or become violent, angry or aggressive. This behavior can be the result of the injury or illness or other factors, such as the effects of drugs, alcohol or medications. Do not take this behavior personally. If you feel threatened by the person's behavior, move away from the person to safety and call 9-1-1 or the designated emergency number, or tell someone to do so.

American Red Cross | First Aid Basics 17

Box 1-7 Strategies for Gathering Information Effectively

Being able to communicate and interact effectively with the person who is injured or ill can increase the person's comfort level with you and makes it more likely that you will be able to get the information you need in order to provide appropriate care.

When the Injured or Ill Person Is a Child

- If the child's parent or guardian is present, remember to get the parent's or guardian's consent to give care.
- Be aware that children often take emotional cues from the adults around them. If the child sees that adults are upset, the child's anxiety and panic may increase. Stay calm and encourage the child's parent or guardian to do the same.
- The child's parent or guardian can be a valuable source of information if the child is not able to speak for themself. However, if the child is old enough to understand and answer your questions, speak directly to the child using age-appropriate language, rather than addressing your questions to the parent or guardian.
- Think about "not being a monster" when talking to children.
  - Don't be loud.
  - Don't tower over them; get on their eye level.
  - Don't be rough; handle them gently.
  - Don't scare them; tell them what you are going to do.
- If the care you need to provide will cause discomfort or pain, describe what the child can expect to feel in terms the child can understand. Never make promises or statements that you cannot support (e.g., do not say that something will not hurt if it will).

When the Injured or Ill Person Is an Older Adult

- Pay attention to how the person introduces themself. If the person gives a last name, consider addressing the person more formally (e.g., "Mr. Johnson" rather than "Bill") as a sign of respect.
- A family member, caregiver or other person who knows the older adult well can be a valuable source of information if the older adult is not able to speak for themself. However, if the older adult is able to understand and answer your questions, speak directly to them, rather than addressing your questions to others who might be present.
- Speak clearly and loudly enough for the person to hear you, but do not shout. If the person does not seem to understand what you are saying, change your words, not the volume of your voice, unless you spoke too softly.
- When interviewing the person, avoid rushing. Allow the person enough time to process your questions and respond.
- Be aware that in older people, the signs and symptoms of a medical emergency may be very general and nonspecific,

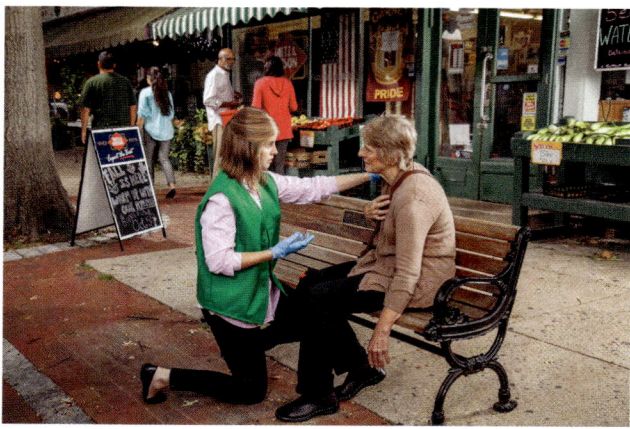

and they may not even be noticeable to someone who does not know the person well. General signs and symptoms that could indicate a medical emergency in an older adult include headache, a change in the person's usual level of activity, a change in mental status (such as agitation, the new onset of confusion, or increased confusion in a person who is already confused), lethargy (extreme drowsiness or sleepiness) and difficulty sleeping.
- Many older adults have impaired hearing, vision or both. If the person seems confused, make sure the "confusion" is not just the result of being unable to hear you or see you clearly. If the person normally wears a hearing aid, make sure it is in place and turned on. If the person usually wears glasses, make sure they have them on.

When the Injured or Ill Person Has a Disability

- Remember, the presence of a physical disability does not mean the person has a cognitive disability. If the person is able to understand and answer your questions, speak directly to them, rather than addressing your questions to others who might be present. However, if they can't speak for themself, a family member, caregiver or other person who knows the injured or ill person well can be a valuable source of information.
- A person with a disability may use a service animal. Be aware that service animals are trained to protect their owners, and both the service animal and the person may become anxious if they are separated. Allow the service animal to stay with the person if possible.
- If the person wears an assistive device (e.g., a leg brace), do not remove the device when you are examining the person unless you have to provide care such as controlling bleeding.
- If the person has an intellectual disability:
  - Address the person as you would any other person in their age group. If the person does not seem to understand you, rephrase your statement or question in simpler terms.

> **Box 1-7** continued
>
> - Be aware that being injured or becoming suddenly ill may make the person very upset, anxious or fearful. Take time to explain who you are and what you intend to do and reassure the person.
> - If the person has impaired hearing:
>   - Approach the person from the front.
>   - Hearing-impaired people who know how to read lips rely on watching your mouth move. Position yourself so that the person can see your mouth and facial expressions. Pronounce your words slowly and clearly and speak in short sentences.
>   - If the person does not seem to understand what you are saying, change your words, not the volume of your voice, unless you spoke too softly. Shouting sometimes causes the person more distress and they still may not understand what you are trying to say.
>   - If the person can't hear you and does not seem to be able to read your lips, you can often communicate by using gestures and writing comments and letting them speak or write their responses.
> - If the person has impaired vision:
>   - Speak in a normal voice. It is not necessary to shout.
>   - As the person may not be able to see what you are doing as you provide care, be sure to describe what you are doing.
>
> **When the Injured or Ill Person Speaks a Different Language**
>
> - Speak in a normal voice. It is not necessary to shout.
> - Find out if any bystanders speak the person's language and can assist by translating.
> - Do your best to communicate nonverbally, using gestures and facial expressions.
> - When you call 9-1-1 or the designated emergency number, explain that you are having difficulty communicating with the person, and tell the dispatcher which language you believe the person speaks. The dispatcher may have someone available who can help with communication.

Do a Focused Check Next, complete a focused check. Before beginning the check, tell the person what you are going to do. The idea of this check is to look for signs of illness or injury based on several factors:

- What the person, a parent/guardian or a bystander has told you
- How the person is acting
- What you see

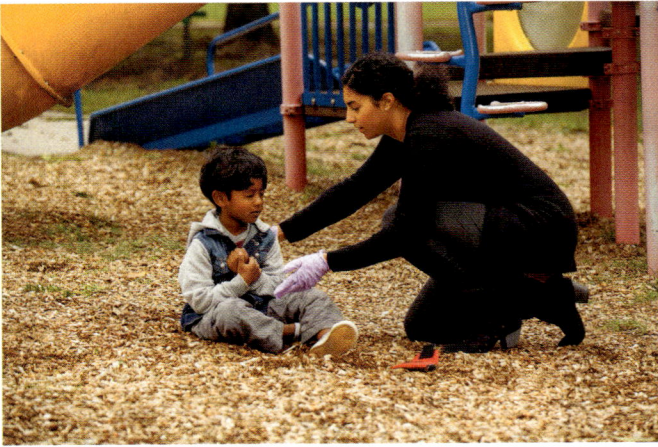

For example, the person may have told you that they have pain in their wrist, so you will want to do a thorough check of their wrist and arm. Or, a child may be moaning and crying and holding their head, so you will want to do a careful check of their head for an injury. Or, a person may not be saying much at all, but you see a lot of blood on the ground that seems to be coming from underneath their leg. In this case you will want to do a careful check for an injury to their leg or back. The person may have multiple signs of an injury or illness in different areas of their body. In this case, be sure to do a focused check in each of these areas.

As you check, take note of any medical identification tags, such as a bracelet or sports band on the person's wrist or ankle, or a necklace around the person's neck. While performing the focused check, look and gently feel for signs of injury, such as bleeding, cuts, burns, bruising, swelling or deformities. Also note if they can't feel you checking or if it is painful. If they experience pain during the focused exam, stop checking that part and note what you find. Think of how the body usually looks. If you are unsure if a body part or limb looks injured, check it against the opposite limb or the other side of the body. Watch the person's face for expressions of discomfort or pain as you check for injuries.

If you detect signs or symptoms of illness or injury:

- Determine whether to call 9-1-1 or the designated emergency number.
- If there is an injury to the head, neck or back, leave the person in the position you found them in unless you need to move them for safety or to control bleeding. If they do not have a head, neck or back injury, help the person rest in a comfortable position.

- Reassure the person by telling them that you will help and that EMS personnel have been called (if appropriate).
- Give care according to the conditions that you find and your level of knowledge and training.
- Be alert to signs that the person's condition is worsening, such as changes in level of consciousness, changes in breathing, changes in skin color or restlessness. These could be signs of shock, a life-threatening condition. (See Chapter 5.)

If the person has no apparent signs or symptoms of injury or illness, have them rest in a comfortable position. Continue to watch for changes in the person's condition. When the person feels ready, help them to stand up.

As part of your check in a first aid situation, you may notice signs and symptoms that suggest abuse or neglect. See Box 1-8 for a discussion of signs and symptoms of abuse and neglect and how you should respond if you suspect this to be the cause of the person's injury or illness. Putting It All Together 1-1 describes and illustrates step-by-step how to check an injured or ill person.

Call 9-1-1 and Get Equipment

If you determine the person is experiencing a life-threatening emergency, immediately activate the EMS system and get equipment.

After check, the next step is call. Of course, you'll want to care for the person right away; but first you want to make sure help is on the way, if necessary, and that you have the equipment you need to help.

Therefore, call may include calling 9-1-1 to activate EMS and getting equipment such as an AED, a first aid kit and a bleeding control kit. Depending on the circumstances, you can either send someone to do this or do it yourself.

Box 1-8 Abuse

Abuse is the willful infliction of injury or harm on another. People who depend on others for care, such as children and the elderly, are at the highest risk for being abused. Abuse can take many forms, including physical abuse (deliberately hurting another person's body), emotional abuse (degrading, belittling or threatening another person), sexual abuse (forcing a person to take part in sexual activities of any kind) and neglect (failing to provide for a dependent person's basic needs).

Signs and symptoms of abuse could include:

- An injury whose cause does not fit its explanation.
- Unexplained fractures or dislocations.
- Unexplained lacerations or abrasions, especially to the mouth, lips and eyes.
- Injuries in various stages of healing, especially bruises and burns.
- Bruises and burns in unusual shapes, such as bruises shaped like belt buckles or handprints, or burns the size of a cigarette tip.
- Bruises, scratches or cuts around the breasts, buttocks or genitals.
- A withdrawn or fearful demeanor, especially in the presence of the person who is causing the abuse.

Signs and symptoms of neglect could include:

- Lack of appropriate supervision.
- Signs of poor personal hygiene.
- Signs of dehydration and malnutrition.
- An unsafe living environment.
- Untreated chronic illness.

In a first aid situation, you may have reason to suspect that the person is a victim of abuse. Your priority is to give first aid care for the person's injury or illness, according to the conditions that you find and your level of training. If you suspect abuse, share your concerns with the responding emergency medical services (EMS) personnel, if possible. You can also report your suspicions to a community or state agency, such as the Department of Social Services, the Department of Child and Family Services, Child Protective Services, or Adult Protective Services.

You may be hesitant to report suspected abuse because you do not wish to get involved or are concerned about legal action. In most states, when you make a report in good faith, you are protected from any civil or criminal liability or penalty, even if the report was made in error. In this instance, good faith means that you honestly believe that abuse has occurred or the potential for abuse exists and that a prudent and reasonable person in the same position would also honestly believe that abuse has occurred or the potential for abuse exists. You may have to identify yourself when you report abuse. In some professions, employees are legally obligated to report suspicions of abuse of a person in their care to their supervisor (or to another person in the organization, per their employer's policy). This does not take the place of any mandatory reporting as required by law or regulation and cannot be used as gatekeeper for mandatory reporting.

Activating the EMS system will send emergency medical help on its way as fast as possible. The sooner emergency personnel arrive, the better the chance for a positive outcome. At times you may be unsure if EMS is needed. You will have to use your best judgment—based on the situation, your assessment of the injured or ill person, and information gained from this course and other training you may have received—to make the decision to call (Box 1-9). When in doubt, make the call. If you didn't find anything or the person has only a minor injury or illness, you *may* not need to call 9-1-1 for help. This may be something that you can handle on your own using your first aid skills and guidance from the Red Cross First Aid app. In this case, get or have someone get a first aid kit and move to care.

Most people in the United States call 9-1-1 for help in emergencies. But in some areas of the United States and in many workplaces, you may need to dial a designated emergency number instead. If you live or work in an area where 9-1-1 is *not* the number you should call in an emergency, make sure you know what the designated emergency number is. Also, in some workplaces and schools there may be an internal number to use in an emergency that not only summons EMS but activates an

Box 1-9 When to Activate the EMS System

Call 9-1-1 or the designated emergency number, or tell someone to do so, for any of the following emergency situations and conditions.

Emergency Situations

- An injured or ill person who needs medical attention and cannot be moved
- Fire or explosion
- Downed electrical wires
- Swiftly moving or rapidly rising flood waters
- Drowning
- Presence of poisonous gas
- Serious motor vehicle collision
- Spilled chemicals

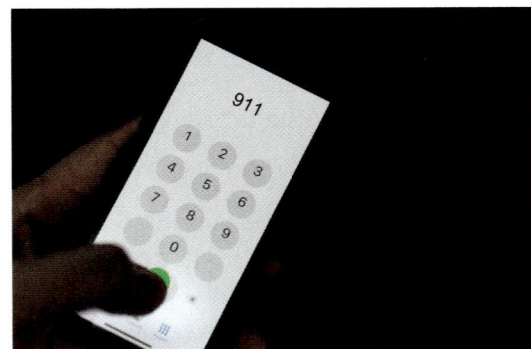

Emergency Conditions

- Unresponsiveness or an altered level of consciousness (LOC), such as drowsiness or confusion
- Cardiac arrest (unresponsive; no breathing or only gasping)
- Choking (cannot cough, cry, speak or breathe; universal sign of choking)
- Anaphylaxis (signs of allergic reaction; history of allergy; swelling of the face, neck, tongue or lips; trouble breathing; shock; change in responsiveness)
- Breathing problems (trouble breathing or no breathing; asthma attack)
- Chest pain, discomfort or pressure lasting more than a few minutes or that radiates to the shoulder, arm, neck, jaw, stomach or back
- Persistent abdominal pain or pressure
- Life-threatening external bleeding (bleeding that spurts or flows continuously from a wound, pools on surfaces, is enough to fill half of a soda can or even less for small children and infants)
- Vomiting blood or passing blood
- Burns
- Suspected poison exposure
- Seizures
- Signs or symptoms of stroke (e.g., drooping of the face on one side; sudden weakness on one side of the body; sudden slurred speech or difficulty speaking; sudden, severe headache)
- Signs or symptoms of shock (e.g., changes in level of responsiveness; rapid breathing; rapid, weak heartbeat; nausea or vomiting; pale, ashen [grayish], cool, moist skin; restlessness or irritability; excessive thirst)
- Opioid overdose (decreased breathing effort and rate; unresponsiveness; bluish or greyish colored skin; small pupils)
- Diabetic emergency (trouble breathing; fast or deep breathing; feeling weak or different; sweating; fast heartbeat)
- Hypothermia (shivering; pale; cold to the touch; disoriented)
- Heat stroke (moist, pale or flushed skin; absence of sweating or some degree of sweating; unresponsive or confused; seizure; headache; nausea; dizziness; weakness; exhaustion)
- Suspected or obvious injuries to the head, neck or spine
- Suspected or obvious broken bone

emergency action plan. In these locations, know how to activate these resources.

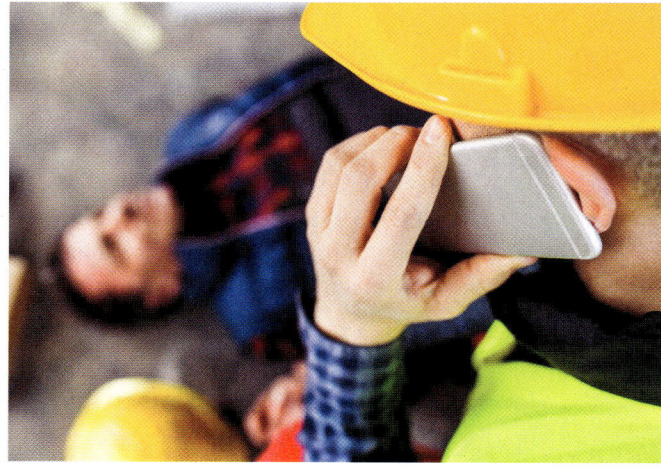

Phone carriers are required to connect 9-1-1 calls made from a mobile phone, even if the phone does not have an active service plan. In most areas, you cannot text 9-1-1. You must call! Unless you have confirmed that the 9-1-1 call center in your area supports texting, you should always call.

If you decide it is necessary to summon EMS, ask someone else to call 9-1-1 so that you can begin giving care. If you ask someone to make the call, always pick someone specific and make sure they come back and let you know they've called. If you just yell, "someone call 9-1-1!" you won't know for sure if it's going to get done. So, instead, look directly at one person and say "You, call 9-1-1." That way you know who made the call and that help is on the way.

If you are alone, make the call quickly using a cell phone preferably so that you can stay by the person's side. Whether you or someone else makes the call, using a cell phone on speaker mode is beneficial. In many areas dispatchers are trained to give instructions on CPR and first aid. Their coaching combined with your training will make you more confident to help. If you need to go to a phone, do so quickly so that you can return to the person. The person making the call should be prepared to give the dispatcher the following information:

- The location of the emergency (the address, or nearby intersections or landmarks if the address is not known)
- The nature of the emergency (e.g., whether police, fire or medical assistance is needed)
- The telephone number of the phone being used
- A description of what happened
- The number of injured or ill people
- What help, if any, has been given so far, and by whom

The caller should stay on the phone until the dispatcher tells them it is all right to hang up. The dispatcher may need more information. Many dispatchers also are trained to give first aid and CPR instructions over the phone, which can be helpful if you are unsure of what to do or need to be reminded of the proper care steps.

If you are alone, do not have a cell phone and there is no one to send to call 9-1-1 or the designated emergency number, you may need to decide whether to call first or give care first (Box 1-10). Call First situations are likely to be cardiac arrest. In cardiac arrest, the priority is getting help on the scene as soon as possible because early access to EMS and an AED increases the person's chances for survival. Care First situations include breathing emergencies and life-threatening bleeding. In these situations, there are immediate actions that you can take at the scene that may prevent the person's condition from worsening. After you take these actions, call 9-1-1 or the designated emergency number to get EMS on the way.

Care for the Person

The final emergency action step is to give care according to the conditions that you find and your level of knowledge and training. First aid care can be the difference between life and death. Often it makes the difference between complete recovery and permanent disability. This manual, the American Red Cross First Aid/CPR/AED courses and the First Aid app provide you with the knowledge, skills and confidence you need to give care to a person in an emergency medical situation. In general, you should give the appropriate care to an injured or ill person until:

- Other trained responders or EMS personnel arrive and begin their care of the person.
- You are too exhausted to continue.
- The scene becomes unsafe.

Follow these general guidelines when giving care:

- Give care consistent with your knowledge and training.
- Offer to assist the person with their own medication, if needed.
- Help the person rest in the most comfortable position.
- Keep the person from getting chilled or overheated.
- Reassure the person by telling the person that you will help and that EMS personnel have been called, if appropriate.
- Continue to watch for changes in the person's condition including breathing and level of responsiveness.

> **Box 1-10 Should You Ever Care First?**
>
> Most of the time, you will call first and then give care. But if you are **alone**, you may have to care first in some situations.
>
>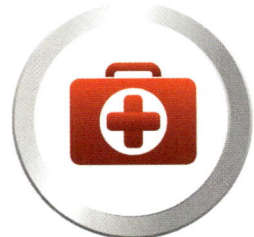
>
> If you are alone and **do not** have a cell phone, you will usually follow the normal steps of check, call and care. However, for a few conditions you will need to give immediate care, then go to call 9-1-1 or the designated emergency number. These conditions include:
>
> - An unresponsive infant or child younger than about 12 years whom you did not see collapse.
> - A person who is choking.
> - A person who is experiencing a severe allergic reaction (anaphylaxis) and has an epinephrine auto-injector.
> - A person who has life-threatening bleeding.

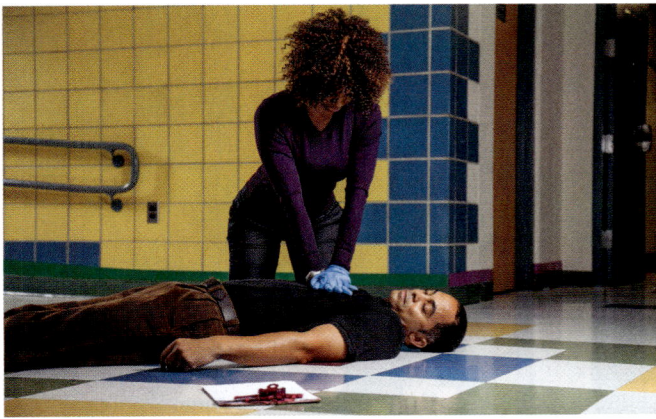

Placing an Injured or Ill Person in a Recovery Position

When a person is unresponsive but breathing or responsive but not fully awake, put the person in a recovery position onto their side if the person has no obvious signs of life-threatening injury or illness (Box 1-11). The recovery position helps to lower the person's risk for choking and aspiration (the inhalation of foreign matter, such as saliva or vomit, into the lungs). You should also use the recovery position if a person with an injury begins to vomit, or if it is necessary to leave the person alone to call 9-1-1 or the designated emergency number.

Moving and Transporting an Injured or Ill Person

Generally speaking, you should avoid moving an injured or ill person to give care. Unnecessary movement can cause additional injury and pain and may complicate the person's recovery. However, under the following three conditions, it would be appropriate to move an injured or ill person:

- You must move the person to protect them from immediate danger (such as fire, flood or poisonous gas). However, you should only attempt this if you can reach the person and remove them from the area without endangering yourself.
- You must move the person to reach another person who may have a more serious injury or illness.
- You must move the person to give proper care. For example, it may be necessary to move a person who needs CPR onto a hard, flat surface or you may need to move a person's extremity to control life-threatening bleeding.

If you must move the person, use one of the techniques described in Appendix A: Emergency Moves.

If the person does not have a life-threatening illness or injury, you may decide to take the injured or ill person to a medical facility yourself instead of calling for EMS personnel. Never transport a person yourself if the person has or may develop a life-threatening condition, if you are unsure of the nature of the injury or illness, or if the trip may aggravate the injury or cause additional injury.

If you decide it is safe to transport the person yourself, which should only be done for non-life-threatening conditions, be sure you know the quickest route to the nearest medical facility capable of handling emergency care. Ask someone to come with you to help keep the person comfortable and monitor the person for changes in condition so that you can focus on driving. Remember to obey traffic laws. No one will benefit if you are involved in a motor-vehicle collision or get a speeding ticket on your way to the medical facility.

Box 1-11 Recovery Position

Placing the Adult, Child or Infant in a Recovery Position

To place an adult, child or infant in a recovery position:

- Extend the person's arm that is closest to you above the person's head.
- Roll the person toward yourself onto their side, so that the person's head rests on their extended arm.
  - Turning the person toward yourself, rather than away from yourself, allows for more control over the movement and helps you monitor the person's airway.
- Bend both of the person's knees to stabilize their body.

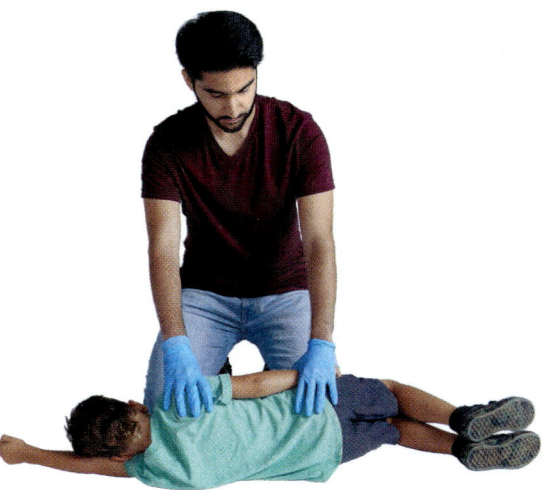

Discourage an injured or ill person from driving themself to the hospital. An injury may restrict movement, or the person may become faint. The sudden onset of pain may be distracting. Any of these conditions can make driving dangerous for the person, passengers, other drivers and pedestrians.

Dealing with Emotional Aspects of Giving Care

Being involved in responding to an emergency situation and giving first aid care to an injured of ill person can cause a wide range of feelings. These feelings are normal. It also is important to know that talking about your feelings is helpful in coping with the stress of responding to someone in an emergency situation. You may wish to talk with family members, consult with your human resources department about your company's employee assistance program, or consult with your personal healthcare provider or clergy for counseling or referral to a professional.

PUTTING IT ALL TOGETHER 1-1

Checking an Injured or Ill Person

Check ✓ 1. Check the scene for safety, form an initial impression, obtain consent and use PPE.

2. If the person appears unresponsive, check for responsiveness, breathing, life-threatening bleeding or other life-threatening conditions.

   - **Shout** to get the person's attention, using the person's name if you know it. If there is no response, **tap** the person's shoulder (if the person is an adult or child) or the bottom of the person's foot (if the person is an infant), and **shout** again while checking for breathing, life-threatening bleeding and other life-threatening conditions.

   Note: *Check for no more than 10 seconds.*
   Note: *Isolated or infrequent gasping is not considered breathing.*

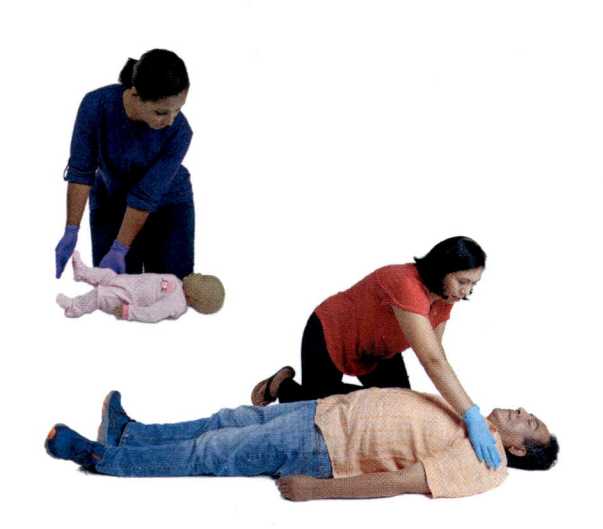

3. If the person does not respond, responds but is not fully awake, is not breathing or is only gasping, or has life-threatening bleeding or another obvious life-threatening condition, move immediately to the CALL and CARE steps.

   Note: *Give care immediately for the condition found and continue your check (as appropriate) to obtain more information and determine whether additional care is needed (see below). For a person who is unresponsive and not breathing, start CPR and use an AED immediately.*

Check ✓ 4. If the person is responsive, or responds to stimulation, and is fully awake and does not appear to have a life-threatening condition:

   - **Interview the person** (or bystanders, if necessary) **using SAM**. This will allow you to get a better understanding of the situation and the nature of the person's illness or injury.
     - ○ **S = Signs and symptoms.** Take note of signs (which you can observe for yourself, using your senses) and ask the person about symptoms (feelings that only the person can describe to you, such as pain, shortness of breath or nausea).
     - ○ **A = Allergies.** Ask the person about allergies, noting causes of allergic reactions in the past and whether the allergic reaction was severe or life-threatening.

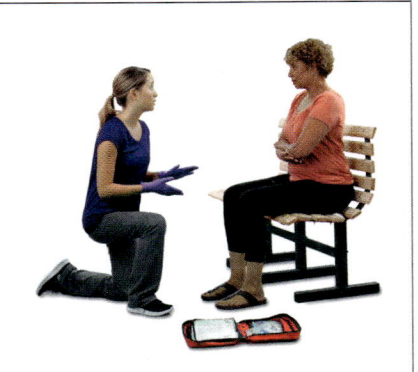

(Continued on next page)

American Red Cross | First Aid Basics

PUTTING IT ALL TOGETHER 1-1

Checking an Injured or Ill Person continued

- ○ **M = Medications and medical conditions.** Ask the person about over-the-counter and prescription medications that they are taking. Ask about the name of the medication and when the person last took it. Ask the person whether they have any medical conditions.

- Do a **focused check**. Check the part or parts of the body that the person is saying hurts, is holding, or where you see obvious signs of injury, including bleeding, cuts, burns, bruising, swelling or deformities. Note if the person has pain or discomfort or is unable or unwilling to move the body part. Record this information. Also notice how the person's skin looks and feels. Is the skin pale, ashen (gray) or flushed? Does it feel moist or dry, cool or hot?

Note: *Do not ask the person to move if you suspect a head, neck or spinal injury. Do not ask the person to move any area of the body that causes discomfort or pain.*

Note: *As you check the person, take note of any medical identification tags (typically worn around the neck, wrist or ankle).*

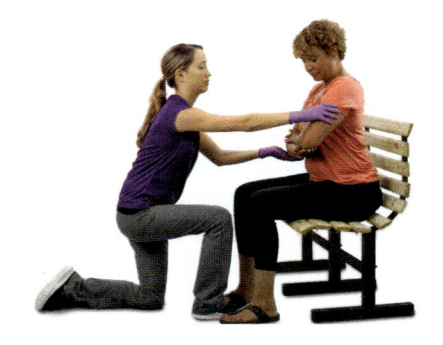

5. After **completing the CHECK step,** move to the **CALL step,** if needed, and then move to **CARE**.

PART 2
First Aid for Cardiac Arrest and Choking

CHAPTER 2: Adult CPR and AED

CHAPTER 3: Pediatric CPR and AED

CHAPTER 4: Choking

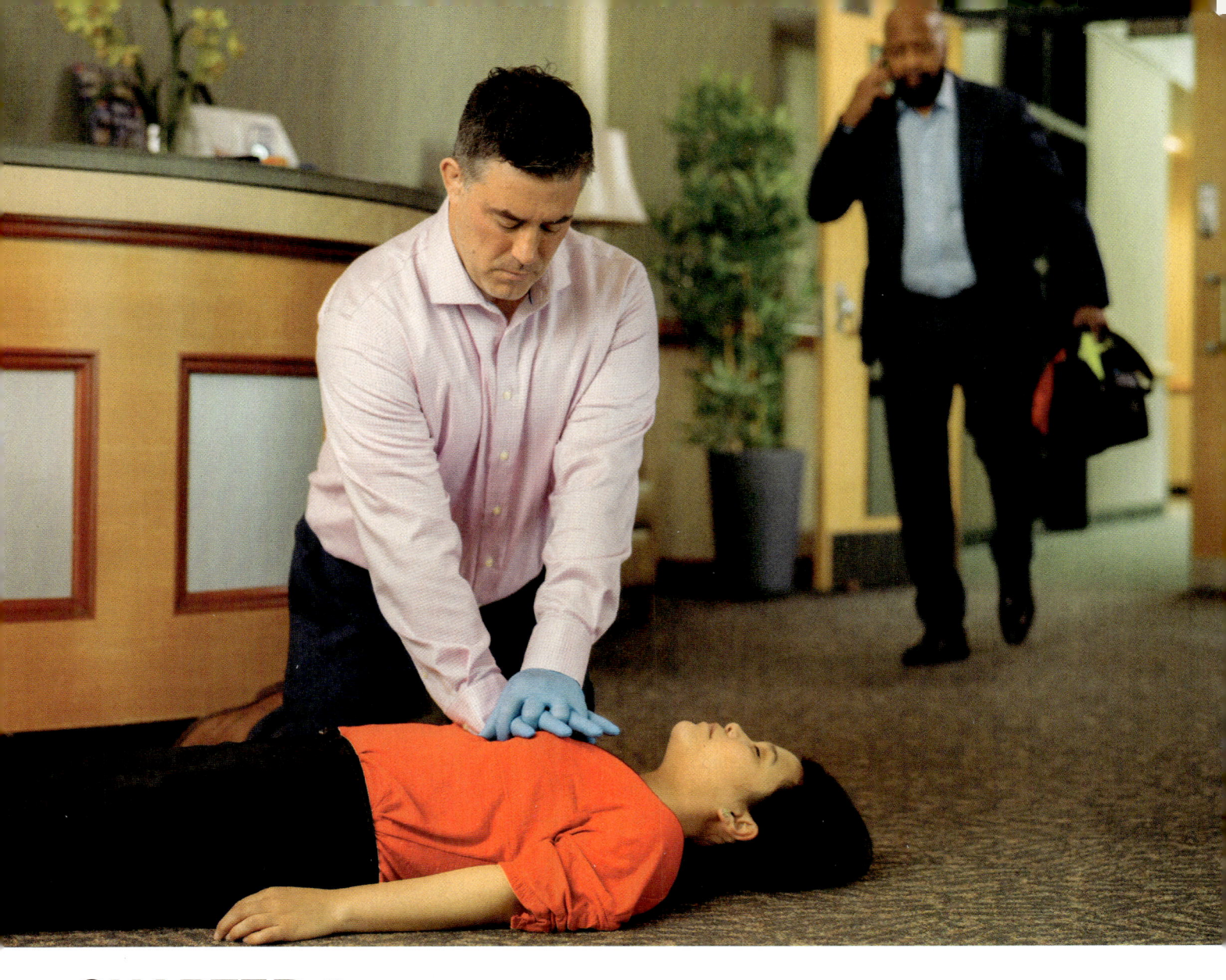

CHAPTER 2
Adult CPR and AED

Life-threatening cardiac arrest often strikes close to home, where we live, work and play. When you know how to recognize and respond to cardiac arrest, the life you could save is likely to be that of someone you know—a family member, co-worker or neighbor. Because every minute counts when a person is experiencing cardiac arrest, the person's survival often depends on lay responders acting quickly and giving appropriate care until EMS personnel arrive and begin their care of the person.

Cardiac arrest occurs when the heart stops beating or beats too ineffectively to circulate blood to the brain and other vital organs. A network of special cells in the heart muscle conducts electrical impulses that coordinate contraction, causing the heart to beat rhythmically. In one of the pathways to cardiac arrest, the electrical impulses become abnormal and chaotic. This causes the heart to lose the ability to beat rhythmically, or to stop beating altogether. Cardiac arrest is not the same thing as a heart attack. A heart attack is a blockage of the blood vessels that supply oxygen to the heart muscle. You will learn about how to recognize if a person is having a heart attack and how to care for a person experiencing a heart attack in Chapter 5: Sudden Illness.

American Red Cross | First Aid for Cardiac Arrest and Choking

Recognizing Cardiac Arrest

The **Cardiac Chain of Survival** describes actions that, when performed in rapid succession, increase the person's likelihood of surviving cardiac arrest and recovering (Box 2-1). In the Cardiac Chain of Survival, each link of the chain depends on, and is connected to, the other links.

Four out of every five cardiac arrests in the United States occur outside of the hospital. That means responders like you are often responsible for initiating the Cardiac Chain of Survival. When you complete the first three links in the Cardiac Chain of Survival—recognizing cardiac arrest and activating the EMS system, immediately beginning CPR, and using an AED as soon as possible—you give the person the best chance for surviving the incident (Figure 2-1).

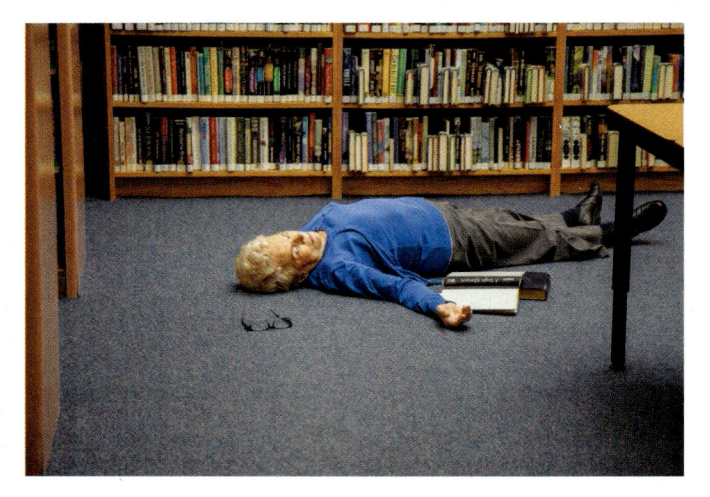

When a person experiences cardiac arrest, you may see the person suddenly collapse. When you check the person who is experiencing cardiac arrest, you will find that the person is not responsive and not breathing, or only gasping. In an unresponsive person, isolated or infrequent gasping in the absence of normal breathing may be **agonal breaths**, which can occur even after the heart has stopped beating. Agonal breaths are not breathing and may be seen early in cardiac arrest. In addition, the person in cardiac arrest has no heartbeat.

Cardiac arrest occurs when the heart stops beating or beats too ineffectively to circulate blood to the brain and other vital organs. Cardiac arrest frequently happens suddenly and without any warning signs or symptoms. When this occurs, the person is said to have experienced **sudden cardiac arrest**. People who have a history of cardiovascular disease or a congenital heart disorder are at higher risk for sudden cardiac arrest. Sudden cardiac arrest can occur due to a heart attack. Also, a heart attack can occur for some time before resulting in cardiac arrest. Sudden cardiac arrest can also happen in people who appear healthy and have no known heart disease or other risk factors for the condition.

Cardiac arrest may also occur after a period of time due to effects of drowning, breathing emergencies or trauma.

Cardiac Chain of Survival

When a person experiences cardiac arrest, quick action on the part of those who witness the arrest is crucial and gives the person the greatest chance for survival.

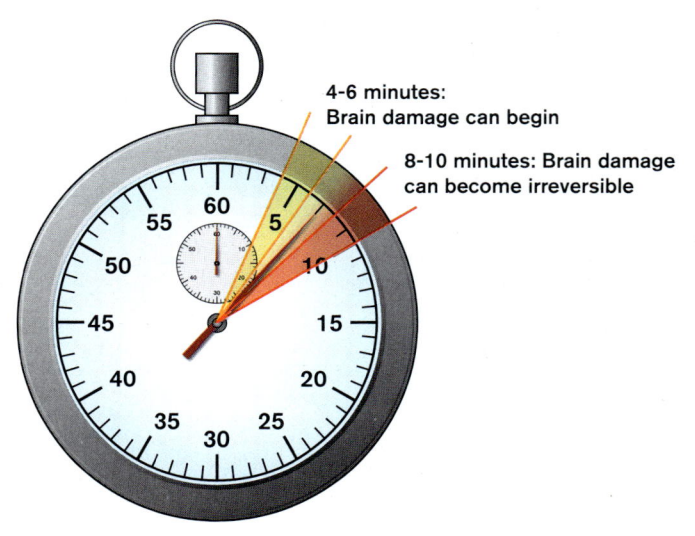

Figure 2-1. Every minute counts in cardiac arrest.

4-6 minutes: Brain damage can begin

8-10 minutes: Brain damage can become irreversible

If you have checked a person and you think that they are in cardiac arrest:

- Call 9-1-1 and get equipment or tell someone to do so.
- Begin CPR immediately.
- Use an AED as soon as possible.

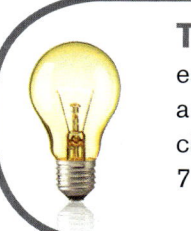

THE PROS KNOW. For each minute that CPR and use of an AED are delayed, a person's chance for survival decreases by 7 to 10 percent.

Box 2-1 The Cardiac Chain of Survival

Adult Out-of-Hospital Cardiac Chain of Survival

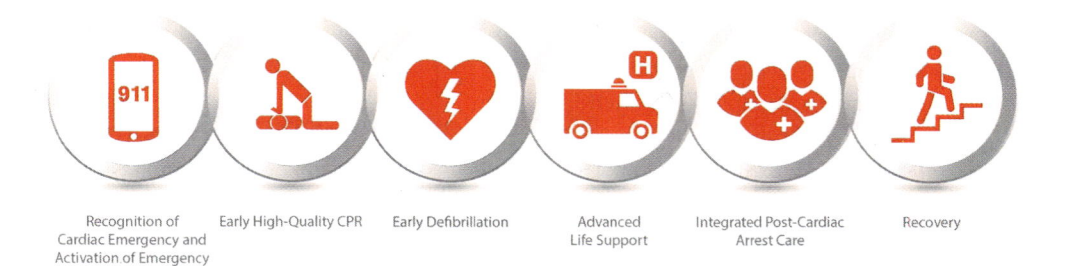

Recognition of Cardiac Emergency and Activation of Emergency Response System | Early High-Quality CPR | Early Defibrillation | Advanced Life Support | Integrated Post-Cardiac Arrest Care | Recovery

- **Recognition of cardiac emergency and activation of emergency response system.** The sooner someone recognizes that a person is in cardiac arrest and calls 9-1-1, the sooner people capable of providing advanced life support will arrive on the scene.
- **Early CPR.** CPR circulates oxygen-containing blood to the brain and other vital organs, helping to prevent brain damage and death.
- **Early defibrillation.** Defibrillation (delivery of an electrical shock using an AED) may restore an effective heart rhythm, significantly increasing the person's chances for survival.
- **Advanced life support.** Provided by EMS personnel at the scene and en route to the hospital, advanced life support gives the person access to emergency medical care delivered by trained professionals.
- **Integrated post–cardiac arrest care.** After the person is resuscitated, an interdisciplinary team of medical professionals works to stabilize the person's medical condition, minimize complications, and diagnose and treat the underlying cause of the cardiac arrest to improve survival outcomes.
- **Recovery.** After the person is discharged from the hospital, it is important that they have continued follow-up during the recovery process in the form of support rehabilitation, therapy and support from family and healthcare providers. This continued follow-up during the recovery process is an important link in the cardiac chain of survival.

Components of High-Quality CPR

You *can* save a life when the heart has stopped beating. **CPR**, or cardiopulmonary resuscitation, is a skill that is used when a person is in cardiac arrest to keep oxygenated blood moving to the brain and other vital organs until EMS arrives (Figure 2-2). CPR consists of giving cycles of 30 compressions followed by giving 2 breaths. High-quality CPR can double or triple a person's chance of survival if it is provided in the first few minutes of a person experiencing cardiac arrest.

Knowing how to perform high-quality CPR ensures you are doing everything you can to save a person's life. **High-quality CPR** includes:

- Using correct hand placement and body position.
- Compressing the chest at a rate of 100 to 120 compressions per minute.
- Compressing the chest to a depth of at least 2 inches.
- Allowing the chest to return to its normal position between each compression.

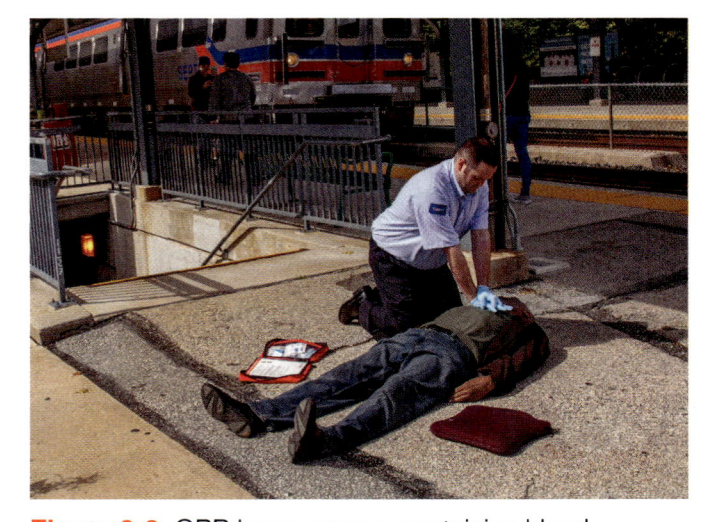

Figure 2-2. CPR keeps oxygen-containing blood circulating to the brain and other vital organs.

- Minimizing necessary interruptions to chest compressions, and if there is an interruption, keeping it to less than 10 seconds.
- Avoiding excessive breaths. Each breath should last about 1 second and cause the chest to begin to rise.

Giving CPR

As stated above, CPR involves giving sets of 30 chest compressions followed by sets of 2 breaths. When you give compressions, you press down on the person's chest. This changes the pressure in the chest, moving blood out of the heart and to the brain and other vital organs. After each compression, you must let the chest return to its normal position. This allows blood to flow back into the heart. The breaths you give after each set of 30 compressions deliver a fresh supply of oxygen into the person's lungs. When you give CPR, you help to keep oxygenated blood moving throughout the body, which can buy the person some time until EMS arrives. If you check a person and find that they are unresponsive and not breathing or only gasping, after calling 9-1-1 and getting equipment or telling someone to do so, begin CPR immediately, starting with chest compressions. Proper technique is important. Table 2-1 summarizes the key steps.

Giving Chest Compressions

First, make sure the person is lying face-up on a firm, flat surface. If the person is on a soft surface like a bed or couch, quickly and carefully move them to the floor before you begin. Kneel beside the person with your knees near their body and your knees spread about shoulder width apart.

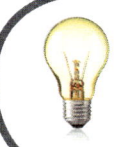

> **THE PROS KNOW.** When drowning is the suspected cause of cardiac arrest, the responder should deliver 2 initial breaths before starting CPR. During the drowning process, water comes into contact with the airway, causing it to spasm. When this occurs, air cannot reach the lungs. Giving breaths first can provide needed oxygen.

TABLE 2-1 CPR Technique for Adults (about age 12 or older)

Positioning 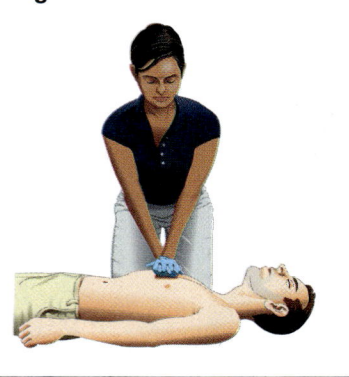	- Kneel beside the person. - Two hands in center of chest; fingers interlaced and off the person's chest - Shoulders directly over hands; elbows locked
Chest Compressions	- Push hard and fast. - Compress **at least 2 inches.** - Rate: 100 to 120 per minute
Breaths Tilt head to **past-neutral position**; pinch nose shut and form seal over mouth 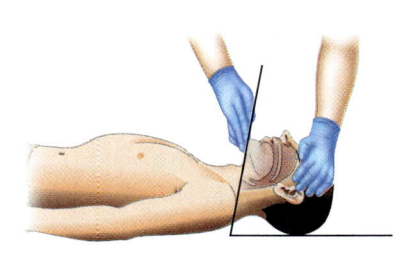	- No barrier/face shield: Open the airway using head-tilt/chin-lift to a **past-neutral position**; pinch nose shut; take a normal breath and form a complete seal over the mouth. - Pocket mask: Seal the mask over the mouth and nose and simultaneously open the airway to a **past-neutral position** using head-tilt/chin-lift technique.
CPR Cycles	One cycle = 30 chest compressions and 2 breaths

Chapter 2 | Adult CPR and AED

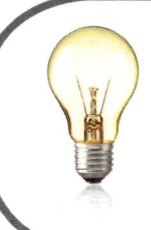

THE PROS KNOW. Many lay responders worry about hurting the person while giving CPR (e.g., breaking the person's ribs or breastbone), but a person who is in need of CPR is clinically dead (i.e., the person has no heartbeat and is not breathing). It is very unlikely that you will injure the person while giving CPR, but even if you do, consider this: any injury you may cause is secondary when compared with the person's current circumstances, and the injury will heal with medical care and time. Remember: The worst thing to do is nothing!

Position Your Hands and Body

Place the heel of one hand in the center of the person's chest on the person's breastbone (sternum). If you feel the notch at the end of the breastbone, move your hand slightly toward the person's head. Place your other hand on top of your first hand and interlace your fingers or hold them up so that your fingers are not on the person's chest. If you have arthritis in your hands, you can grasp the wrist of the hand positioned on the chest with your other hand instead. The person's clothing should not interfere with finding the proper hand position or your ability to give effective compressions. If it does, loosen or remove enough clothing to allow deep compressions in the center of the person's chest.

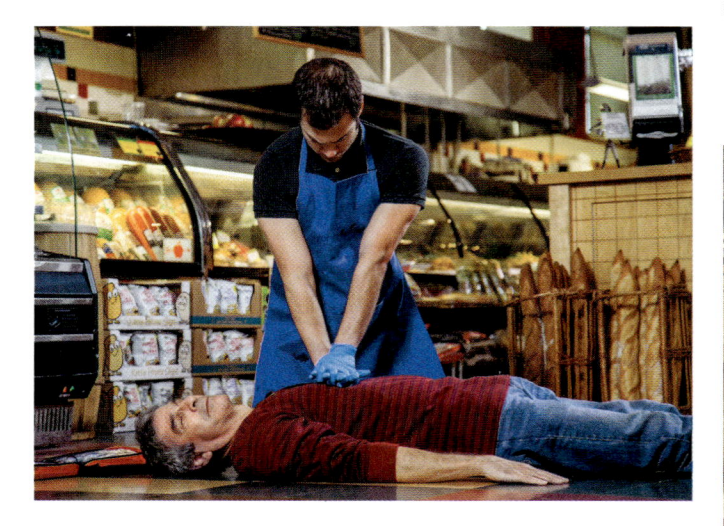

THE PROS KNOW. Incorrect technique or body position can cause your arms and shoulders to tire quickly when you are giving compressions. Use the weight of your upper body to compress the chest, not your arm muscles. Avoid rocking back and forth, because rocking makes your compressions less effective and wastes your energy. Also avoid leaning on the chest, because leaning prevents the chest from returning to its normal position after each compression, limiting the amount of blood that can return to the heart.

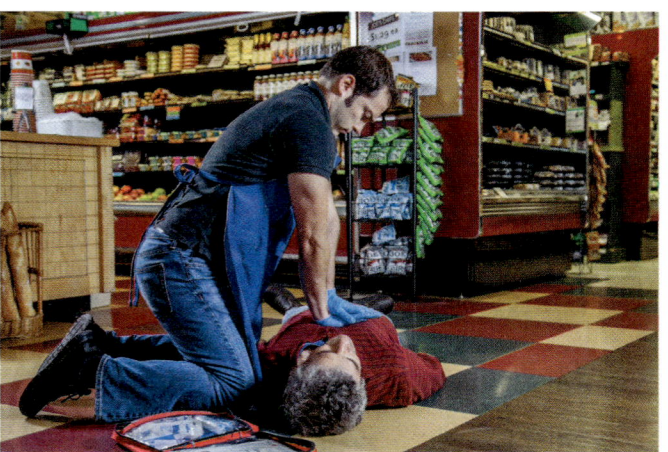

Position your body so that your shoulders are directly over your hands and lock your elbows to keep your arms straight. This technique allows you to use your body weight to help compress the center of the chest. It will also let you push on the chest using a straight up-and-down motion, which moves the most blood with each push and is also less tiring.

Give a Set of 30 Compressions

Keeping your arms straight, push down at least 2 inches, and then let the chest completely return to its normal position. Push hard and push fast! You want to go at a rate of 100 to 120 compressions per minute or about one compression every half second. As you give compressions, count out loud up to 30.

After each compression, let the chest return to its normal position. Maintain a smooth, steady down-and-up rhythm and do not pause between compressions.

American Red Cross | First Aid for Cardiac Arrest and Choking

> **THE PROS KNOW.** Counting out loud as you give compressions can help you to keep a steady, even rhythm. For compressions 1 through 12, say "one and two and three and four and five and six and . . ." up to 12. When you get to 13, just say the number: "thirteen, fourteen, fifteen, sixteen . . ." up to 30. Push down as you say the number and come up as you say "and" (or the second syllable of the number). This will help you to keep a steady, even rhythm.

> **THE PROS KNOW.** When giving breaths, keep the person's head tilted back and avoid taking too large of a breath or blowing too forcefully. Failing to keep the person's head tilted back, taking too large of a breath, or blowing too forcefully can force air into the person's stomach instead of into their lungs, which can make the person vomit and cause other complications. Remember: Keep the head tilted back, take a normal breath, and blow just enough to make the chest begin to rise.

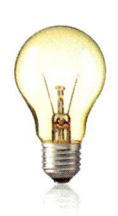

Do not interrupt chest compressions unless it is necessary to do so, for example, to give breaths, apply the AED pads, or move the person because the situation becomes dangerous. In those cases, minimize interruptions to chest compressions to as short as possible, but less than 10 seconds.

Giving Breaths

After giving 30 chest compressions, you will give a set of 2 breaths. Giving breaths is an essential part of CPR and supplies oxygen to a person who is not breathing. Studies have shown that breaths in combination with chest compressions increase a person's chance of survival and minimize brain injury.

While the risk of infection is extremely low, and data show you will most likely use your training for family or a friend, CPR breathing barriers, such as face shields and pocket masks, are available to further lower your risk of infectious disease. These devices protect you from contacting saliva and other body fluids, and from breathing the air that the person exhales.

While giving breaths improves the person's chance of survival, please remember if you are unwilling to give breaths, you can give compression-only CPR. This still helps the person and will be discussed later in the chapter.

Key points to remember when giving breaths are that each breath should last about 1 second and make the chest begin to rise, and it is important to pause between the breaths to allow for exhalation. This allows air to exit so that the next breath can effectively enter. After you finish giving 2 breaths, return to giving compressions as quickly as possible. The process of giving 2 breaths and getting back to compressions should take less than 10 seconds. Never give more than 2 breaths per set. Table 2-2 describes how to troubleshoot special situations when giving breaths.

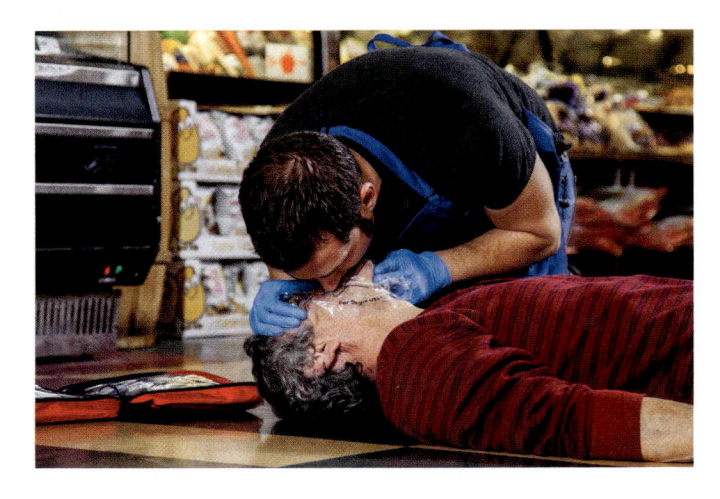

To give breaths, open the person's airway using the **head-tilt/chin-lift maneuver**. Place one of your hands on the person's forehead and two fingers of your other hand on the bony part of the person's chin. Tilt the person's head back and lift the chin. For an adult, tilt the head to a past-neutral position (see Table 2-1).

Pinch the person's nose shut. Take a normal breath, make a complete seal over the person's mouth with your mouth, and blow into the person's mouth to give the 1st breath. Take another breath, make a seal, and give the 2nd breath. Each breath should last about 1 second and make the person's chest begin to rise. Allow the air to leave the chest while you take another breath, make a seal and give a 2nd breath.

TABLE 2-2 Special Situation: Giving Breaths

SPECIAL SITUATION	SOLUTION
The breaths do not make the chest rise.	If the 1st breath does not cause the chest to begin to rise, reopen the airway to a past-neutral position using the head-tilt/chin-lift technique and ensure that the person's nose and mouth are properly sealed before giving the 2nd breath.
	If the 2nd breath does not make the chest rise when beginning CPR, an object may be blocking the person's airway, that is, the person may be in cardiac arrest due to choking. When clearing a blockage in an unresponsive person, you will use the CPR technique with one additional step.
	First, immediately begin chest compressions. The chest compressions used in CPR may dislodge the object. Then, before attempting breaths again, add the additional step of opening the mouth and looking for an object in the person's mouth; if you see it, remove it with a finger sweep using your index finger.
	You should never do a finger sweep if you don't see an object because you might push the object farther into the person's airway.
	If breaths go in, that is, the chest begins to rise, resume the normal CPR sequence of 30 compressions and 2 breaths with an AED.
	If breaths do not go in, that is, the chest does not begin to rise, continue with cycles of compressions followed by looking in the mouth and then trying to give breaths.
	Never attempt more than 2 breaths during each cycle of CPR.
The person vomits or there is fluid in the mouth. 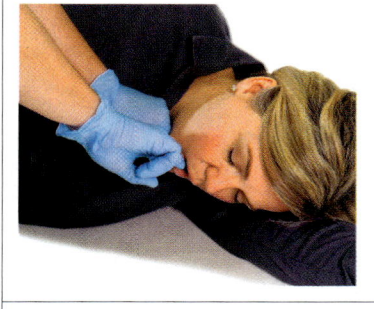	Roll the person onto their side and clear the mouth of fluid using a gloved finger or a piece of gauze. Then roll the person onto their back and resume giving care.
You are unable to form a tight seal over the person's mouth (e.g., due to an injury). 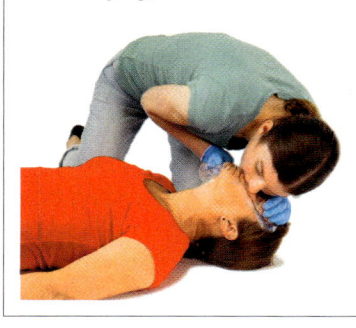	Use mouth-to-nose breathing instead. With the person's head tilted back, close the person's mouth by pushing on the person's chin. Make a complete seal over the person's nose with your mouth and blow in for 1 second to make the chest rise.

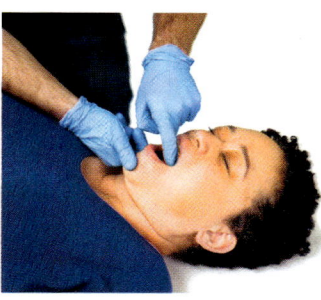

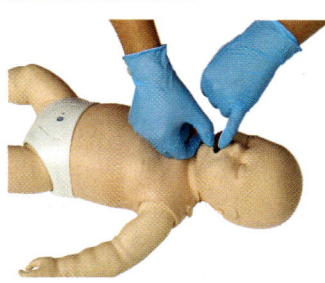

(Continued)

TABLE 2-2 Special Situation: Giving Breaths continued

SPECIAL SITUATION	SOLUTION
The person has a **tracheostomy** or "stoma," a surgically created opening in the front of the neck that opens into the trachea (windpipe) to form an alternate route for breathing when the upper airway is blocked or damaged.	Use mouth-to-stoma breathing instead. Expose the person's neck down to the breastbone and remove anything covering the stoma (e.g., a filter or stoma cover). Wipe away any secretions from the stoma. Make a complete seal over the person's stoma or tracheostomy tube with your mouth and blow in for 1 second to make the chest rise. ■ If the chest does not rise, the tracheostomy tube may be blocked. Remove the inner tube and try breaths again. ■ If you hear or feel air escaping from the person's mouth or nose, the person is a partial neck breather. (This means there is still a connection between the trachea and the upper airway, and although the person breathes mainly through the stoma, he or she is also able to breathe to some extent through the mouth and nose). Seal the person's mouth and nose with your hand or a tight-fitting mask so that air does not escape out of the mouth or nose when you give breaths into the stoma.

Giving Breaths with a Barrier Device

If available, use a CPR breathing barrier, such as a face shield or a pocket mask when you are giving breaths, but do not delay breaths to find a breathing barrier or learn how to use it.

Face Shield

A face shield is a flat piece of thin plastic that is placed over the person's face with the opening over the person's mouth. It has a valve that you give breaths through without making mouth-to-mouth contact.

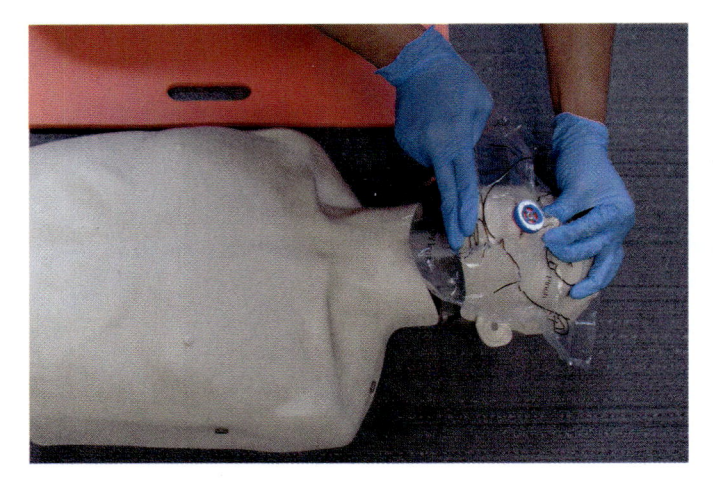

First, place the face shield over the person's face, ensuring the one-way valve is over their mouth. This is the most important step when using a face shield; ensuring that the opening or valve is over the mouth. Then, open the person's airway using the head-tilt/chin-lift technique. Put one hand on the forehead and two fingers on the bony part of the chin and tilt the head back to a past-neutral position. Next, pinch the person's nose shut, take a normal breath, and make a complete seal over the person's mouth with your mouth. Then, blow into their mouth for about 1 second, while looking to see that the chest begins to rise. Allow the person's chest to fall and the air to exit while you take another breath. Then make a seal and give the person a 2nd breath.

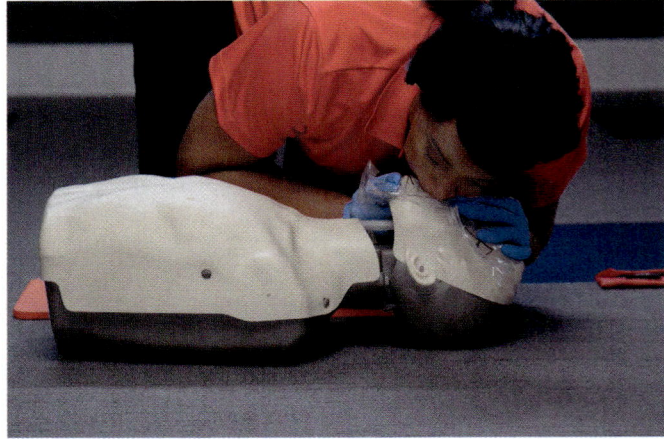

Pocket Mask

A pocket mask is a transparent flexible device that can be sealed to the face, covering the person's nose and mouth. It has a one-way valve that you give breaths through without making mouth-to-mouth contact or inhaling air exiting from the person's lungs.

Place the mask at the bridge of the nose and then lower it over the person's nose and mouth, making sure it doesn't go past the chin.

Seal the mask by placing the space of your hand between your thumb and index finger at the top of the mask above the valve. Place your remaining fingers on the side of the person's face. Then, place the thumb of your other hand along the base of the mask and place your bent index finger under the person's chin. Lift the person's face into the mask and open the airway to a past-neutral position by tilting the head back. This ensures both that there is a good seal between the mask and the face, and that the airway is in the open position.

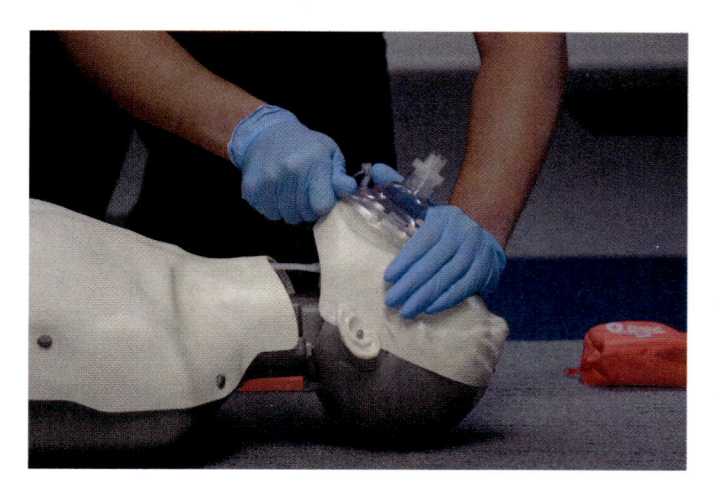

Gently but firmly hold the pocket mask in place to form and maintain a good seal so air does not leak out of the sides when you give breaths.

Then, take a normal breath, make a complete seal over the mask valve with your mouth, and give 2 breaths. Each breath should last about 1 second and make the person's chest begin to rise. Allow the air to leave the chest while you take another breath, make a seal and give a 2nd breath.

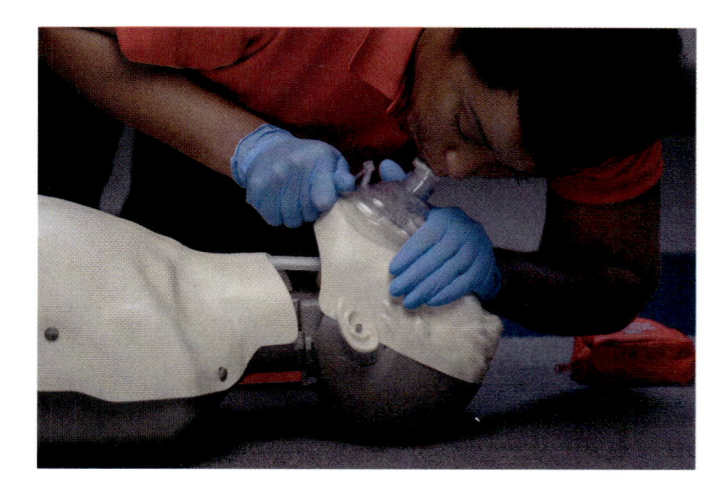

With a pocket mask the most important points are to ensure you have a good seal and that you maintain the seal. In addition, maintain an open airway in the past-neutral position, being careful not to push the head down.

Giving CPR Cycles

Once you begin CPR, continue giving cycles of chest compressions and breaths. One cycle of CPR is 30 compressions and 2 breaths.

It is important to begin each CPR cycle by giving 30 chest compressions. However, if drowning is the suspected cause of cardiac arrest, deliver 2 initial breaths before starting CPR cycles. Compress the chest at a rate of 100 to 120 per minute and at a depth of at least 2 inches. Remember, the goal is to push hard and fast!

Also, be sure to use correct hand placement and allow the chest to return to its normal position between compressions. Then give 2 breaths. Remember each breath should last about 1 second each and make the chest begin to rise. Allow the chest to fall before the next breath. Make sure you smoothly transition between chest compressions and breaths and minimize interruptions to chest compressions (to give breaths) to less than 10 seconds.

Continue cycles of CPR until:

- You notice an obvious sign of life, such as movement. (If the person shows an obvious sign of life, stop CPR, place the person in the recovery position and continue to monitor the person's condition until EMS personnel take over.)
- An AED is ready to use and no other trained responders are available to assist you with the AED.
- You have performed approximately 2 minutes of CPR (five sets of 30:2) and another trained responder is available to take over compressions. Giving chest compressions correctly is physically tiring. If more than one responder is available and trained in CPR, the responders should switch responsibility for compressions every 2 minutes, or whenever the responder giving compressions indicates that they are tiring. Switching responsibility for giving chest compressions frequently reduces responder fatigue, which improves the quality of chest compressions and leads to a better chance of survival for the person.
- You have performed approximately 2 minutes of CPR (five sets of 30:2), you are alone and caring for a child, and you need to call 9-1-1.
- EMS personnel arrive and begin their care of the person.
- You are alone and too tired to continue.
- The scene becomes unsafe.

American Red Cross | First Aid for Cardiac Arrest and Choking

CPR Special Considerations

Telephone CPR

When CPR is started before EMS personnel arrive, the person's chance of survival increases. Your decision to call 9-1-1 and take action makes a difference in saving lives!

As you learned in Chapter 1, many dispatchers are trained to give instructions for CPR over the phone. They can give instructions to an untrained person on the scene or remind a first aid responder what to do. When you call 9-1-1 on a mobile phone, put the phone on "speaker mode" and put the phone down beside you. This frees up both of your hands so that you can perform CPR and follow the directions of the dispatcher.

Compression-Only CPR

Although full CPR (compressions and breaths) is preferred, if you are unable or unwilling for any reason to give full CPR, you can give **compression-only CPR** instead. In compression-only CPR, you give continuous chest compressions with no breaths. After checking the scene for safety, checking the person, and calling 9-1-1 and getting equipment, or telling someone to do so, give chest compressions without stopping at a rate of 100 to 120 per minute. Continue giving chest compressions until the person shows an obvious sign of life like breathing, the scene becomes unsafe, an AED is ready, you're too exhausted to continue, another trained responder takes over, or EMS personnel arrive and begin their care of the person.

Using an AED

While CPR can help to prevent brain damage and death by keeping oxygenated blood moving throughout the body, an AED can correct the underlying problem for some people who go into sudden cardiac arrest. Two abnormal heart rhythms in particular, **ventricular fibrillation (V-fib)** and **ventricular tachycardia (V-tach)**, can lead to sudden cardiac arrest. In V-fib, the heart muscle simply quivers (fibrillates) weakly instead of contracting strongly. In V-tach, the heart muscle contracts too fast (*tachy-* means "fast"). Both abnormal rhythms impair the heart's ability to pump and circulate blood throughout the body and are life-threatening. However, in many cases, V-fib and V-tach can be corrected by an electrical shock delivered by an AED. This shock disrupts the heart's electrical activity long enough to allow the heart to spontaneously develop an effective rhythm on its own.

Starting CPR immediately and using an AED as soon as possible gives the person the best chance for surviving cardiac arrest (Figure 2-3).

Different types of AEDs are available, but all are simple to use and similar to operate and use visual displays, voice prompts, or both, to guide the responder. If your place of employment has an AED on site, know where it is located, how to operate it and how to maintain it (Box 2-2). Also take note of the location of AEDs in public places that you frequent, such as shopping centers, airports, recreation centers and sports arenas.

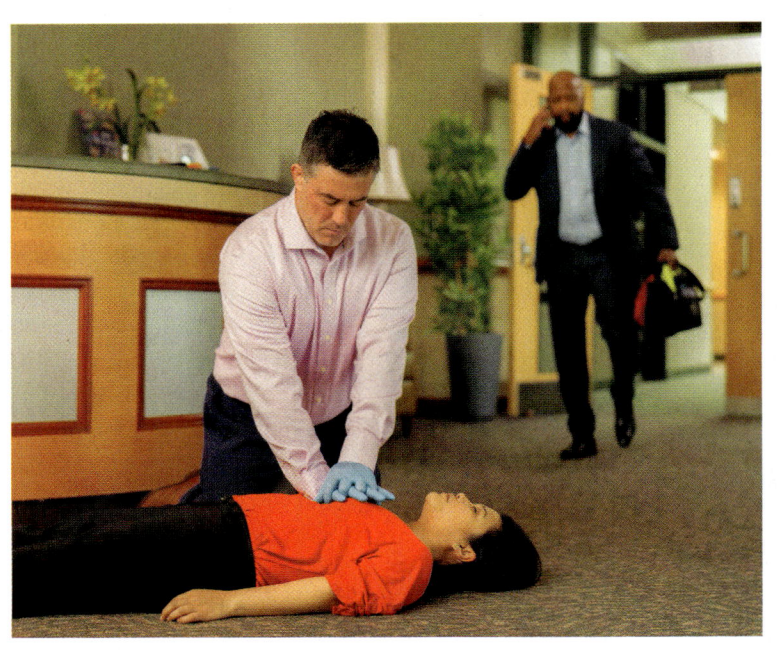

Figure 2-3. Immediately beginning CPR and using an AED as soon as possible gives the person the best chance for survival.

Box 2-2 AED Maintenance

AEDs require minimal maintenance, but it is important to check them regularly according to the manufacturer's instructions or your employer's policy to ensure that they are in good working order and ready for use whenever they are needed.

- Familiarize yourself with the owner's manual and follow the manufacturer's instructions for maintaining the equipment.
- Familiarize yourself with the method the AED uses to indicate the status of the device. Many AEDs have a status indicator that displays a symbol or illuminates to indicate that the AED is in proper working order and ready to respond. The status indicator may also display symbols indicating that routine maintenance (e.g., a battery change) is needed or that a problem with the device has been detected. Some AEDs have a warning indicator that will illuminate or beep if the AED is not in proper working order and ready to respond.
- Check to make sure the battery is properly installed and within its expiration date.
- Make sure AED pads are adequately stocked, stored in a sealed package, and within their expiration date.
- After using the AED, make sure that all supplies are restocked and that the device is in proper working order.
- If at any time the AED fails to work properly, or warning indicators illuminate, take the AED out of service and contact the manufacturer or the appropriate person at your place of employment, according to your employer's policy. You may need to return the AED to the manufacturer for service. If the AED stops working during an emergency, continue giving CPR until EMS personnel arrive and begin their care of the person.

When a person is in cardiac arrest, use an AED as soon as possible. Environmental and person-specific considerations for safe and effective AED use are given in Box 2-3. Table 2-3 provides useful facts regarding use of an AED.

Using an AED: One First Aid Responder

To use an AED if you are the only responder, first turn the device on. Remove or cut away clothing and undergarments to expose the person's chest. The shock should be delivered from the pads directly to the person's skin.

If the person's chest is wet, dry it using a towel or gauze pad. Dry skin helps the AED pads to stick properly. Do not use an alcohol wipe to dry the skin because alcohol is flammable. Next, place the AED pads. Always use adult AED pads on anyone older than 8 years old and/or weighing more than 55 pounds (25 kilograms). Do *not* use pediatric AED pads or the pediatric AED setting in these age/weight groups because the shock delivered will not be sufficient.

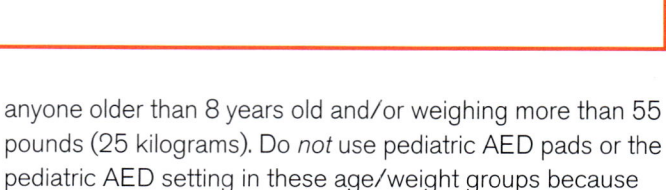

Peel the backing off the pads as directed, one at a time, to expose the adhesive. Place one pad on the upper right side of the person's chest and the other pad on the lower left side of the person's chest, a few inches below the left armpit, pressing firmly to adhere (Figure 2-4). This is best position for delivery of the shock to the heart. Follow the diagrams and labeling of where each pad goes.

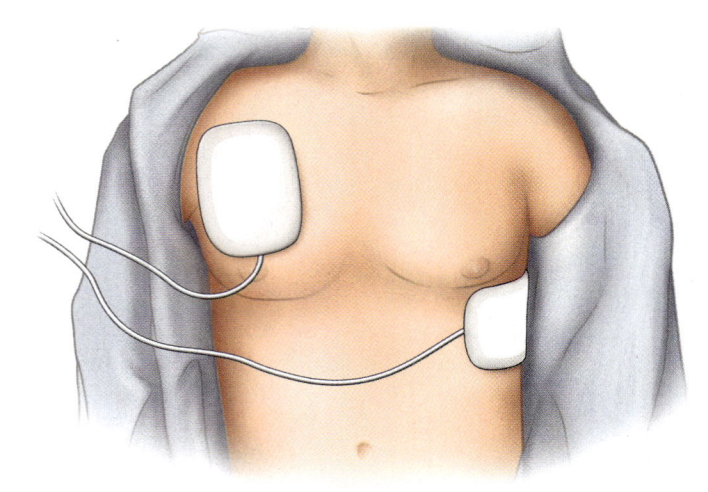

Figure 2-4. Place one AED pad on the upper right side of the chest and the other on the lower left side of the chest, below the left armpit.

American Red Cross | First Aid for Cardiac Arrest and Choking 39

Box 2-3 Considerations for Safe and Effective AED Use

Environmental Considerations

- **Flammable or combustible materials.** Do not use an AED around flammable or combustible materials, such as gasoline or free-flowing oxygen.
- **Metal surfaces.** It is safe to use an AED when the person is lying on a metal surface, as long as appropriate precautions are taken. Do not allow the AED pads to contact the metal surface, and ensure that no one is touching the person when the shock is delivered.
- **Water.** If the person is in water, remove him or her from the water before using the AED. Once you have removed the person from the water, be sure there are no puddles of water around you, the person or the AED.
- **Inclement weather.** It is safe to use AEDs in all weather conditions, including rain and snow. Provide a dry environment if possible, for example, by sheltering the person with umbrellas, but do not delay defibrillation to do so. Remove wet clothing and wipe the person's chest dry before placing the AED pads. Avoid getting the AED or AED pads wet.

Person-Specific Considerations

- **Pregnancy.** It is safe to use an AED on a woman who is pregnant.
- **Pacemakers and implantable cardioverter-defibrillators (ICDs).** A person who has a known arrhythmia (irregular heartbeat) may have a pacemaker or an ICD. These are small devices that are surgically implanted under the skin to automatically prevent or correct an irregular heartbeat. You may be able to see or feel the outline of the pacemaker or ICD in the area below the person's collarbone, or the person may wear medical identification indicating that he or she has a pacemaker or ICD. If the implanted device is visible or you know that the person has a pacemaker or ICD, adjust pad placement as necessary to avoid placing the AED pads directly over the device because doing so may interfere with the delivery of the shock. However, if you are not sure whether the person has an implanted device, place the pads as you normally would.
- **Transdermal medication patches.** Some types of medications, including nitroglycerin (used to relieve chest pain caused by cardiovascular disease) and smoking cessation medications, are delivered through patches applied to the skin. Remove any medication patches that you see before applying AED pads and using an AED. Wear gloves to prevent absorption of the drug through your own skin.
- **Chest hair.** Time is critical in a cardiac arrest situation and chest hair rarely interferes with pad adhesion, so in most cases, you should proceed as you normally would—attach the AED pads, pressing firmly to attach them. However, if the person has a great deal of thick chest hair and it seems like the chest hair could interfere with pad-to-skin contact, quickly shave the areas where the pads will be placed and then attach the pads.
- **Jewelry and body piercings.** You do not need to remove the person's jewelry or body piercings before using an AED, but you should avoid placing the AED pads directly over any metallic jewelry or piercings. Adjust pad placement if necessary.

TABLE 2-3 AED Fact or Fiction

STATEMENT	FACT OR FICTION	EXPLANATION
Cardiac arrest is the same as a heart attack and an AED should be used for both conditions.	Fiction	Although a heart attack can lead to cardiac arrest, the two conditions are different. With cardiac arrest the heart has stopped or is not pumping blood, but with a heart attack the heart may not be functioning normally but it is still PUMPING blood. An AED should only be used on a person who is in cardiac arrest.
AED pads must be removed before giving CPR.	Fiction	AED pads should not be removed before giving CPR, nor should the AED be turned off. It is possible that the AED will tell you that additional shocks are needed.

TABLE 2-3 AED Fact or Fiction continued

STATEMENT	FACT OR FICTION	EXPLANATION
It doesn't matter which AED pad is placed on the upper right side of the chest and which one is placed on the lower left side of the chest. The lower left side of the chest the placement of the AED pads is reversed, the AED will still work.	Fact	It is best to place pads as indicated, but if pad placement is reversed, the AED will still work.
If adult AED pads are not available, it is OK to use pediatric pads on an adult or on a child older than 8 years or weighing more than 55 pounds (25 kilograms).	Fiction	Do not use pediatric AED pads on an adult or on a child older than 8 years or weighing more than 55 pounds (25 kilograms) because the shock delivered will not be sufficient. However, adult AED pads can be used on a child up to 8 years of age or weighing less than 55 pounds (25 kilograms) if pediatric AED pads are not available.
It is safe to use an AED when the person is in a pool or lying in a puddle of water.	Fiction	If the person is in water, remove them from the water before using the AED.
It is safe to use an AED in rain or snow.	Fact	It is safe to use AEDs in all weather conditions. Provide for a dry environment if possible, but do not delay defibrillation to do so. Remove wet clothing and wipe the person's chest dry before placing the electrode pads.
It is OK to use an AED on a pregnant woman.	Fact	An AED is safe to use on a pregnant woman and offers the best chance of survival for both the mother and the fetus.
Shave a man's chest hair before applying the AED pads.	Fiction	Time is critical in a cardiac arrest situation and chest hair rarely interferes with pad adhesion, so in most cases, you should proceed as you normally would—attach the AED pads, pressing firmly to attach them. However, if the person has a great deal of thick chest hair and it seems like the chest hair could interfere with pad-to-skin contact, quickly shave the areas where the pads will be placed and then attach the pads.
Remove the person's jewelry and/or body piercings before using an AED.	Fiction	Do not delay the use of an AED to remove jewelry or body piercings. However, you should avoid placing the AED pads directly over metallic jewelry or body piercings. Adjust AED pad placement if necessary.
Never use an AED on a person who has an implantable cardioverter-defibrillator (ICD) or pacemaker device.	Fiction	It is safe to use an AED on a person with an ICD or pacemaker device. However, if you can see the implanted device or you know that the person has one, do not place the AED pads directly over the device because doing so may interfere with the delivery of the best shock. Adjust AED pad placement if necessary.
It is safe to use an AED when a person is lying on a metal surface.	Fact	It is safe to deliver a shock to a person in cardiac arrest on a metal surface as long as appropriate safety precautions are taken. Avoid allowing the defibrillation electrodes to contact the metal surface and ensure that no one is touching the person when the shock button is pushed.

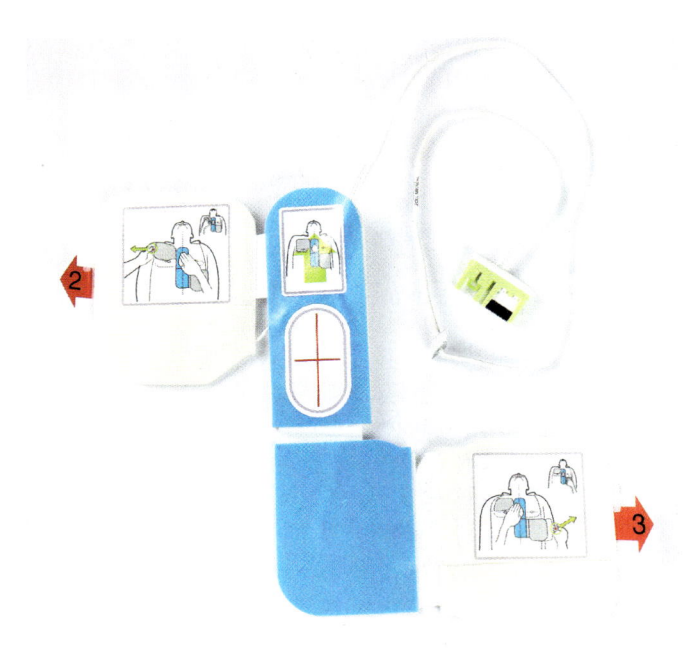

Figure 2-5. AED pads with feedback device.

If the AED pad has a feedback device (Figure 2-5), follow the manufacturer's instructions for use. Plug the pad connector cable into the AED (if necessary) and follow the device's directions. Most AEDs will begin to analyze the heart rhythm automatically, but some may require you to push an "analyze" button to start this process. No one should touch the person while the AED is analyzing the heart rhythm because this could result in a faulty reading. Say "CLEAR!" in a loud, commanding voice and be ready to deliver a shock if the AED determines one is needed. Next, the AED will tell you to push the "shock" button if a shock is advised. Again, avoid touching the person, because anyone who is touching the person while the device is delivering a shock is at risk for receiving a shock as well. Say "CLEAR!" in a loud, commanding voice and, if a shock is advised, push the shock button to deliver the shock. After a shock is delivered (or if the AED determines that no shock is necessary), immediately start CPR, beginning with compressions. Even after a successful shock, a person will still have low flow so starting CPR immediately will help.

The AED will continue to check the heart rhythm every 2 minutes. Listen for prompts from the AED.

Continue giving CPR until:

- You notice an obvious sign of life.
- The AED prompts you to analyze again.
- Another trained responder is available to take over compressions.
- EMS personnel arrive and begin their care of the person.
- You are alone and too tired to continue.
- The scene becomes unsafe.

If you notice an obvious sign of life, stop CPR but leave the AED turned on and the pads in place on the person's chest, and continue to follow the AED's prompts.

Putting It All Together 2-1 describes and illustrates step-by-step how to give CPR and use an AED for an adult.

Using an AED: Two or More First Aid Responders

Remember, when you are giving CPR, you want to give high-quality compressions at the appropriate depth and rate. You also want to minimize interruptions to chest compressions to less than 10 seconds. If you are the only trained responder at the scene, you will begin to tire as you give CPR, and the quality of your compressions will diminish. You will also need to stop CPR to prepare the AED for use when it arrives, which means that during that time there is no oxygenated blood moving through the person's body.

If you have another CPR- and AED-trained person with you, working as a team to provide CPR and use an AED can lead to a better chance of survival for the person in cardiac arrest. This teamwork reduces responder fatigue and minimizes interruptions to chest compressions when the AED arrives.

When there are two or more trained responders, the steps for using an AED are the same, but one person does CPR while the other operates the AED. Trained responders can share the responsibility for giving compressions, switching off every 2 minutes, which reduces fatigue and leads to better quality compressions.

When two or more responders trained in CPR and using an AED are at the scene, all should identify themselves as being trained. The first responder should begin CPR and tell the second responder to call 9-1-1 and get the AED and first aid kit. When the second responder returns with the AED, they will set it up by turning the device on, applying the pads to the person's chest and plugging in the connector cable, if necessary. The first responder should not pause CPR until the device is ready to analyze the person's heart rhythm and the second responder tells everyone to stand clear.

After the second responder delivers the shock, or if no shock is advised, the responders should switch roles so that the second responder can take over giving chest compressions. When responders switch roles, they should remain positioned on either side of the person with the AED at the head of the person so that both responders can easily operate it (Figure 2-6). The responders then switch roles about every 2 minutes. This role switch should take less than 10 seconds in order to minimize interruptions to chest compressions.

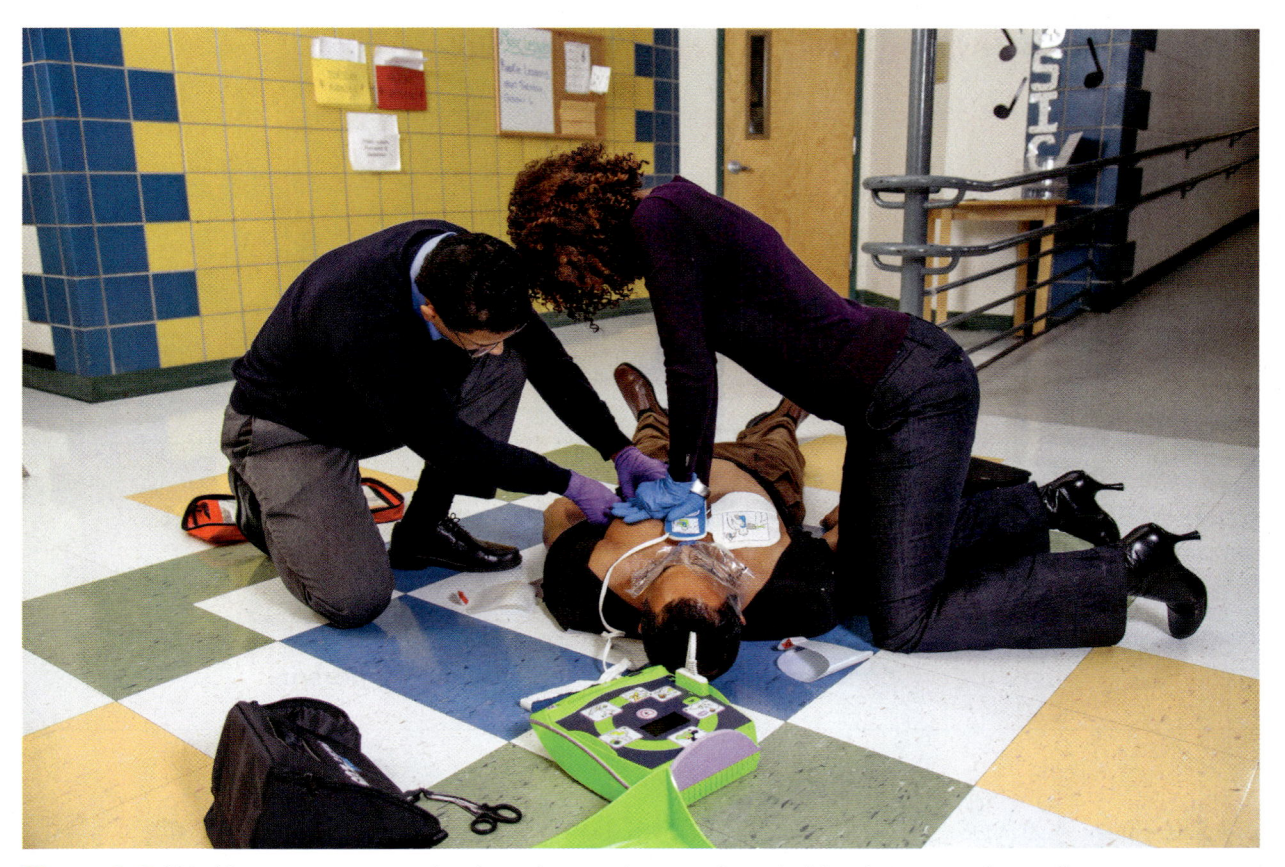

Figure 2-6. Working as a team can lead to a better chance of survival for the person in cardiac arrest.

PUTTING IT ALL TOGETHER 2-1

Giving CPR and Using an AED for an Adult

1. Check the scene for safety, form an initial impression, and use PPE.

2. If the person appears unresponsive, check the person for responsiveness (shout-tap-shout). 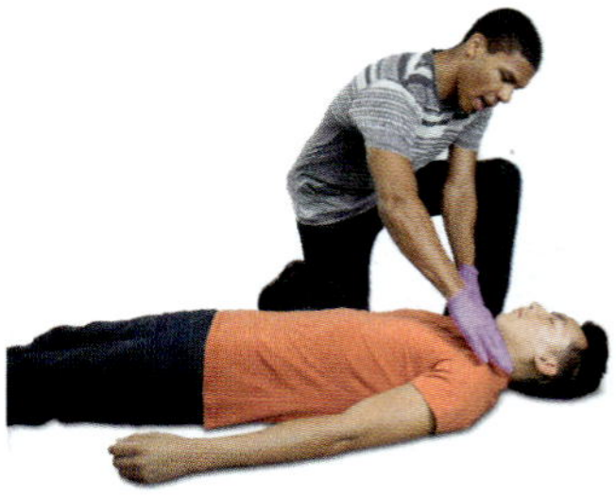
- Shout to get the person's attention, using the person's name if you know it. If the person does not respond, tap the person's shoulder and shout again while checking for breathing, life-threatening bleeding or another obvious life-threatening condition.

3. If the person does not respond and is not breathing or only gasping, call 9-1-1 and get equipment, or tell someone to do so, and continue to step 4.

4. Place the person on their back on a firm, flat surface. Kneel beside the person.

5. Give 30 chest compressions. 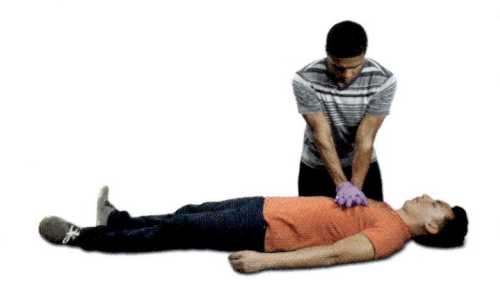
- Place the heel of one hand in the center of the person's chest, with your other hand on top and your fingers interlaced and off the person's chest.
- Position your body so that your shoulders are directly over your hands; lock your elbows.
- Keeping your arms straight, push down at least 2 inches, and then let the chest return to its normal position.
- Push hard and push fast! Give compressions at a rate of 100 to 120 compressions per minute.

6. Give 2 breaths. 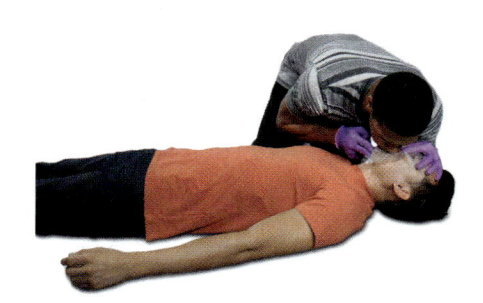
- If using a face shield:
  - Place the face shield over the person's nose and mouth, ensuring the one-way valve is over their mouth.
  - Open the airway to a past-neutral position using the head-tilt/chin-lift technique. (Put one hand on the forehead and two fingers on the bony part of the chin and tilt the head back.)
  - Pinch the nose shut, take a normal breath, and make a complete seal over the person's mouth with your mouth.

PUTTING IT ALL TOGETHER 2-1

6. Give 2 breaths (continued).

- If using a pocket mask:
  - Place the mask at the bridge of the nose and lower it over the person's nose and mouth.
  - Seal the mask and open the airway.
    - Place the space of your hand between your thumb and index finger at the top of the mask above the valve.
    - Place your remaining fingers on the side of the person's face.
    - Place the thumb of your other hand along the base of the mask and place your bent index finger under the person's chin.
    - Lift the person's face into the mask and open the airway to a past-neutral position by tilting the head back.
    - Take a normal breath and make a complete seal over the mouth valve.
- Give 1st breath.
  - Blow into the person's mouth for about 1 second, looking to see that the chest begins to rise.
  - Pause between breaths to allow for exhalation.
- Give 2nd breath.
  - Take another breath, make a seal, then give the 2nd breath.
- Minimize interruptions to chest compressions to less than **10 seconds**.

Note: *If the 1st breath does not cause the chest to rise, retilt the head and ensure a proper seal before giving the 2nd breath. If the 2nd breath does not make the chest rise, an object may be blocking the airway. After the next set of chest compressions and before attempting breaths, open the mouth, look for an object and, if seen, remove it using a finger sweep. Continue to check the person's mouth for an object after each set of compressions until the breaths go in, and then resume CPR.*

7. Continue giving sets of 30 chest compressions and 2 breaths until:

- You notice an obvious sign of life.
- An AED is ready to use and no other trained responders are available to assist you with the AED.
- You have performed approximately 2 minutes of CPR (5 sets of 30:2) and another responder is available to take over compressions.
- EMS personnel arrive and begin their care of the person.
- You are alone and too tired to continue.
- The scene becomes unsafe.

Use an AED as soon as one is available!

8. Turn on the AED and follow the voice prompts.

9. Remove all clothing covering the chest and, if necessary, wipe the chest dry.

(Continued on next page)

American Red Cross | First Aid for Cardiac Arrest and Choking

PUTTING IT ALL TOGETHER 2-1

Giving CPR and Using an AED for an Adult continued

10. Attach pads correctly.
- Place one pad on the upper right side of the chest and the other on the lower left side of the chest, a few inches below the left armpit.
- If the pads may touch, place one pad in the middle of the chest and the other pad on the back, between the shoulder blades.

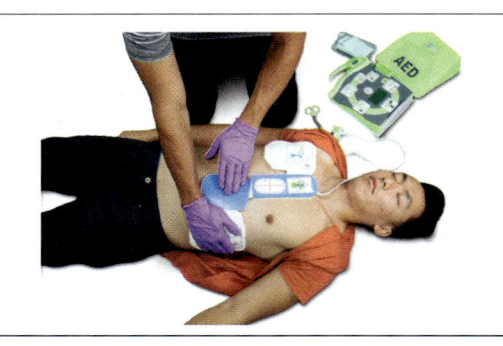

11. Plug the pad connector cable into the AED, if necessary.

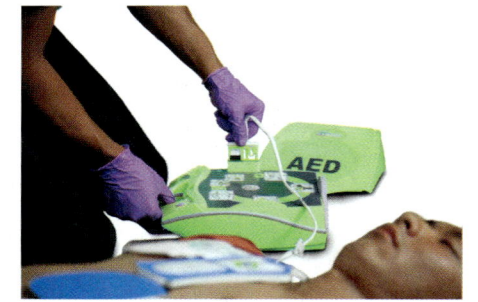

12. Prepare to let the AED analyze the heart's rhythm.
- Make sure no one, including you, is touching the person. Say, "CLEAR!" in a loud, commanding voice.
- If the AED tells you to, push the "analyze" button to start this process.

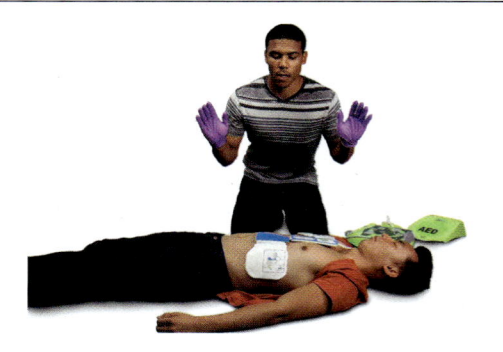

13. Deliver a shock, if the AED determines one is needed.
- Make sure no one, including you, is touching the person. Say, "CLEAR!" in a loud, commanding voice.
- Push the "shock" button to deliver the shock.

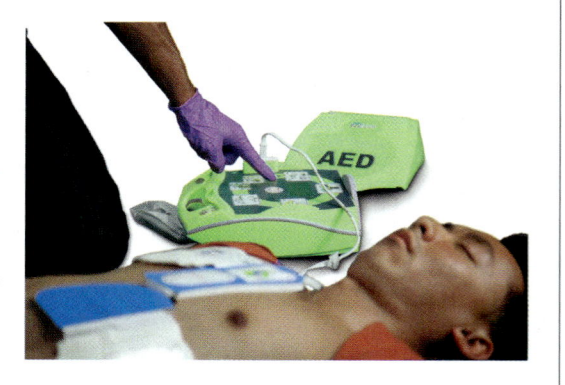

pediatric advanced life support gives the child or infant access to emergency medical care delivered by trained professionals.

- **Integrated post–cardiac arrest care.** After the child or infant is resuscitated, an interdisciplinary team of medical professionals works to stabilize the person's medical condition, minimize complications, and diagnose and treat the underlying cause of the cardiac arrest to improve survival outcomes.
- **Recovery.** After the child or infant is discharged from the hospital, recovery continues in the form of rehabilitation, therapy and support from family and healthcare providers. This continued follow-up during the recovery process is an important link in the cardiac chain of survival.

Components of High-Quality CPR

Knowing how to perform high-quality CPR ensures you are doing everything you can to save a child's or infant's life. High-quality CPR for children and infants includes:

- Using correct hand placement and body position.
- Compressing the chest at a rate of 100 to 120 compressions per minute.
- Compressing the chest to a depth of *about* 2 inches for children and *about* 1½ inches for infants.
- Allowing the chest to return to its normal position between each compression.
- Minimizing necessary interruptions to chest compressions and if there is an interruption, keep it to less than 10 seconds.
- Avoiding excessive breaths. Each breath should last about 1 second and cause the chest to begin to rise.

CPR and AED Differences Among Adults, Children and Infants

Responding to a cardiac arrest for a child or an infant is similar to responding to a cardiac arrest for an adult and uses all the skills you have already learned with a few key differences.

These key differences include compression technique, compression depth, opening the airway position, use of appropriately sized breathing barriers, and, when using an AED, AED pad selection and pad placement differences.

See Table 3-1 for a comparison of CPR technique among adults, children and infants.

Giving CPR to a Child

Giving CPR to a child is very similar to giving CPR to an adult with a few key differences in depth of compressions, opening the airway position, and the size of breathing barriers used for giving breaths.

Giving Chest Compressions Differences

Giving chest compressions to children is similar to giving compressions to an adult with a key difference in the depth of compressions. Position one hand on top of the other in the center of the chest with your fingers interlaced and off the chest.

The compression rate of 100 to 120 per minute is the same for a child as for an adult. The depth of the compression, however, is different. For an adult, compress the chest *at least* 2 inches; however, for a child, compress only slightly less, *about* 2 inches.

For a smaller child, you may use one hand, instead of two hands, to give compressions. When using one hand, be sure you're able to compress the chest about 2 inches. Simply place the heel of one hand in the center of the chest and give compressions.

Giving Breaths Differences

Giving breaths to children is similar to giving breaths to an adult with a few differences. Subtle differences in positioning are applied when opening the airway of a child compared with an adult. For a child, open the airway using the head-tilt/chin-lift technique by putting one hand on the forehead and two fingers on the bony part of the chin and

> **THE PROS KNOW.** When drowning is the suspected cause of cardiac arrest, the responder should deliver 2 initial breaths before starting CPR. During the drowning process, water comes into contact with the airway, causing it to spasm. When this occurs, air cannot reach the lungs. Giving breaths first can provide needed oxygen.

TABLE 3-1 Comparison of CPR Technique in Adults, Children and Infants

ADULT	CHILD	INFANT
About 12 years or older	Between the ages of 1 and 12 years	Younger than 1 year

Positioning

■ Kneel beside the person. ■ Two hands in center of chest; fingers interlaced and off the person's chest ■ Shoulders directly over hands; elbows locked	■ Kneel beside the person. ■ Two hands in center of chest; fingers interlaced and off the person's chest ■ Shoulders directly over hands; elbows locked **Note:** *Alternatively, you can use the one-hand technique.*	■ Stand or kneel to the side of the infant, with your hips slightly angled. ■ Both thumbs (side-by-side) on the center of the infant's chest, just below the nipple line ■ Other fingers encircle the infant's chest toward the back, providing support **Note:** *Alternatively, you can use the two-finger technique or one-hand technique.*

Chest Compressions

■ Push hard and fast. ■ Compress **at least 2** inches. ■ Rate: 100 to 120 compressions/min	■ Push hard and fast. ■ Compress **about 2** inches. ■ Rate: 100 to 120 compressions/min	■ Push hard and fast. ■ Compress **about 1½** inches. ■ Rate: 100 to 120 compressions/min

Breaths

■ No breathing barrier/**face shield**: Place face shield (if using) over face, ensuring the one-way valve is over the mouth. Open the airway using head-tilt/chin-lift to a **past-neutral position**; pinch nose shut; take a normal breath and form a complete seal over the mouth. ■ **Pocket mask**: Seal the mask over the mouth and nose and simultaneously open the airway using head-tilt/chin-lift technique to a **past-neutral position**.	■ No breathing barrier/**face shield**: Place face shield (if using) over face, ensuring the one-way valve is over the mouth. Open the airway using head-tilt/chin-lift to a **slightly past-neutral position**; pinch nose shut; take a normal breath and form a complete seal over the mouth. ■ **Pocket mask**: Seal the mask over the mouth and nose and simultaneously open the airway using head-tilt/chin-lift technique to a **slightly past-neutral position**.	■ No breathing barrier/**face shield**: Place face shield (if using) over face, ensuring the one-way valve is over the mouth. Open the airway using head-tilt/chin-lift to a **neutral position**; take a normal breath and form a complete seal over the mouth *and* nose. ■ **Pocket mask**: Seal the mask over the mouth and nose and simultaneously open the airway using head-tilt/chin-lift technique to a **neutral position**.

TABLE 3-1 Comparison of CPR Technique in Adults, Children and Infants continued

ADULT	CHILD	INFANT
Tilt head to **past-neutral position**; pinch nose shut and form seal over mouth	Tilt head to **slightly past-neutral position**; pinch nose shut and form seal over mouth	Tilt head to **neutral position**; form seal over mouth and nose

CPR Cycles

| One cycle = 30 chest compressions and 2 breaths | One cycle = 30 chest compressions and 2 breaths | One cycle = 30 chest compressions and 2 breaths |

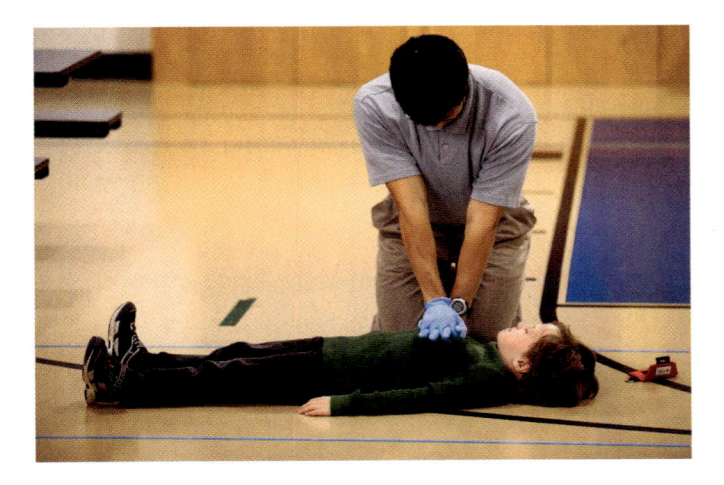

---

tilting the head back to a *slightly past-neutral* position, which is a little less than for an adult (see Table 3-1).

The technique for giving breaths to a child in cardiac arrest is the same for adults. Give smooth, effortless breaths that last about 1 second and make the chest begin to rise. As children's lungs are smaller, it will take less air to begin chest rise.

When providing care to a child, it is essential that you use appropriately sized equipment. If you are using a pocket mask, make sure it is sized appropriately. Some pocket masks come in different sizes and some are one-size-fits-all for adults and children. If one size, the mask can be rotated so that the narrow end fits over the child's chin. In other instances, separate pocket masks are available for use with children.

Giving CPR to an Infant

The general principles of giving CPR to an infant are the same as they are for children and adults with several key differences in the techniques of giving chest compressions, the depth of compressions, opening the airway position, and size of breathing barriers used for giving breaths.

First, ensure that the infant is on their back on a firm, flat surface such as the ground or a stable tabletop. If the infant is in a stroller or on a soft surface, carefully move them to a firm, flat surface.

If they are in a crib with padding but no soft mattress, you can perform CPR there, but if there is a thick soft mattress, it is better to move the infant to a hard surface or remove the mattress.

Giving Chest Compressions Differences

The technique of giving compressions to an infant is the same sequence of steps with differences in technique from an adult and child because of the infant's smaller size. Because the infant's body is smaller, you will position your body and hands differently to deliver compressions. Compressions are delivered using the encircling thumbs technique (also known as the two-thumb/encircling hands technique). Using this technique makes it easier to compress the infant's chest, which results in less fatigue.

- Stand or kneel to the side of the infant, with your hips at a slight angle.

American Red Cross | First Aid for Cardiac Arrest and Choking

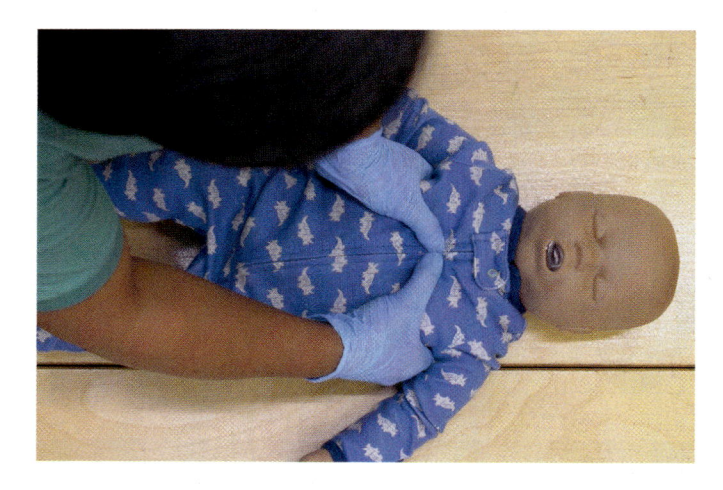

- Place both thumbs (side-by-side) on the center of the infant's chest, just below the nipple line.
- Use the other fingers to encircle the infant's chest toward the back, providing support.
- Using both thumbs at the same time, compress the chest about 1½ inches at a rate of at least 100 but no more than 120 compressions per minute. Let the chest return to its normal position after each compression.

Alternatively, you can use the two-finger technique to give compressions to an infant.

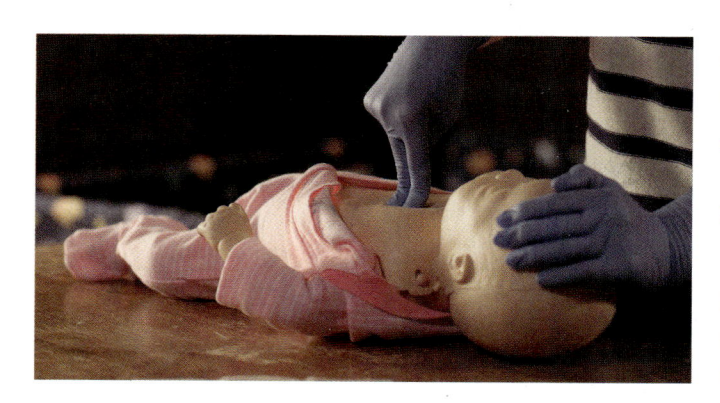

- Stand or kneel to the side of the infant and, using your hand that is closest to the infant's feet, place two fingers in the center of the chest, just below the nipple line. If you feel the notch at the end of the infant's breastbone, move your fingers slightly toward the infant's head.
- The fingers should be oriented so that they are parallel, not perpendicular, to the chest.
- You can use your index and middle fingers or your middle and fourth fingers to give compressions. Fingers that are more similar in length tend to make compressions easier to perform.
- Place your other hand on the infant's forehead to help keep the airway open while you give compressions.

If you are not able to compress the infant's chest about 1½ inches using either the encircling thumbs technique or the two-finger technique, you can use the one-hand technique that was described previously.

The **rate of compression** of 100 to 120 per minute is the same for an infant as for an adult or child. The **depth of compression**, however, is different. For an infant compress the chest about 1½ inches.

Giving Breaths Differences

Giving breaths to an infant is similar to giving breaths to an adult or child with a few differences.

Subtle differences in positioning are applied when opening the airway of an infant compared with an adult or child. For an infant, open the airway using the head-tilt/chin-lift technique by putting one hand on the forehead and two fingers on the bony part of the chin and tilting the head back to a *neutral* position (see Table 3-1). Do not tilt their head back too far; overextending their airway can block it.

The technique for giving breaths to an infant in cardiac arrest depends on whether you are using no breathing barrier or a face shield or a pocket mask.

- No breathing barrier or face shield: Cover the infant's mouth *and* nose with your mouth and give breaths.
- Pocket mask: Use the same technique as you would use for an adult or child.

In both cases, give smooth, effortless breaths that last about 1 second and make the chest begin to rise. As with a child, the amount of air needed to begin chest rise is far less than you would need for an adult.

When providing care to an infant, it is essential that you use appropriately sized equipment. If you are using a pocket mask, make sure it is a specifically sized infant pocket mask so that you can make a good seal.

Using an AED on a Child or Infant

Although cardiac arrest in children and infants is less common than in adults, the use of an AED remains a critical component of child and infant cardiac arrest care and can be lifesaving.

AEDs work the same way regardless of the patient's age. The procedure for using an AED on a child or infant is the same as the procedure for using an AED on an adult.

However, there are differences in AED pad selection and differences in pad placement that are important to keep in mind when giving care to younger or smaller children and infants.

AED Pad Differences

Some AEDs come with pediatric AED pads that are smaller and designed specifically to analyze a child's heart rhythm and deliver a lower level of energy. Other AEDs have a key or switch that configures the AED for use on a child up to 8 years of age or weighing less than 55 pounds (25 kilograms). These pediatric pads or pediatric settings change the amount of energy delivered to children up to 8 years of age and infants. However, if all you have is an AED with adult pads or adult settings, use these. It is safe to do so, and they have the ability to save the child's or infant's life.

Keep the following guidelines in mind when using an AED on a child or an infant (Figure 3-3).

- Use **pediatric** AED pads for children up to 8 years of age (including infants) or weighing less than 55 pounds (25 kilograms), if available.
  - If pediatric AED pads are not available, it is safe to use adult AED pads on a child or infant.
- Use **adult** AED pads for children older than 8 years of age and/or weighing more than 55 pounds (25 kilograms).
- Do *not* use pediatric AED pads or the pediatric setting on an adult or a child older than 8 years of age and/or weighing more than 55 pounds (25 kilograms) because the shock delivered will not be sufficient. In these cases, always use adult AED pads.

AED Pad Placement Differences

Just as when you are using an AED on an adult, apply the AED pads to the child's bare, dry chest. For a **child**, position the pads in the same way you would for an adult, placing one pad on the upper right side of the chest and the other pad on the lower left side of the chest a few inches below the left armpit. The AED pads should *never* touch each other when applied.

If you cannot position the pads this way without them touching, position one pad in the middle of the chest and the other pad on the back between the shoulder blades (Figure 3-4, A–B). When using an AED on an **infant**, *always* use the front/back pad placement. Then follow the standard procedure for using an AED.

Putting It All Together 3-1 and Putting It All Together 3-2 describe and illustrate step-by-step how to give CPR and use an AED for a child and for an infant.

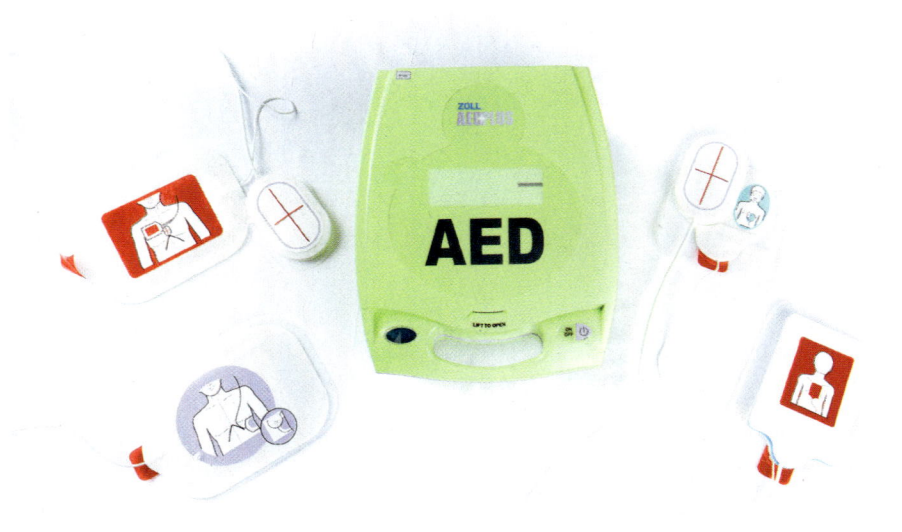

Figure 3-3. AED pad differences.

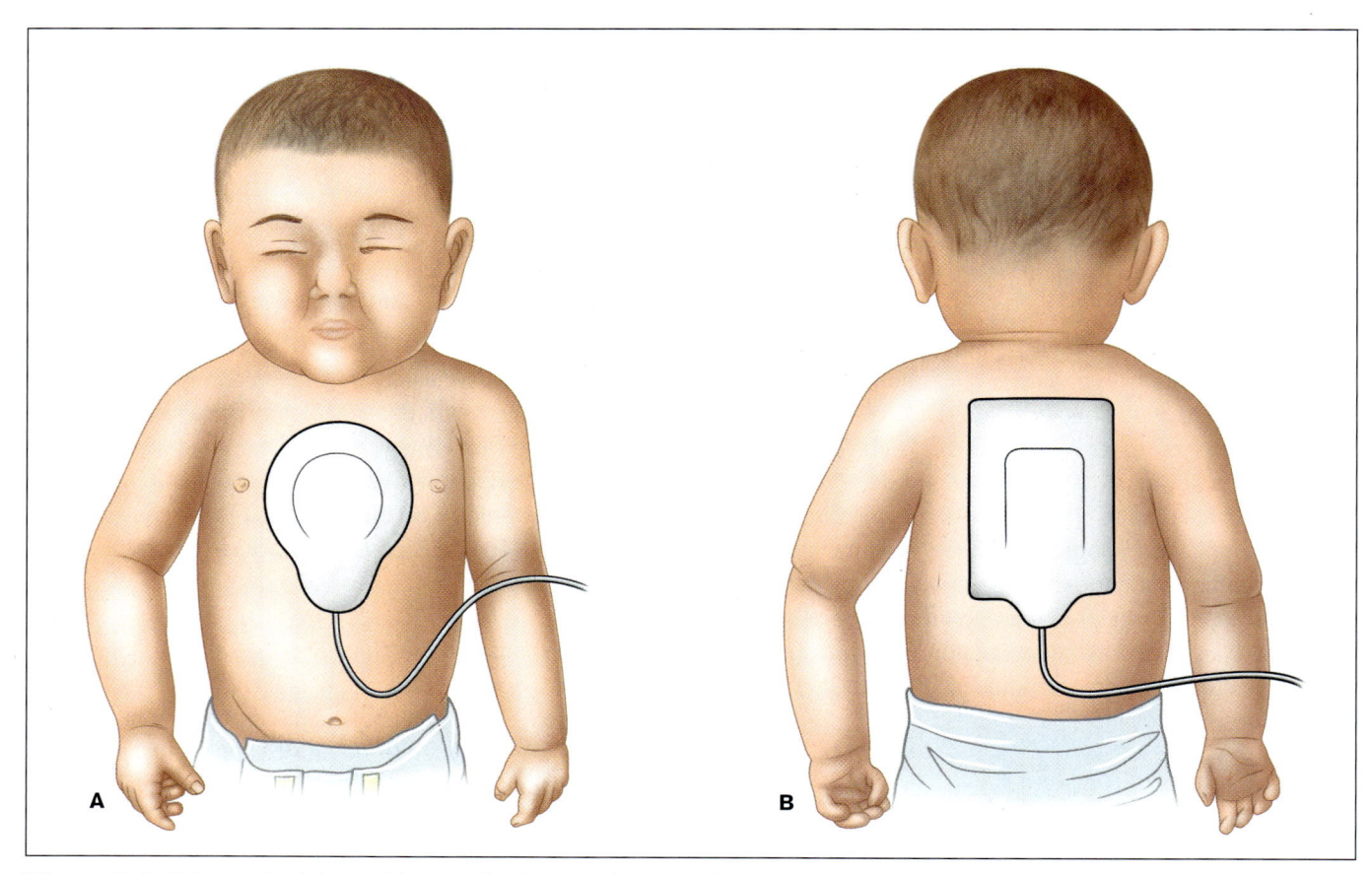

Figure 3-4. If the pads risk touching on the front of the chest in a small child, and always in infants, place one pad on the middle of the chest (A) and the other pad on the back between the shoulder blades (B).

PUTTING IT ALL TOGETHER 3-1

Giving CPR and Using an AED for a Child

Check

1. **Check the scene** for safety, **form an initial impression, obtain consent** from the parent or guardian, and **use PPE**.

2. If the child appears unresponsive, **check the child** for responsiveness (**shout-tap-shout**).
   - Shout to get the child's attention, using the child's name if you know it. If the child does not respond, tap the child's shoulder and shout again while checking for breathing, life-threatening bleeding or another obvious life-threatening condition.

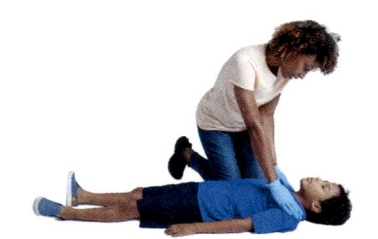

Call

3. If the child does not respond and is not breathing or only gasping, **call 9-1-1** and get equipment, or tell someone to do so, and continue to step 4.

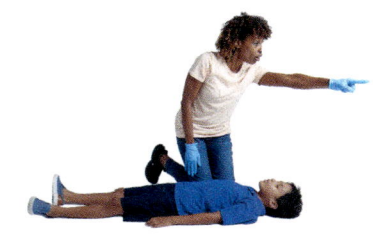

Care

4. **Place the child on their back** on a firm, flat surface. Kneel beside the child.

5. **Give 30 chest compressions.**
   - Place the heel of one hand in the center of the child's chest, with your other hand on top and your fingers interlaced and off the child's chest.
   - Position your body so that your shoulders are directly over your hands; lock your elbows. (Alternatively, in a small child, you can use a one-handed CPR technique: place the heel of one hand in the center of the child's chest.)
   - Keeping your arms straight, push down about 2 inches, and then let the chest return to its normal position.
   - Push hard and push fast! Give compressions at a rate of 100 to 120 compressions per minute.

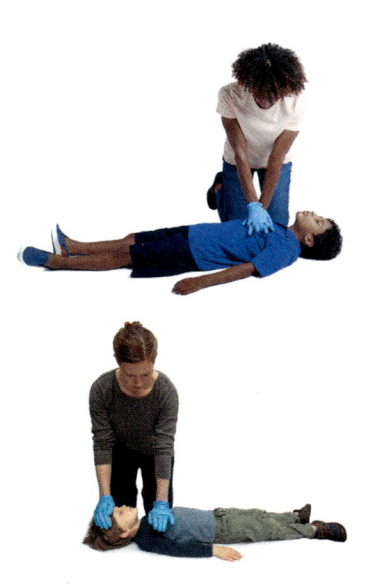

(Continued on next page)

American Red Cross | First Aid for Cardiac Arrest and Choking

PUTTING IT ALL TOGETHER 3-1

Giving CPR and Using an AED for a Child continued

6. Give 2 breaths.

- If using a face shield:
  - Place the face shield over the child's nose and mouth, ensuring the one-way valve is over their mouth.
  - Open the airway to a slightly past-neutral position using the head-tilt/chin-lift technique. (Put one hand on the forehead and two fingers on the bony part of the chin and tilt the head back.)
  - Pinch the nose shut, take a normal breath, and make a complete seal over the child's mouth with your mouth.
- If using a pocket mask:
  - Place the mask at the bridge of the nose and lower it over the child's mouth and nose.
  - Seal the mask and open the airway.
    - Place the space of your hand between your thumb and index finger at the top of the mask above the valve.
    - Place your remaining fingers on the side of the child's face.
    - Place the thumb of your other hand along the base of the mask and place your bent index finger under the child's chin.
    - Lift the child's face into the mask and open the airway to a slightly past-neutral position by tilting the head back.
  - Take a normal breath and make a complete seal over the mouth valve.
- Give 1st breath.
  - Blow into the child's mouth for about 1 second, looking to see that the chest begins to rise.
  - Pause between breaths to allow for exhalation.
- Give 2nd breath.
  - Take another breath, make a seal, then give the 2nd breath.
- Minimize interruptions to chest compressions to **less than 10 seconds**.

Note: *If the 1st breath does not cause the chest to rise, retilt the head and ensure a proper seal before giving the 2nd breath. If the 2nd breath does not make the chest rise, an object may be blocking the airway. Performing the same techniques as CPR with one slight change will help to clear this obstruction. After the next set of chest compressions and before attempting breaths, open the mouth, look for an object and, if seen, remove it using a finger sweep. Continue to check the child's mouth for an object after each set of compressions until the breaths go in.*

7. Continue giving sets of 30 chest compressions and 2 breaths until:

- You notice an obvious sign of life.
- An AED is ready to use and no other trained responders are available to assist you with the AED.
- You have performed approximately 2 minutes of CPR (5 sets of 30:2) and another responder is available to take over compressions.
- You have performed approximately 2 minutes of CPR (5 sets of 30:2), you are alone and caring for a child, and you need to call 9-1-1.
- EMS personnel arrive and begin their care of the child.
- You are alone and too tired to continue.
- The scene becomes unsafe.

Use an AED as soon as one is available!

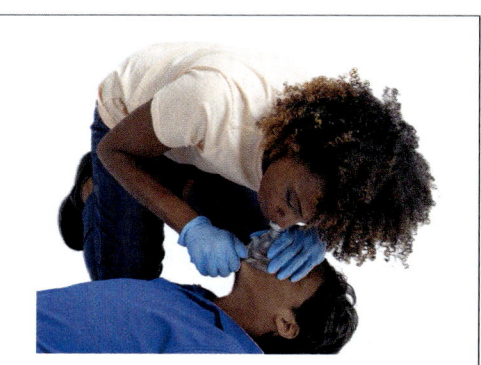

PUTTING IT ALL TOGETHER 3-1

8. Turn on the AED and follow the voice prompts.

9. Remove all clothing covering the chest and, if necessary, wipe the chest dry.

10. Choose appropriate pads.
- Use pediatric pads or pediatric settings for children and infants up to 8 years of age/weighing less than 55 pounds (25 kilograms).
- Use adult pads for children older than 8 years of age/weighing more than 55 pounds (25 kilograms).

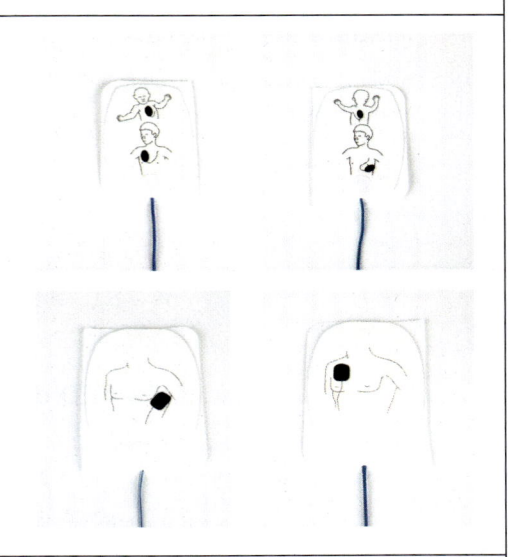

11. Attach pads correctly.
- Place one pad on the upper right side of the chest and the other on the lower left side of the chest, a few inches below the left armpit.
- If the pads may touch, place one pad in the middle of the chest and the other pad on the back, between the shoulder blades.

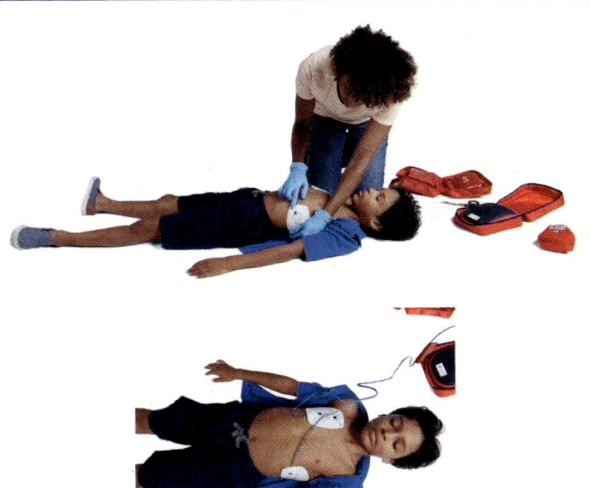

12. Plug the pad connector cable into the AED, if necessary.

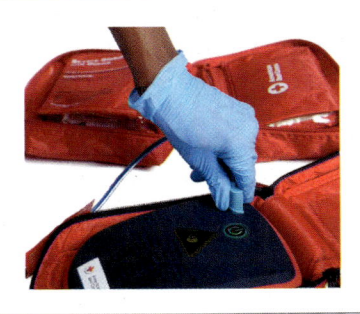

(Continued on next page)

American Red Cross | First Aid for Cardiac Arrest and Choking

PUTTING IT ALL TOGETHER 3-1

Giving CPR and Using an AED for a Child continued

13. Prepare to let the AED analyze the heart's rhythm.
- Make sure no one, including you, is touching the child. Say, "CLEAR!" in a loud, commanding voice.
- If the AED tells you to, push the "analyze" button to start this process.

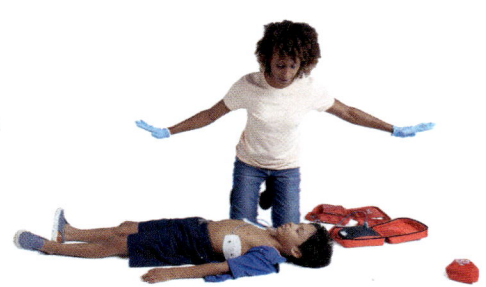

14. Deliver a shock, if the AED determines one is needed.
- Make sure no one, including you, is touching the child. Say, "CLEAR!" in a loud, commanding voice.
- Push the "shock" button to deliver the shock.

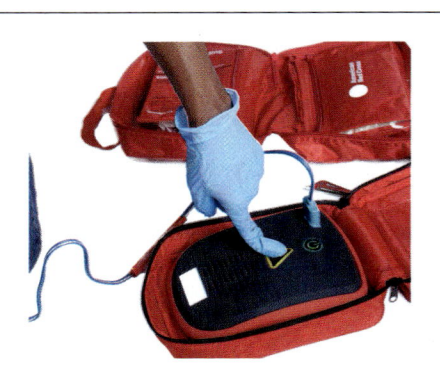

15. After the AED delivers the shock, or if no shock is advised, immediately start CPR, beginning with compressions and continue until:
- You notice an obvious sign of life.
- The AED prompts you to analyze again.
- Another trained responder is available to take over compressions.
- EMS personnel arrive and begin their care of the child.
- You are alone and too tired to continue.
- The scene becomes unsafe.

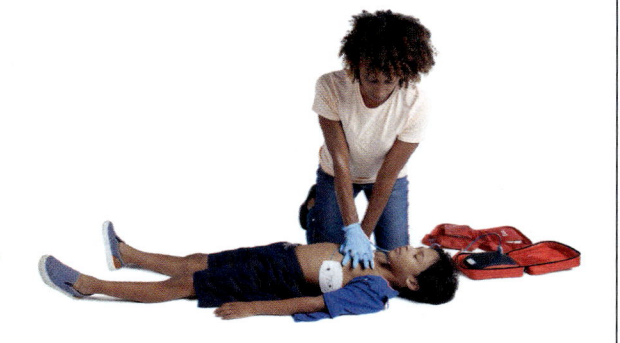

Note: *Do not use pediatric AED pads on an adult or on a child older than 8 years of age and/or weighing more than 55 pounds (25 kilograms). However, adult AED pads can be used on a child up to 8 years of age or weighing less than 55 pounds (25 kilograms) if pediatric AED pads are not available.*

PUTTING IT ALL TOGETHER 3-2

Giving CPR and Using an AED for an Infant

Check

1. **Check the scene** for safety, **form an initial impression, obtain consent** from the parent or guardian and **use PPE**.

2. If the infant appears unresponsive, **check the infant** for responsiveness (**shout-tap-shout**).
   - Shout to get the infant's attention, using the infant's name if you know it. If the infant does not respond, **tap the bottom of the infant's foot** and shout again while checking for breathing, life-threatening bleeding or another obvious life-threatening condition.

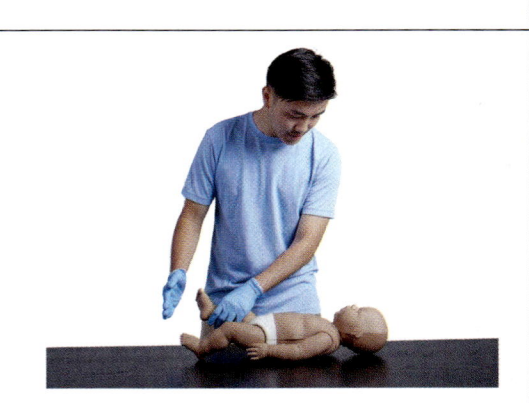

Call

3. If the infant does not respond and is not breathing or only gasping, **call 9-1-1** and get equipment, or tell someone to do so, and continue to step 4.

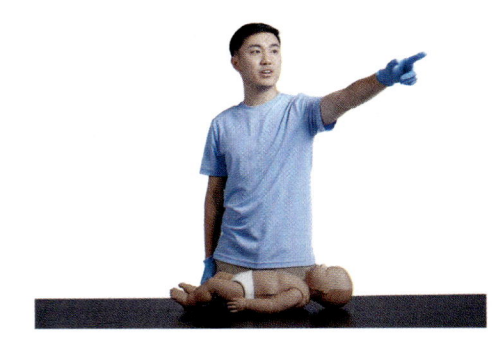

Care

4. **Place the infant on their back** on a firm, flat surface.

5. **Give 30 chest compressions** using the encircling thumbs technique.
   - Stand or kneel to the side of the infant, with your hips at a slight angle.
   - Place both thumbs (side-by-side) on the center of the infant's chest, just below the nipple line.
   - Use the other fingers to encircle the infant's chest toward the back, providing support.
   - Push hard and push fast! Using both thumbs at the same time, compress the chest about 1½ inches at a rate of at least 100 but no more than 120 compressions per minute. Let the chest return to its normal position after each compression.

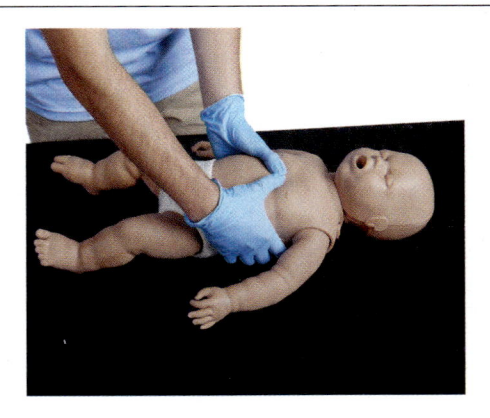

   Note: *Alternatively, you can use the two-finger technique. Stand or kneel to the side of the infant and give compressions using two fingers placed parallel to the chest, in the center of the chest. If the required depth cannot be achieved with either the encircling thumbs technique or two-finger technique, you may consider using a one-hand technique.*

(Continued on next page)

American Red Cross | First Aid for Cardiac Arrest and Choking 61

PUTTING IT ALL TOGETHER 3-2

Giving CPR and Using an AED for an Infant continued

6. Give 2 breaths.

- If using a face shield:
  - Place the face shield over the infant's nose *and* mouth, ensuring the one-way valve is over their mouth.
  - Open the airway to a neutral position using the head-tilt/chin-lift technique. (Put one hand on the forehead and two fingers on the bony part of the chin and tilt the head back.)
  - Take a normal breath, and make a complete seal over the infant's mouth *and* nose with your mouth. 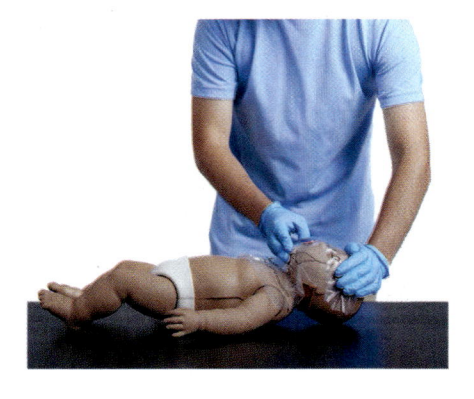
- If using a pocket mask:
  - Place the mask at the bridge of the nose and lower it over the infant's mouth and nose.
  - Seal the mask and open the airway.
    - Place the space of your hand between your thumb and index finger at the top of the mask above the valve.
    - Place your remaining fingers on the side of the infant's face.
    - Place the thumb of your other hand along the base of the mask and place your bent index finger under the infant's chin.
    - Lift the infant's face into the mask and open the airway to a neutral position by tilting the head back.
  - Take a normal breath and make a complete seal over the mouth valve. 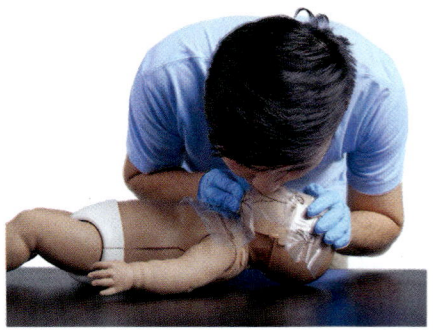 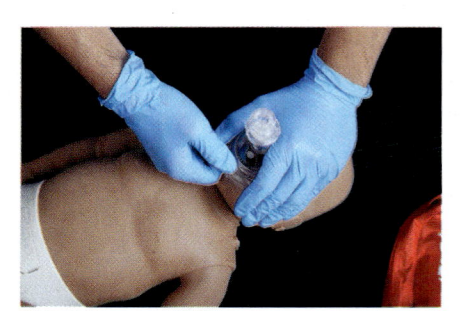
- Give 1st breath.
  - Blow into the infant's mouth for about 1 second, looking to see that the chest begins to rise.
  - Pause between breaths to allow for exhalation.
- Give 2nd breath.
  - Take another breath, make a seal, then give the 2nd breath.
- Minimize interruptions to chest compressions to **less than 10 seconds**.

Note: *If the 1st breath does not cause the chest to rise, retilt the head and ensure a proper seal before giving the 2nd breath. If the 2nd breath does not make the chest rise, an object may be blocking the airway. Performing the same techniques as CPR with one slight change will help to clear this obstruction. After the next set of chest compressions and before attempting breaths, open the mouth, look for an object and, if seen, remove it using a finger sweep using your pinky finger. Continue to check the infant's mouth for an object after each set of compressions until the breaths go in.*

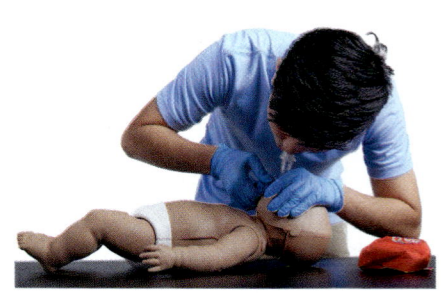

PUTTING IT ALL TOGETHER 3-2

7. Continue giving sets of 30 chest compressions and 2 breaths until:
- You notice an obvious sign of life.
- An AED is ready to use and no other trained responders are available to assist you with the AED.
- You have performed approximately 2 minutes of CPR (5 sets of 30:2) and another responder is available to take over compressions.
- You have performed approximately 2 minutes of CPR (5 sets of 30:2), you are alone and caring for an infant, and you need to call 9-1-1.
- EMS personnel arrive and begin their care of the infant.
- You are alone and too tired to continue.
- The scene becomes unsafe.

Use an AED as soon as one is available!

---

8. Turn on the AED and follow the voice prompts.

---

9. Remove all clothing covering the chest and, if necessary, wipe the chest dry.

---

10. Choose appropriate pads.
- Use pediatric pads or pediatric settings for children and infants up to 8 years of age or weighing less than 55 pounds (25 kilograms).

---

11. Attach pads correctly.
- Place one pad in the middle of the chest and the other pad on the back, between the shoulder blades.

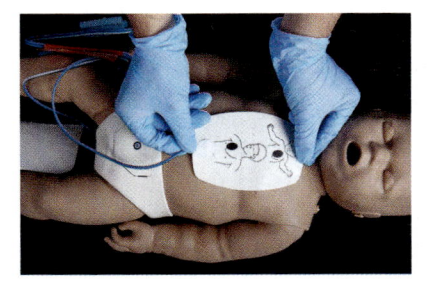

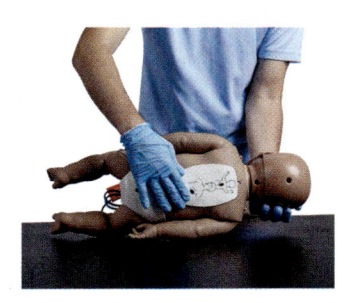

(Continued on next page)

American Red Cross | First Aid for Cardiac Arrest and Choking

PUTTING IT ALL TOGETHER 3-2

Giving CPR and Using an AED for an Infant continued

12. **Plug the pad connector cable into the AED,** if necessary.

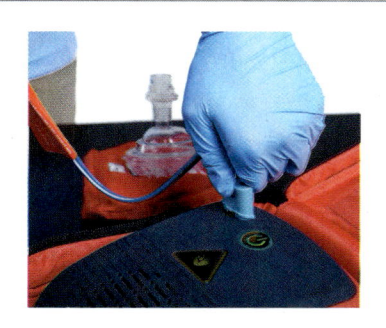

13. **Prepare to let the AED analyze the heart's rhythm.**
- Make sure no one, including you, is touching the infant. Say, "CLEAR!" in a loud, commanding voice.
- If the AED tells you to, push the "analyze" button to start this process.

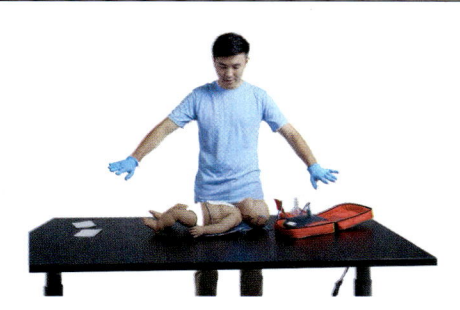

14. **Deliver a shock,** if the AED determines one is needed.
- Make sure no one, including you, is touching the infant. Say, "CLEAR!" in a loud, commanding voice.
- Push the "shock" button to deliver the shock.

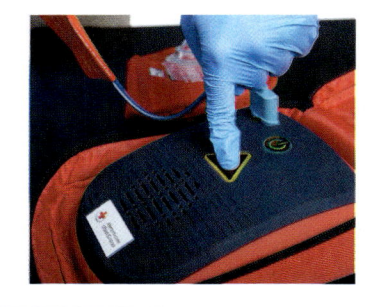

15. After the AED delivers the shock, or if no shock is advised, **immediately start CPR,** beginning with compressions and continue until:
- You notice an obvious sign of life.
- The AED prompts you to analyze again.
- Another trained responder is available to take over compressions.
- EMS personnel arrive and begin their care of the infant.
- You are alone and too tired to continue.
- The scene becomes unsafe.

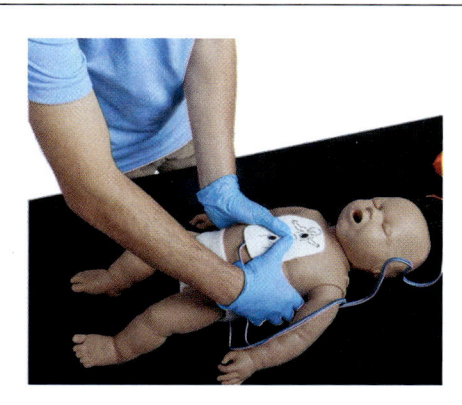

Note: *Adult AED pads can be used on a child up to 8 years of age or weighing less than 55 pounds (25 kilograms) if pediatric AED pads or pediatric settings are not available.*

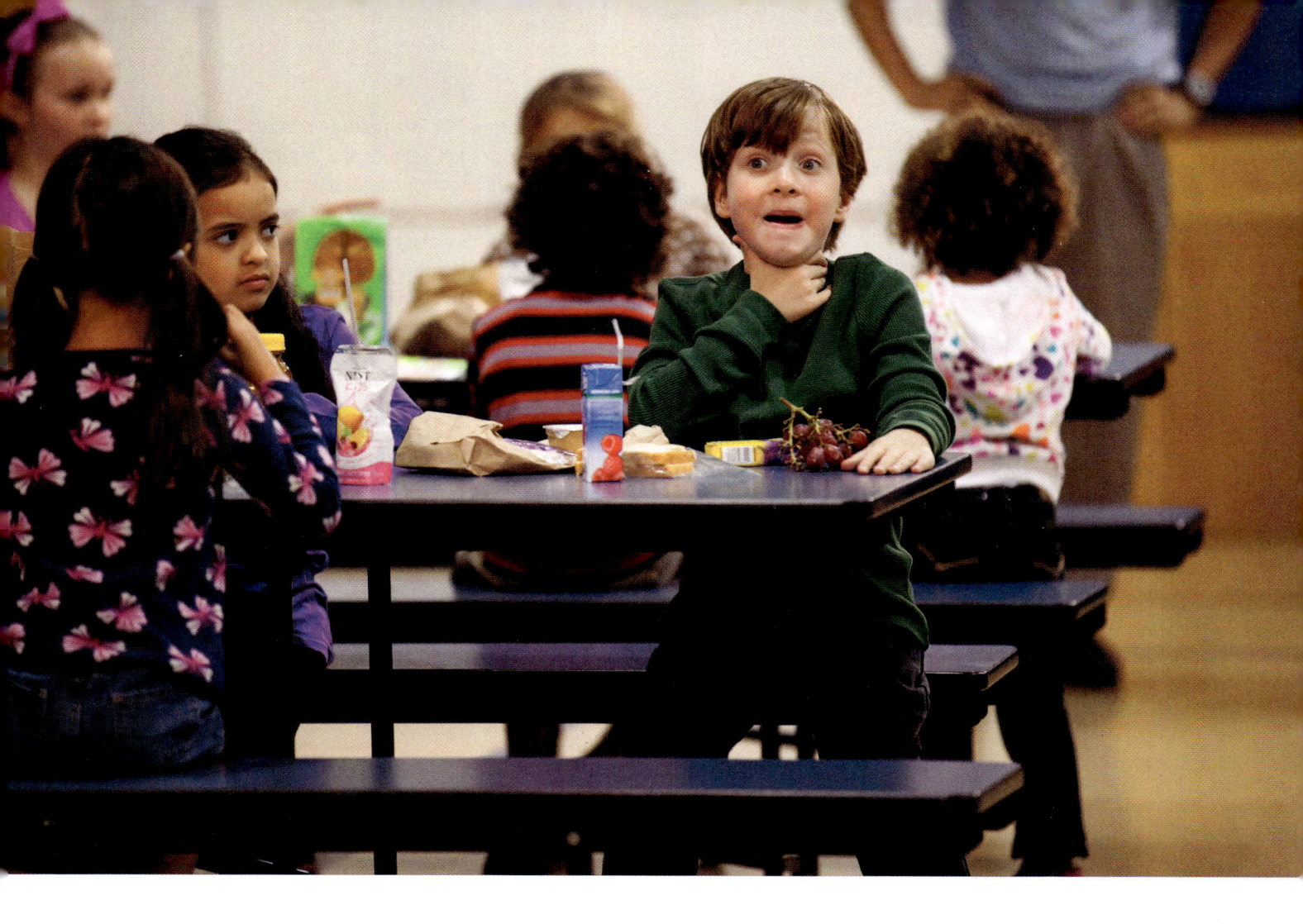

CHAPTER 4
Choking

Choking occurs when the airway becomes either partially or completely blocked by a foreign object, such as a piece of food or a small toy; by swelling in the mouth or throat; or by body fluids, such as vomit or blood. Choking is especially common in young children and older adults, but a person of any age can choke. A person who is choking can quickly become unresponsive and, if unresponsive and if left untreated, can go into cardiac arrest before EMS arrives. By taking action and providing immediate care, you can save a life. It is important to recognize when a person is choking and act quickly.

Risk Factors for Choking

Certain behaviors can put a person at risk for choking, such as talking or laughing with the mouth full or eating too fast. Medical conditions (such as a neurological or muscular condition that affects the person's ability to chew, swallow, or both) can increase risk for choking. Likewise, dental problems or poorly fitting dentures can affect the person's ability to chew food properly.

Children younger than 5 years are at particularly high risk for choking (Box 4-1). Infants and toddlers explore by putting things in their mouths and can easily choke on them. Even some common foods can be choking hazards in young children. For example, a young child can choke on small foods (such as nuts and seeds); round, firm foods (such as grapes, hot dogs and hard candies); and sticky foods (such as peanut butter). This is because young children do not have the skills needed to chew these foods thoroughly, so they often try to just swallow them whole. Laughing, talking or running with the mouth full can also lead to choking.

Recognizing Choking

As in all life-threatening emergencies, first check the scene, form an initial impression as you are approaching the person and obtain consent.

Box 4-1 Choking Hazards

In children younger than 5 years, the following foods, household objects and toys may be choking hazards.

Foods

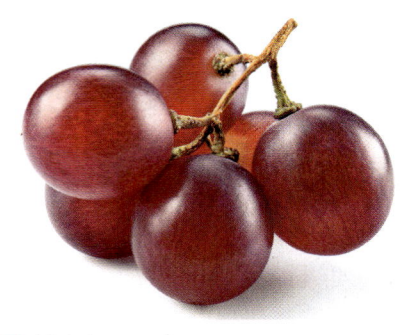

- Hot dogs and sausages
- Nuts and seeds
- Chunks of meat or cheese
- Chunks of fruit (such as apples) and whole grapes
- Raw vegetables (such as carrots and celery)
- Popcorn
- Peanut butter
- Hard, gooey or sticky candy (such as peppermint candies, fruit strips, marshmallows, gummy bears and chewing gum)

Household Objects and Toys

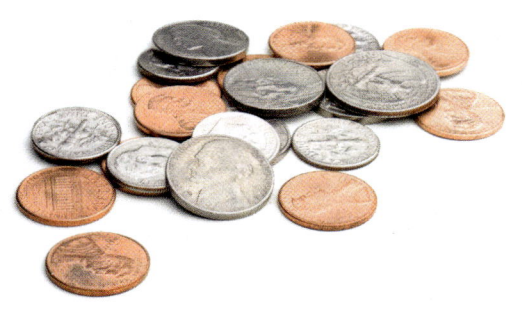

- Plastic bags, broken or uninflated balloons, and disposable gloves (the thin material can block the airway)
- Coins
- Buttons
- Small "button" batteries (found inside watches, car key fobs, singing greeting cards, hearing aids and other electronics)
- Magnets
- Marbles
- Beads
- Pebbles
- Pen or marker caps
- Safety pins and hairpins
- Jewelry
- Baby powder
- Vitamins
- Items from the trash (such as eggshells or the pull tabs from soda cans)
- Toys meant for older children, which may be small or have small parts*

*For infants and toddlers, no toy should be smaller than 1-inch in diameter. If you can fit the toy through a toilet paper tube, then it is too small and not safe for a young child.

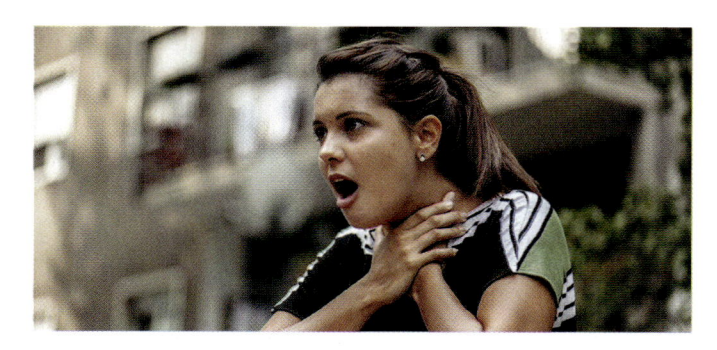

When forming an initial impression, you may notice that the person has a panicked, confused or surprised facial expression. Some people may place one or both hands on their throat. The person may cough (either forcefully or weakly), or they may not be able to cough at all. You may hear high-pitched squeaking noises as the person tries to breathe, or nothing at all. If the person is not able to speak, cry or cough, assume the airway is blocked. The person's skin may initially appear flushed (red) but will become pale or bluish in color as the body is deprived of oxygen.

If you notice any of these signs or symptoms, ask the person if they are choking, or check to see if an infant is crying or making other noises.

If the person is making only high-pitched noises or is unable to speak, cry or cough forcefully, the airway is blocked. This is a life-threatening emergency and the person will soon become unresponsive unless the airway is cleared.

Call 9-1-1 and get equipment, or tell someone to do so. Then, immediately begin to give care according to your level of training.

A person who can speak, cry or cough forcefully is getting enough air and the body is trying to clear the obstruction. The body's mechanism to clear the airway does a better job than we can do, so only intervene when the person is unable to clear the object. If the person can speak or cry and is coughing forcefully, encourage them to keep coughing. However, it is important to keep checking them and be prepared to act if the person's condition changes. Do not allow the person to leave your presence and do not leave the person alone because their condition may change for the worse.

Giving First Aid Care for an Adult or Child Who Is Choking

When an adult or child is choking, give a combination of 5 **back blows** (blows between the shoulder blades) followed by 5 **abdominal thrusts** (inward and upward thrusts just above the navel). The goal of giving back blows and abdominal thrusts is to force the object out of the airway, allowing the person to breathe.

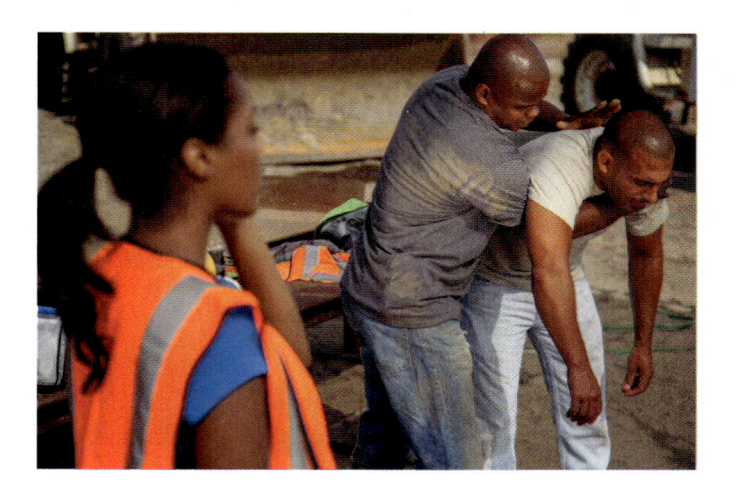

Giving Back Blows

To give back blows, position yourself to the side and slightly behind the choking person. For a small child, you may need to kneel. Place one arm diagonally across the person's chest (to provide support) and bend the person forward at the waist so that the person's upper body is as parallel to the ground as possible. This position helps both to remove the object and helps you to brace yourself if the person becomes unresponsive.

Firmly strike the person between the shoulder blades with the heel of your other hand. Each of the 5 back blows should be separate from the others (Figure 4-1, A).

Giving Abdominal Thrusts

After the 5th back blow, if the person is unable to cough or speak, give abdominal thrusts. To give abdominal thrusts, have the person stand up straight. Find the

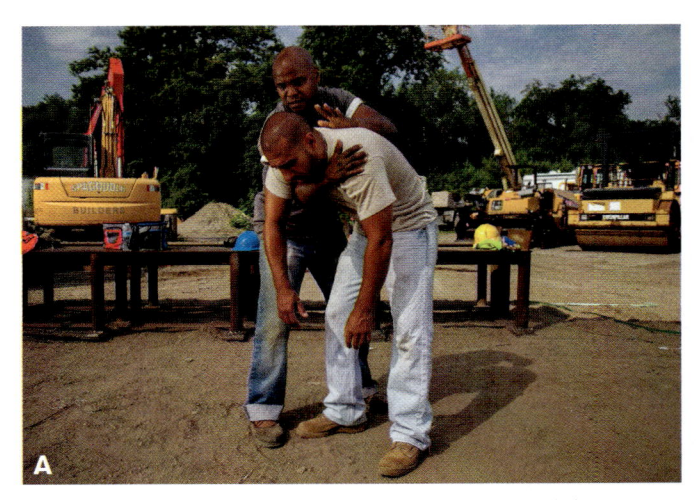

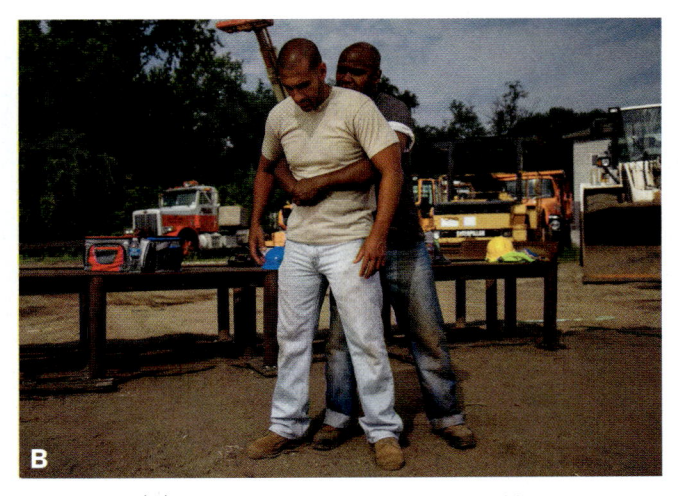

Figure 4-1. Use a combination of back blows (A) and abdominal thrusts (B) when an adult or child is choking.

person's navel with two fingers, then move behind the person and place your front foot in between the person's feet. Bend your knees slightly to provide balance and stability. For a small child, you may need to kneel behind them rather than stand.

Make a fist with your other hand and place the thumb side against the person's abdomen, right above your fingers. Take your first hand and cover your fist with that hand.

Pull inward and upward to give an abdominal thrust. Each of the 5 abdominal thrusts should be separate from the others (Figure 4-1, B).

You should continue giving sets of 5 back blows and 5 abdominal thrusts until the person can cough or speak or the person becomes unresponsive. After the choking incident is over, even if the person seems fine, they should still be evaluated by a healthcare provider to make sure there is no damage to the airway and there are no other internal injuries. For step-by-step instructions on giving first aid to an adult or child who is choking, see Putting It All Together 4-1.

Chest Thrusts

In certain special situations, you may need to give **chest thrusts** instead of abdominal thrusts (Table 4-1). To give chest thrusts for a responsive person, position yourself behind the person as you would for abdominal thrusts. Make a fist with one hand, place the thumb side of your fist on the center of the

> **THE PROS KNOW.** It is important to know that back blows, abdominal thrusts and chest thrusts are all equally effective, but it may take more than one technique to clear the airway.

person's chest, grab your fist with the other hand and give quick thrusts into the chest.

If the Adult or Child Becomes Unresponsive

If a person who is choking becomes unresponsive, carefully lower the person to a firm, flat surface and immediately begin CPR, starting with chest compressions. The chest compressions used in CPR may dislodge the object.

After each set of chest compressions and before attempting breaths, open the person's mouth and look for the object. If you see an object in the person's mouth, remove it with a finger sweep (Figure 4-2, A–B). However, never do a finger sweep if you don't see an object because you might accidentally push the object deeper into the person's throat.

If breaths go in, that is, the chest begins to rise, resume the normal CPR sequence of 30 compressions and 2 breaths and use of an AED. If breaths do not go in, that is, the chest does not begin to rise, continue with cycles of compressions followed by looking in the mouth and then trying to give breaths. You should never attempt more than 2 breaths during each cycle.

TABLE 4-1 Special Situation: Choking in an Adult or Child

SPECIAL SITUATION	SOLUTION
The person is too large for you to wrap your arms around to give abdominal thrusts.	Give **chest thrusts** instead of abdominal thrusts.
The person is obviously pregnant or known to be pregnant.	Give **chest thrusts** instead of abdominal thrusts.
The person is in a wheelchair. 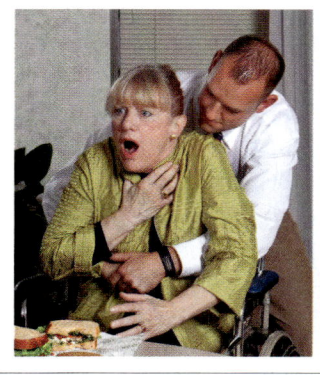	If you can, give **abdominal thrusts** in the same way that you would for a person who is standing. It may be necessary to kneel behind the wheelchair. If the features of the wheelchair make it difficult to give abdominal thrusts, give **chest thrusts**. You may need to remove the armrests of the wheelchair to give chest thrusts or abdominal thrusts. If, after removing the armrests, you are *still* unable to physically reach around the person to give chest thrusts or abdominal thrusts, then a last option is to remove the person from the wheelchair in order to give care for choking.
You are choking and alone. 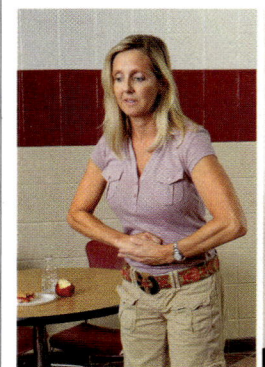 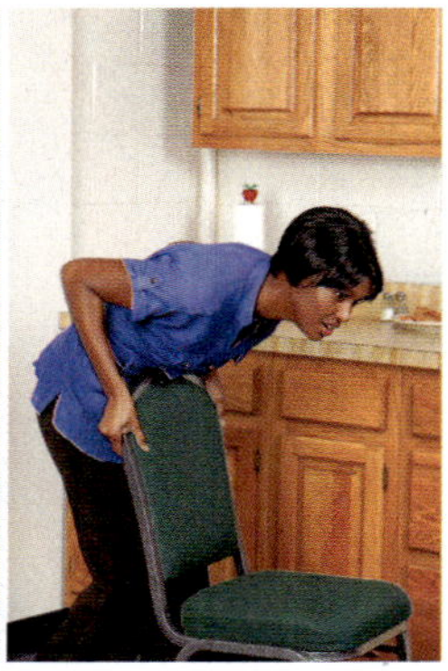	Call 9-1-1 using a landline or a GPS-enabled mobile phone. Even if you are not able to speak, the open line will cause the dispatcher to send help. Give yourself **abdominal thrusts**, using your hands, just as if you were giving abdominal thrusts to another person. Alternatively, bend over and press your abdomen against any firm object, such as the back of a chair or a railing. Do not bend over anything with a sharp edge or corner that might hurt you, and be careful when leaning on a railing that is elevated.

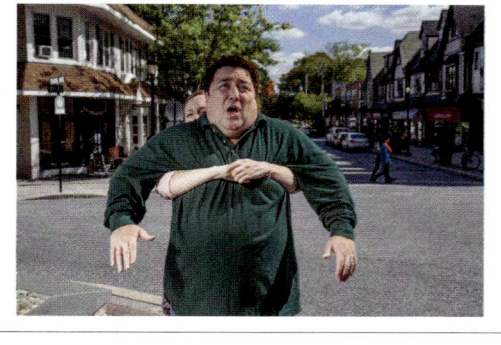

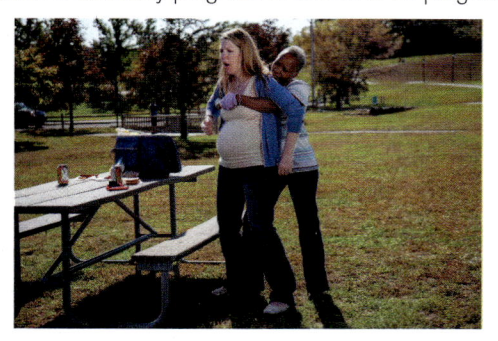

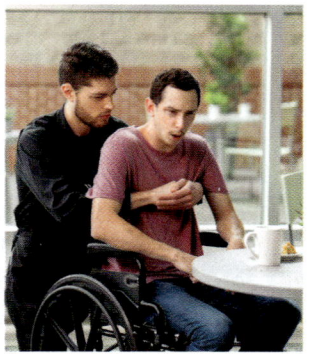

American Red Cross | First Aid for Cardiac Arrest and Choking

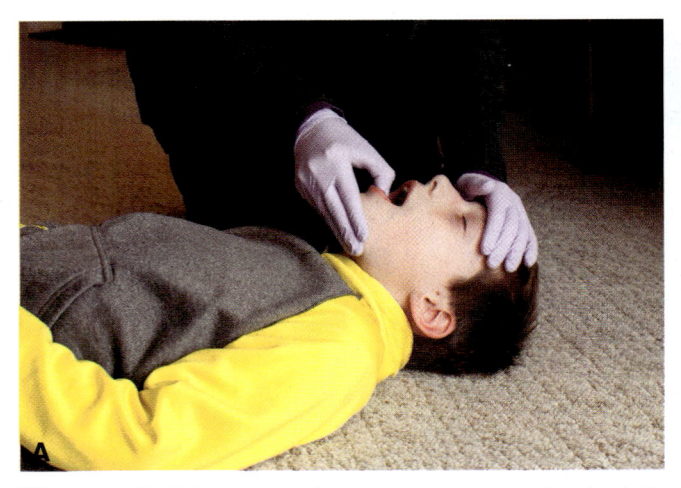

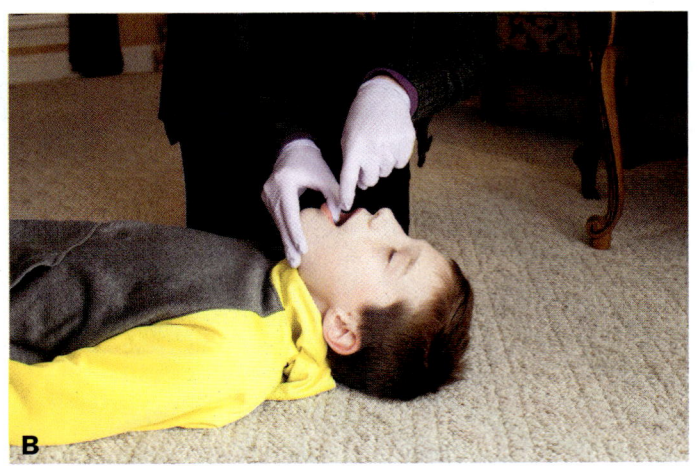

Figure 4-2. If the person becomes unresponsive, look for the object in the person's mouth (A), and if you see it, use a finger sweep to remove it (B).

Giving First Aid Care for an Infant Who Is Choking

When an infant is choking, give a combination of 5 back blows followed by 5 chest thrusts (instead of abdominal thrusts) (Figure 4-3, A–B). You can sit, kneel or stand to give first aid care to a choking infant, as long as you are able to support the infant along your arm braced on your thigh with the infant's head lower than their chest. If the infant is large or your hands are small, you may find it easier to sit or kneel.

Giving Back Blows

First, get the infant into position for back blows. Place the infant's back along your forearm, cradling the back of the infant's head with your hand. Place your other forearm on the infant's front, supporting the infant's jaw with your thumb and fingers. (Be careful not to cover the infant's mouth with your hand while you are supporting the infant's jaw.) Turn the infant to a face-down position and hold them along your forearm, using your thigh for support and keeping the infant's head lower than their body. Continue to support the infant's jaw with the thumb and fingers of one hand, but make sure your fingers are on the sides of the head and not blocking the mouth. Firmly strike the infant between the shoulder blades with the heel of your other hand. Keep your fingers up to avoid hitting the infant's head or neck.

Each of the 5 back blows should be separate from the others.

Giving Chest Thrusts

If back blows don't dislodge the object so that the infant can cough or cry, give chest thrusts. First, position the infant between your forearms, supporting the head and neck, and turn the infant face-up. Then lower the infant onto your thigh with their head lower than their chest. Place two

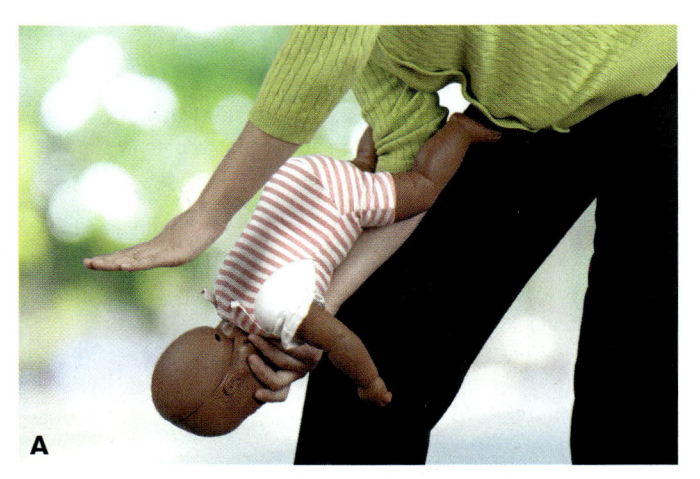

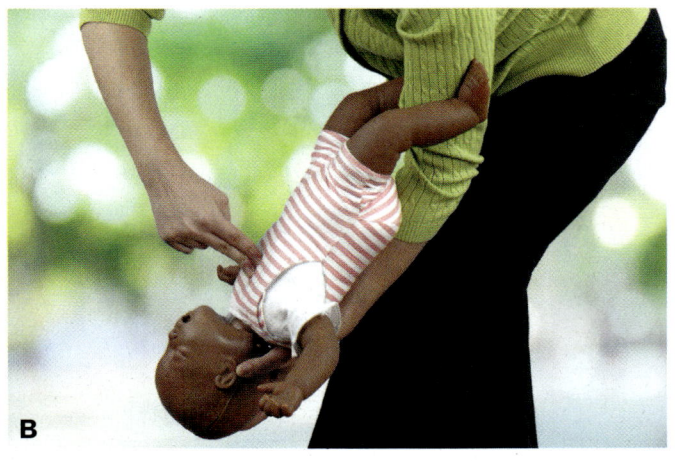

Figure 4-3. Use a combination of back blows (A) and chest thrusts (B) when an infant is choking.

fingers in the center of the infant's chest, just below the nipple line. Give 5 quick chest thrusts about 1½ inches deep and then let the chest return to its normal position, keeping your fingers in contact with the chest.

Each chest thrust should be separate from the others. Remember to support the infant's head, neck and back while giving chest thrusts.

Continue sets of 5 back blows and 5 chest thrusts until the infant can cough forcefully or cry, or the infant becomes unresponsive. After the choking incident is over, even if the infant seems fine, they should still be evaluated by a healthcare provider to make sure there is no damage to the airway and there are no other internal injuries. For step-by-step instructions on giving first aid to an infant who is choking, see Putting It All Together 4-2.

If the Infant Becomes Unresponsive

If an infant who is choking becomes unresponsive, carefully lower them to a firm, flat surface and begin CPR, starting with chest compressions. When giving chest compressions for an infant, be sure to use the encircling thumbs technique (alternatively, you can use the two-finger technique). After each set of chest compressions and before attempting breaths, open the infant's mouth and look for the object. If you see an object in the infant's mouth, remove it with a finger sweep using your pinky finger (Figure 4-4, A–B). However, never do a finger sweep if you don't see an object because you might accidentally push the object deeper into the infant's throat.

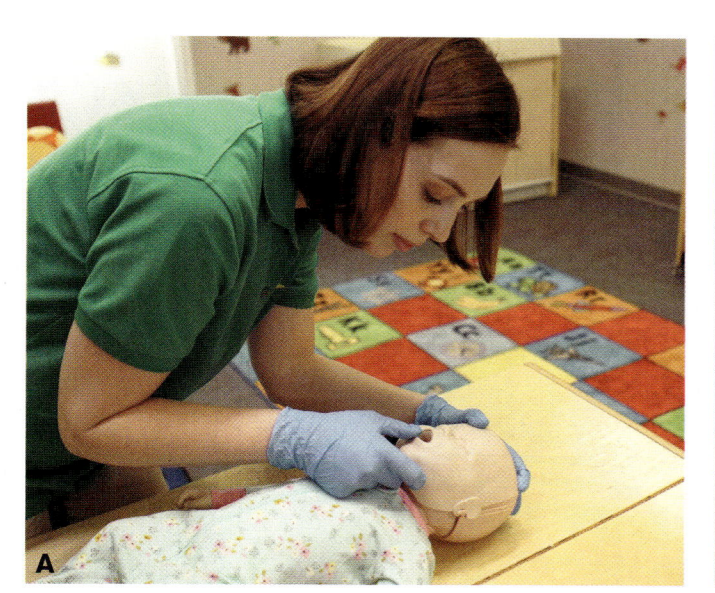

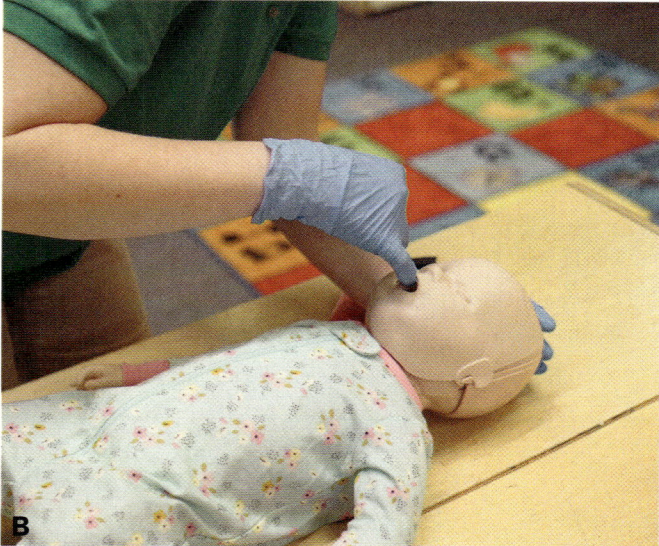

Figure 4-4. If the infant becomes unresponsive, look for the object in the infant's mouth (A), and if you see it, remove it with a finger sweep using your pinky finger (B).

PUTTING IT ALL TOGETHER 4-1

Caring for an Adult or Child Who Is Choking

Check

1. **Check the scene** for safety, **form an initial impression, obtain consent** and **use PPE**.

2. **Verify that the person is choking** by asking the person to speak to you.
   - If the person is able to speak to you or is coughing forcefully: If coughing, encourage the person to keep coughing. Keep observing the person and be prepared to give first aid for choking if the person's condition changes.

Call

3. If the person is unable to speak, cry or cough: **Call 9-1-1** and get equipment or tell someone to do so. Continue to step 4.

Care

4. **Give 5 back blows.**
   - Position yourself to the side and slightly behind the choking person.

   Note: *For a small child, you may need to kneel behind them rather than stand.*

   - Place one arm diagonally across the person's chest (to provide support) and bend them forward at the waist so that the person's upper body is as parallel to the ground as possible.
   - Firmly strike the person between the shoulder blades with the heel of your hand.
     - Each of the 5 back blows should be separate from the others.

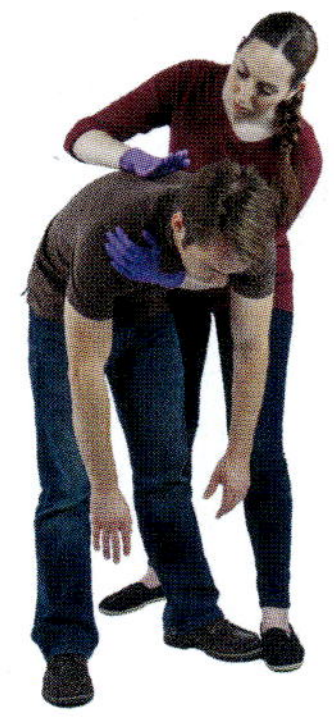

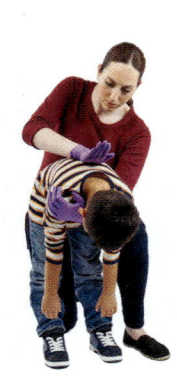

5. **Give 5 abdominal thrusts.**
   - Have the person stand up straight. Find the person's navel with two fingers.
   - Move behind the person and place your front foot in between the person's feet and bend your knees slightly to provide balance and stability. 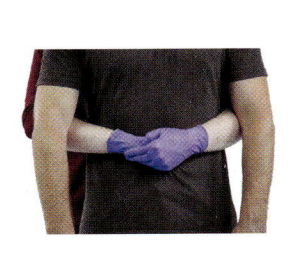 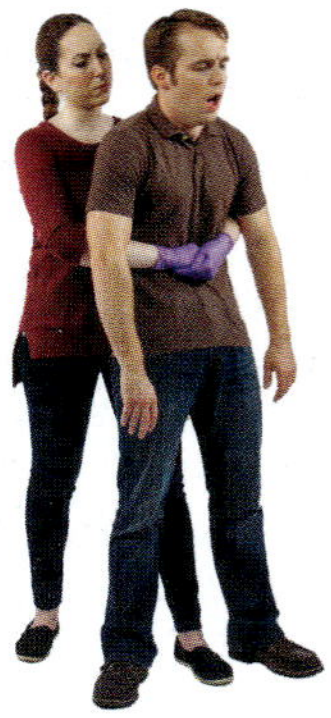

   Note: *For a small child, you may need to kneel behind them rather than stand.*

   - Make a fist with your other hand and place the thumb side against the person's stomach, right above your fingers.
   - Take your first hand and cover your fist with that hand.
   - Pull inward and upward to give an abdominal thrust.
     - Each of the 5 abdominal thrusts should be forceful and separate from the others.

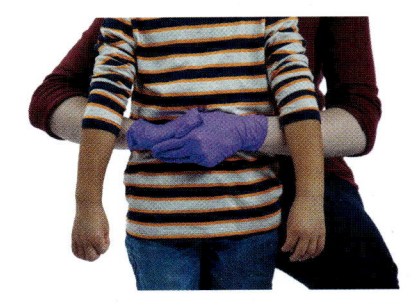

PUTTING IT ALL TOGETHER 4-1

6. Continue giving sets of 5 back blows and 5 abdominal thrusts until:
- The person can cough forcefully, speak, cry or breathe.
- The person becomes unresponsive.

Note: *If the person becomes unresponsive, gently lower them to the floor and begin CPR, starting with compressions. After each set of compressions and before attempting breaths, open the person's mouth, look for the object and, if seen, remove it with a finger sweep. Never do a finger sweep unless you actually see the object.*

PUTTING IT ALL TOGETHER 4-2

Caring for an Infant Who Is Choking

Check
1. **Check the scene** for safety, **form an initial impression, obtain consent** from the parent or guardian and **use PPE**.

2. **Verify that the infant is choking** by checking to see if the infant is crying or coughing forcefully.
   - If the infant is crying or coughing forcefully: If coughing, allow the infant to keep coughing. Continue to observe the infant and be prepared to give first aid for choking if the infant's condition changes.

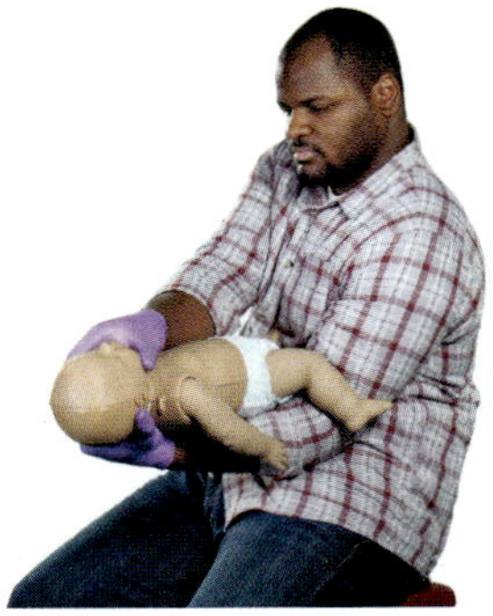

Call
3. If the infant is unable to cry or cough: **Call 9-1-1** and get equipment or tell someone to do so. Continue to step 4.

Care
4. **Give 5 back blows.**
   - Place the infant's back along your forearm, cradling the back of the infant's head with your hand.
   - Place your other forearm on the infant's front, supporting the infant's jaw with your thumb and fingers; do not cover the infant's face.
   - Turn the infant to a face-down position and hold them along your forearm using your thigh for support. Keep the infant's head lower than their body.
   - Use the heel of your hand to give a back blow between the infant's shoulder blades. Keep your fingers up to avoid hitting the infant's head or neck.
   - Give 5 firm back blows, with each one separate from the others.

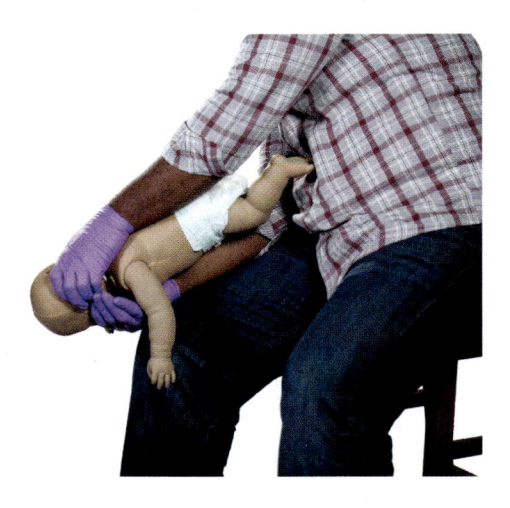

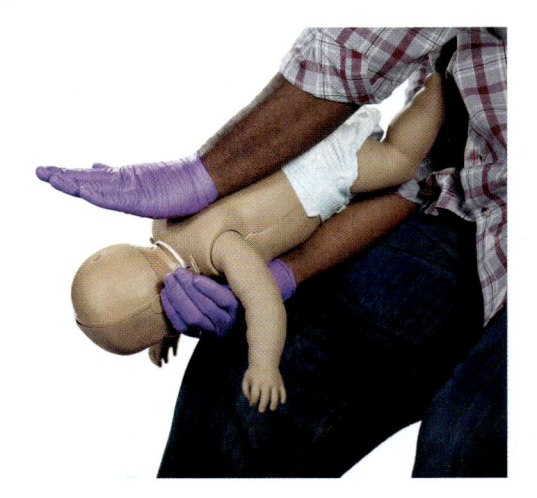

PUTTING IT ALL TOGETHER 4-2

5. Give 5 chest thrusts.

- Position the infant between your forearms:
  - Support the head and neck.
  - Turn the infant face-up.
  - Lower the infant onto your thigh with their head lower than their chest.
- Place two fingers in the center of the infant's chest, just below the nipple line.
- Give 5 quick chest thrusts about 1 ½ inches deep.
- Let the chest return to its normal position, keeping the fingers in contact with the chest:
  - Each chest thrust should be separate from the others.
  - Support the infant's head, neck and back while giving chest thrusts.

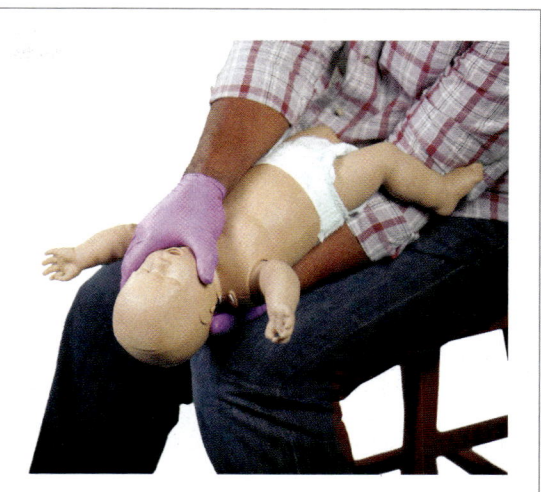

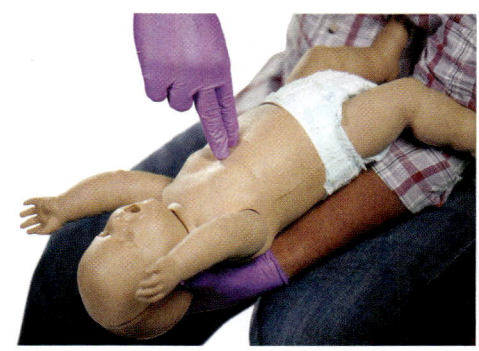

6. Continue giving sets of 5 back blows and 5 chest thrusts until:

- The infant can cough forcefully or cry.
- The infant becomes unresponsive.

Note: *Always support the infant's head and neck while giving back blows and chest thrusts.*

Note: *If the infant becomes unresponsive, lower them to a firm, flat surface and begin CPR, starting with compressions using the encircling thumbs technique. After each set of compressions and before attempting breaths, open the infant's mouth, look for the object and, if seen, remove it with a finger sweep using your pinky finger. Never do a finger sweep unless you actually see the object.*

American Red Cross | First Aid for Cardiac Arrest and Choking

PART 3
First Aid for Sudden Illnesses and Injuries

CHAPTER 5: Sudden Illness

CHAPTER 6: Wounds and Bleeding

CHAPTER 7: Injuries and Environmental Emergencies

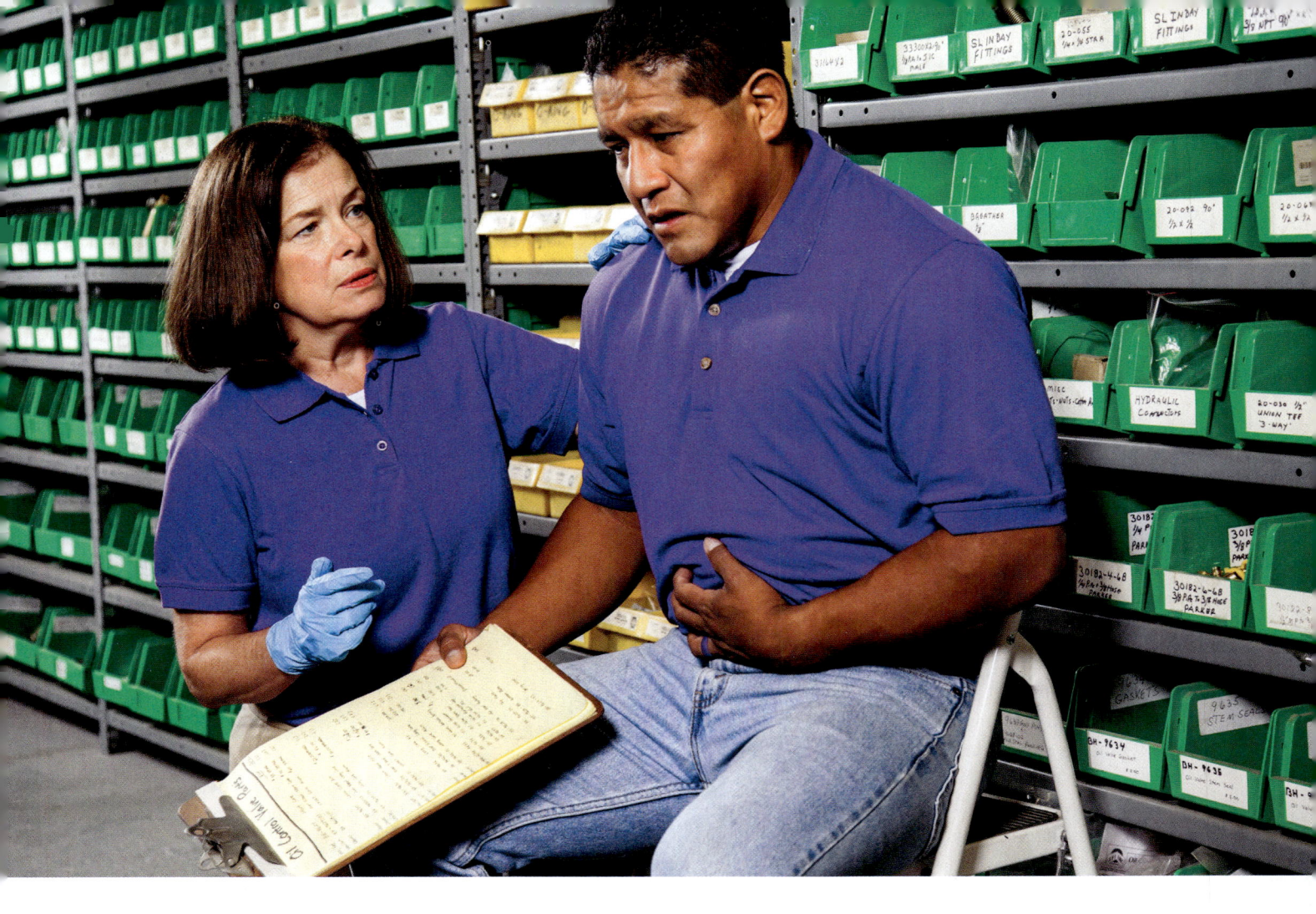

CHAPTER 5
Sudden Illness

Illness often strikes with little to no warning at work, at school, at home or while we are out having fun. When a person becomes suddenly ill, you can help by following the emergency action steps, CHECK—CALL—CARE, as you have learned to do for any emergency situation.

General Approach to Sudden Illness

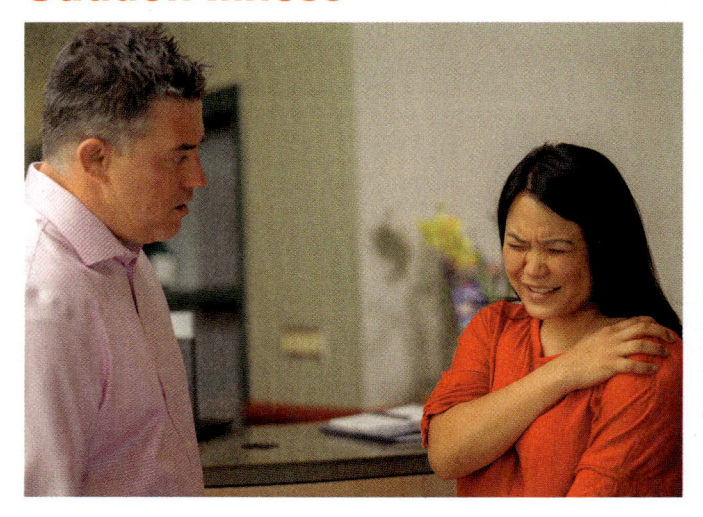

An **acute illness** is an illness that strikes suddenly and usually only lasts for a short period of time. A **chronic illness** is an illness that a person lives with on an ongoing basis and that often requires continuous treatment to manage. When a person becomes suddenly ill, it may be the result of an acute illness, it may be an acute flare-up of a chronic condition, or it may be due to increased susceptibility to acute illnesses due to a chronic illness.

Recognizing Sudden Illness

Fortunately, you do not need to know exactly what is wrong to provide appropriate first aid care. First, check that the scene is safe for you to enter before rushing to give care. Then check the person by forming an initial impression of the person and the situation, obtain consent and then continue checking the person.

Note: *If, during the initial impression, you determine that the person appears to be experiencing a life-threatening emergency, immediately go to the call step and give general care for the condition found. Then, continue your check (as appropriate) to determine if additional care is needed.*

If the person is responsive and experiencing a non-life-threatening emergency, continue the check by asking them (or bystanders, if necessary) questions using SAM (**S**igns and symptoms, **A**llergies, **M**edications and medical conditions) to gain a better understanding of the situation. Then do a focused check, focusing in on the area of concern (see Chapter 1).

Signs and Symptoms of Sudden Illness

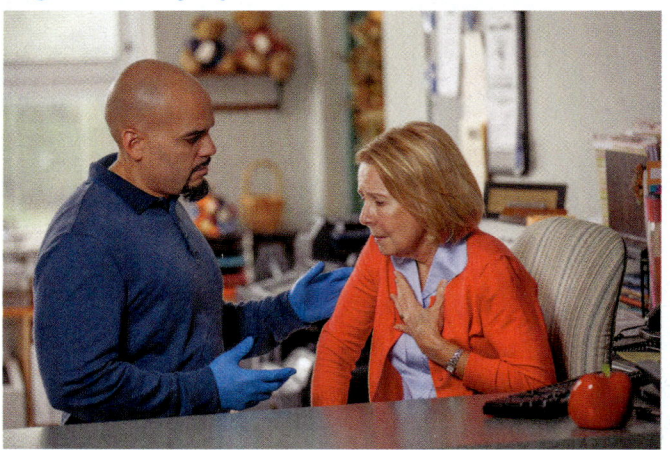

Signs and symptoms of sudden illness vary widely, depending on the cause of the illness. The person may have:

- Trouble breathing.
- Pain, such as chest pain, abdominal pain or a headache.
- Changes in level of responsiveness, such as being confused or unaware of one's surroundings, or becoming unresponsive.
- Extreme fatigue.
- Light-headedness or dizziness.
- Nausea, vomiting, diarrhea or stomach cramps.
- A fever.
- Pale, ashen (gray) or very flushed skin, which may be excessively sweaty or dry, or excessively hot or cold.

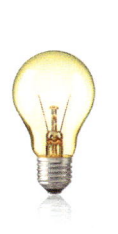

THE PROS KNOW. Be sure to look for a medical identification tag on the person or a digital medical identification on the person's phone when you are checking the person. It may offer a valuable clue as to the cause of the person's sudden illness.

THE PROS KNOW. Changes in skin color, including pale, gray (ashen) or flushed skin, happens in all people and is simply a degree of change from the person's baseline skin color. To look for changes in skin color, it can be helpful to look at less pigmented areas of the skin, such as lips or mucous membranes. In addition, a person with a sudden illness will just not "look right" and will have other signs and symptoms of sudden illness, such as sweating, trouble breathing, nausea, and so on, in addition to skin color changes.

- Problems seeing or speaking (e.g., blurred vision or slurred speech).
- Numbness, weakness or paralysis.
- Seizures.

Call 9-1-1

If you recognize at any time that the person is unresponsive, is not breathing or is having trouble breathing, is experiencing life-threatening bleeding or pain that is persistent or severe, is having problems seeing, speaking, feeling or moving, or if you recognize signs and symptoms of a sudden illness that is potentially life-threatening, such as a heart attack, asthma attack, anaphylaxis, opioid overdose, diabetic emergency, seizures, stroke, shock, or, in young children and infants, a high fever or dehydration, which can be caused by vomiting, diarrhea or other conditions, call 9-1-1 and get an AED and first aid kit or tell someone to do so. If you are unsure about the severity of the illness, it is better to call for help early than to wait for the illness to progress. Even if you don't need to call 911, it is still important that you get an AED and a first aid kit, or send someone to do so.

Giving General Care for Sudden Illness

Follow the same general guidelines as you would for any emergency:

- Give care consistent with the condition found and your knowledge and level of training and continue to watch for changes in the person's condition including breathing and responsiveness.
- Ask SAM questions and do a focused check, if not already done.
- Keep the person from getting cold or overheated.
- Treat for shock.
- Monitor the person's breathing and level of responsiveness.
- Reassure the person that you will help and that EMS personnel have been called (if appropriate).

In addition, positioning and assisting with medications may be necessary as part of general care for sudden illness.

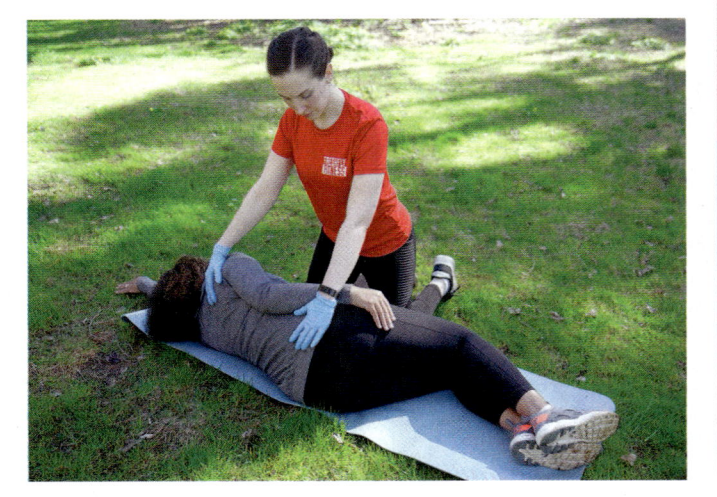

Positioning

An unresponsive person who is breathing or a person who responds but is not fully awake should be placed in the recovery position while waiting for EMS to arrive. A responsive person who is fully awake should be allowed to assume a position of comfort, such as sitting upright and leaning forward (if they wish) and loosening any tight clothing.

A person who is actively seizing should be monitored until the seizing has stopped. Turn them onto their side into a recovery position if it is possible to do so without injury. If they become unresponsive, position them in the recovery position. (See the section on Seizures for more information.)

Assisting with Medications

For some sudden illnesses, giving first aid care may involve *assisting* a person or their family member with medication. Assist the person with any of their medications they request or if it is indicated.

When assisting with medication, follow these general guidelines:

- Explain to the person or family member what you are going to do.
- Offer to get their medication.
- Ask the person to confirm that you have the right medication.
- Assemble the medication device, if necessary.
- Give the person or their family member the medication to self-administer.

Examples of medications that you may assist with when the person is experiencing a sudden illness include aspirin for heart attack; quick-relief (rescue) medications for asthma; epinephrine for anaphylaxis; naloxone for an opioid overdose; and sugar or glucose tablets, liquid or gel for diabetes.

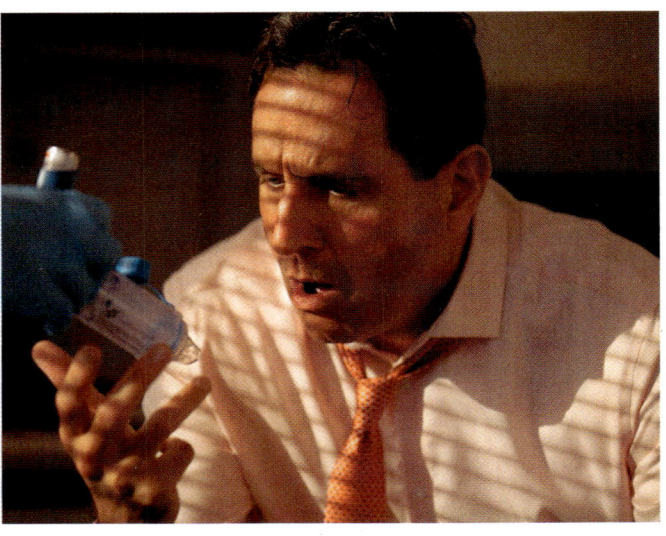

Administering Medications

You may administer medications that are stocked at your facility, if it is allowable by state laws and regulations and you are trained and authorized to do so. If this is done at your facility, there will be a specific plan in place for you to follow. Under some state laws and regulations, you may also administer a person's prescribed medication to them.

> **ALERT!**
>
> You should *not administer* medications unless it is allowable by state laws and regulations and you are trained and authorized to do so. Additional training on medication administration is available through the American Red Cross, if you need it.

When administering medications, follow these general guidelines:

- Explain to the person or family member what you are going to do.
- Get the stocked medication from the storage location at your facility or the prescribed medication from the person if allowed.
- Check the label for the medication name and expiration date.
- Assemble the medication device, if necessary.
- Administer the medication as you have been taught.

More information on administering medications can be found in Appendix D: Skill Practice Sheets for Skill Boosts.

Heart Attack

A **heart attack** occurs when blood flow to part of the heart muscle is blocked. Because the cells in the affected area of the heart muscle are not receiving the oxygen and nutrients they need, they become damaged and can die, causing the heart to not pump normally and if untreated, stop pumping blood. Calling 9-1-1 as soon as you recognize the signs and symptoms of a heart attack can minimize the damage to the heart and may save the person's life.

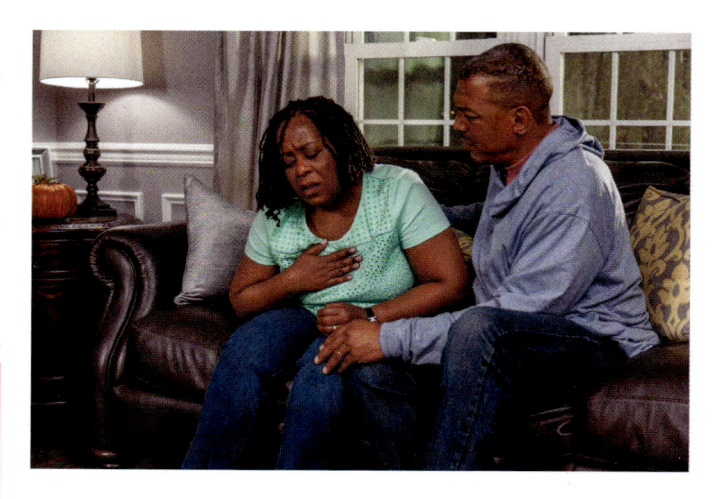

Recognizing a Heart Attack

Signs and symptoms of a heart attack vary from person to person and can be different in women than they are in men. Even people who have had a heart attack before may not experience the same signs and symptoms if they have a second heart attack. If you suspect a heart attack, always respond as if it is one. A person who is having a heart attack may show any of the following signs and symptoms:

- Chest pain, which can range from mild to unbearable. The person may complain of pressure, squeezing, tightness, aching or heaviness in the chest. The pain or discomfort is persistent, usually lasts longer than 3 to 5 minutes, or goes away and then comes back. It is not relieved by resting, changing position or taking medication. It may be difficult to distinguish the pain of a heart attack from the pain of indigestion, heartburn or a muscle spasm.
- Isolated or unexplained discomfort or pain that spreads to one or both arms, the back, the shoulder, the neck, the jaw or the upper part of the stomach
- Dizziness or light-headedness
- Trouble breathing, including noisy breathing, shortness of breath or breathing that is faster than normal
- Nausea or vomiting
- Pale, ashen (gray) or slightly bluish skin
- Sweating
- A feeling of anxiety or impending doom
- Extreme fatigue (tiredness)
- Unresponsiveness

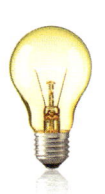

> **THE PROS KNOW.** Signs and symptoms of heart attack include chest pain, pressure, squeezing, tightness, aching or heaviness that lasts longer than 3 to 5 minutes or goes away and comes back, and isolated, unexplained discomfort in the arm(s), neck, jaw, back or stomach.
>
> In addition, more general signs and symptoms may be present and include shortness of breath, dizziness, unresponsiveness, sweating, nausea, vomiting or diarrhea, extreme fatigue, shortness of breath.

Although men often have the "classic" signs and symptoms of a heart attack, such as chest pain that radiates down one arm, women may have more subtle signs and symptoms or experience the signs and symptoms of a heart attack differently than men do. For example, in women, the "classic" signs and symptoms may be milder or accompanied by more general signs and symptoms such as back pain, shortness of breath, nausea or vomiting, extreme fatigue, and dizziness or light-headedness. Because these signs and symptoms are so general and nonspecific, women may experience them for hours, days or even weeks leading up to the heart attack but dismiss them as nothing out of the ordinary.

The signs and symptoms of a heart attack may also be more subtle in people with certain medical conditions, such as diabetes.

If you think that a person is having a heart attack, immediately call 9-1-1 and get an AED and first aid kit or tell someone to do so. Trust your instincts. Many people who are having a heart attack delay seeking care because they hope they are experiencing signs and symptoms of a more minor condition that will go away with time, such as indigestion, heartburn, a muscle strain or the flu. People often worry about calling an ambulance and going to the emergency room for a "false alarm." However, most people who die of a heart attack die within 2 hours of first experiencing signs or symptoms. Early advanced medical care can help to minimize the damage to the heart. *Always* seek advanced medical care as soon as signs and symptoms of a heart attack are noticed.

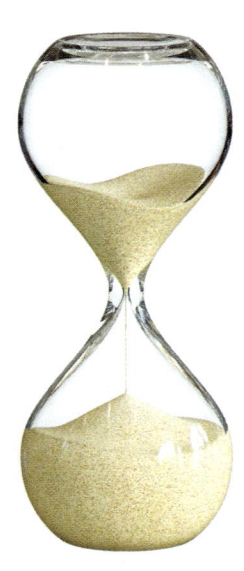

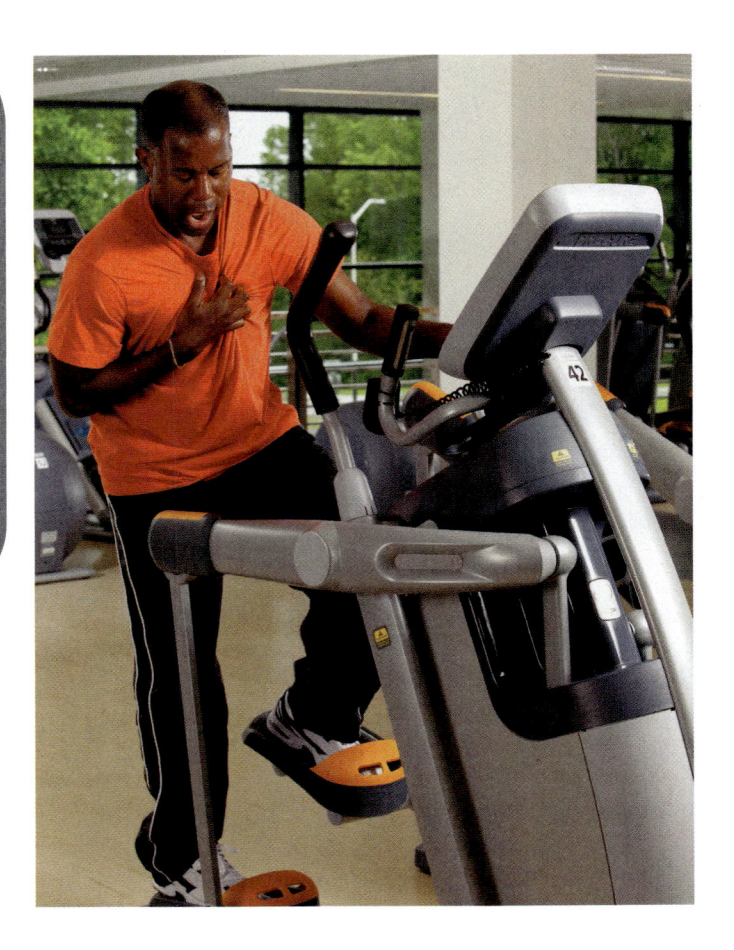

Therefore, if you think that someone might be having a heart attack, you should call 9-1-1 immediately and get an AED and a first aid kit or tell someone to do so. Never try to drive a person who is experiencing signs and symptoms of a heart attack to the hospital yourself. EMS personnel can transport the person to the hospital safely while initiating care.

Giving First Aid Care for a Heart Attack

If you are trained in giving CPR and using an automated external defibrillator (AED), be prepared to give CPR and use an AED if the person becomes unresponsive and is not breathing.

After calling 9-1-1, have the person stop what they are doing and rest in a comfortable position to reduce the heart's need for oxygen. Many people experiencing a heart attack find it easier to breathe while sitting.

Closely monitor the person's condition until EMS personnel arrive and begin their care of the person. Notice any changes in the person's appearance or behavior.

Respiratory Distress

Respiratory distress, or difficulty breathing, is evidenced by signs and symptoms such as shortness of breath, gasping for breath, breathing that is faster than normal, or breathing that is uncomfortable or painful. Respiratory distress can lead to **respiratory arrest** (absence of breathing) and even cardiac arrest.

Causes of Respiratory Distress

A number of different conditions can cause respiratory distress, including but not limited to acute flare-ups of chronic respiratory conditions such as asthma or chronic obstructive pulmonary disease (COPD); bronchopulmonary dysplasia (BPD) in infants; lung and respiratory tract infections (such as pneumonia, bronchitis, croup or bronchiolitis); severe allergic reactions (anaphylaxis); heart conditions (such as a heart attack or heart failure); trauma; poisoning; drug overdose; and mental health conditions (such as panic disorder).

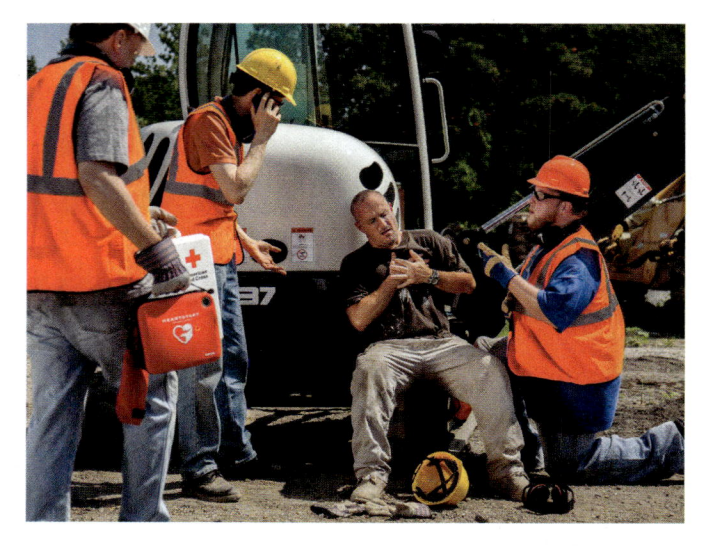

If the person is awake, can follow simple commands, can chew and swallow, and is allowed to have aspirin, you may assist the person with taking two to four low-dose (81-mg) aspirin tablets (162 to 324 mg) or one regular-strength (325-mg) aspirin tablet (Box 5-1).

If the person has a history of heart disease and takes a prescribed medication to relieve chest pain (e.g., nitroglycerin), offer to assist with the medication.

Then, loosen any tight or uncomfortable clothing and reassure the person. Anxiety increases the person's discomfort.

Box 5-1 Aspirin for a Heart Attack

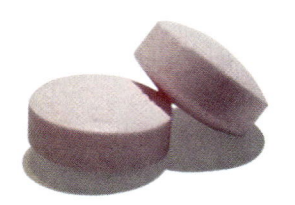

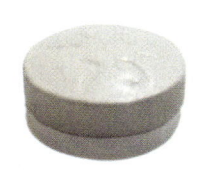

You may be able to help a person who is showing signs and symptoms of a heart attack by offering the person an appropriate dose of aspirin. Aspirin can help and is most effective when given soon after the onset of signs and symptoms of a heart attack. However, you should never delay calling 9-1-1 or getting equipment to find or offer aspirin.

Before assisting with aspirin, make sure the person is responsive, able to chew and swallow, and allowed to have aspirin. Ask the person:

- Are you allergic to aspirin?
- Have you ever been told by a healthcare provider to avoid taking aspirin?

If the person answers "no" to each of these questions, you may offer the person two to four 81-mg low-dose aspirin tablets (162 to 324 mg) or one 325-mg regular-strength aspirin tablet. The aspirin may be enteric-coated or non-enteric-coated. Have the person chew the aspirin completely. Chewing the aspirin speeds its absorption into the bloodstream.

Do not offer the person an aspirin-containing combination product meant to relieve multiple conditions, or non-aspirin other type of pain medication, such as acetaminophen (Tylenol®), ibuprofen (Motrin®, Advil®) or naproxen (Aleve®). These medications do not work the same way aspirin does and are not beneficial for a person who is experiencing a heart attack.

---

84 Chapter 5 | Sudden Illness

Recognizing Respiratory Distress

When a person is experiencing a breathing emergency, it is important to act at once. In some breathing emergencies, the oxygen supply to the body is greatly reduced and/or carbon dioxide is increased. If breathing stops or is restricted long enough, the person will become unresponsive, the heart will stop beating and body systems will quickly fail. Recognizing that a person is having trouble breathing and giving appropriate first aid care can save the person's life.

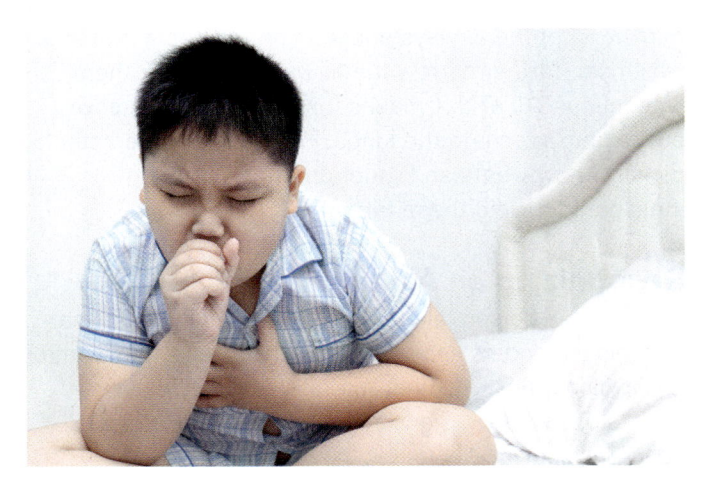

A person who is experiencing respiratory distress is, understandably, often very frightened. The person may feel like they cannot get enough air and may gasp for breath. Because the person is struggling to breathe, speaking in complete sentences may be difficult. You might hear wheezing, gurgling, high-pitched noises as the person tries to breathe, or for infants and young children, changes in sound or a weak cry. You may also notice that the person's breathing is unusually slow or fast, unusually deep or shallow, or irregular. The person's skin may feel moist or cool, and it may be pale, ashen (gray), bluish or flushed. Lack of oxygen can make the person feel dizzy, light-headed, confused, unresponsive, or give them a headache. High carbon dioxide can make the person drowsy, tired or unresponsive.

You usually can identify a breathing problem by watching and listening to any abnormal sounds you can hear as the person breathes and by asking them how they feel. If a person is having trouble breathing, do not wait to see if the person's condition improves. Call 9-1-1 and get equipment or tell someone to do so. Then give first aid care according to your training until help arrives.

Giving First Aid Care for Respiratory Distress

After calling 9-1-1, be prepared to give CPR and use an AED if the person becomes unresponsive and is not breathing, and you are trained in these skills.

If you know the cause of the respiratory distress (for example, an asthma attack or anaphylaxis) and the person carries medication used for the emergency treatment of the condition, offer to assist the person take their medication.

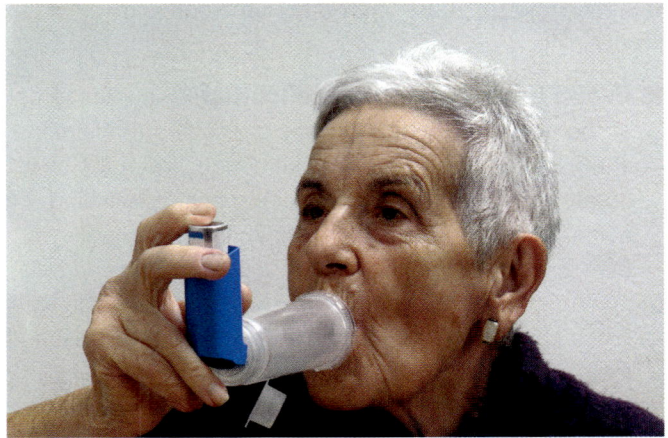

Encourage the person to sit down and assume a position of comfort. Most people will naturally assume a position that helps to make breathing easier. Providing reassurance can reduce anxiety, which may also help to make breathing easier.

If the person is responsive, gather additional information by interviewing the person using SAM and doing a focused check after assisting with medications, if needed, and while waiting for EMS to arrive. Remember that a person having breathing problems may find it difficult to talk. Try phrasing your questions as "yes" or "no" questions so the person can nod or shake their head in response instead of making the effort to speak. You may also be able to ask bystanders what they know about the person's condition.

Pediatric Considerations

For children, respiratory distress is a common sudden illness. Children are more susceptible than adults to respiratory distress because their airways are smaller, narrower and less rigid. In addition to the signs and symptoms of respiratory distress seen in adults, children may have the following signs and symptoms:

- Nasal flaring (widening of the nostrils when breathing in)
- More pronounced use of the chest and neck muscles to breathe (muscles pull in around the collarbone and ribs)
- Grunting

The most common respiratory emergency in kids often involves bronchospasm and can be due to a chronic condition called asthma. Two common infections associated with respiratory distress in children are croup and bronchiolitis.

- **Croup (laryngotracheobronchitis)** is an infection of the upper airway that causes difficulty breathing and a harsh, repetitive, bark-like cough. When the child breathes in, they may make a high-pitched whistling noise. Croup is most common in children younger than 5 years. Croup usually is not serious and can be managed at home; however, in some cases, a child with croup can progress quickly from respiratory distress to respiratory arrest.
- **Bronchiolitis** is an infection of the lower airway that can cause difficulty breathing. Symptoms include common cold symptoms (fever, runny nose, congestion, cough), decreased appetite, irritability and vomiting. More severe symptoms include fast, labored breathing or **wheezing** (a high-pitched, noisy breathing and/or whistling sound during exhalation) and troubling drinking or eating. Bronchiolitis is most common in infants and can also occur in young children up to about 2 years of age. Bronchiolitis can range from minor to life-threatening, depending on the symptoms.

Asthma and Asthma Attack

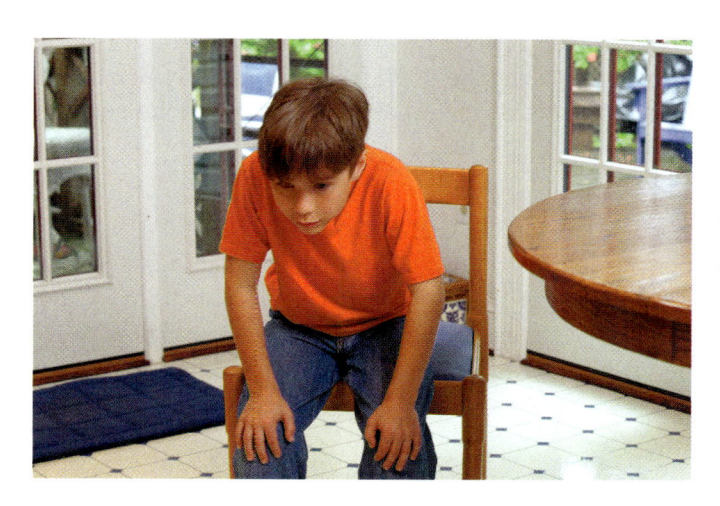

Many people have **asthma**, a chronic illness in which certain substances or conditions, called **triggers**, cause inflammation and narrowing of the airways, making breathing difficult. This is called an asthma attack. Some people, especially young children and infants, may not know they have asthma and only find out when they have their first asthma attack. Common triggers for an asthma attack include exercise, temperature extremes, allergies, respiratory infections, stress or anxiety, air pollution and strong odors (such as perfume, cologne and scented cleaning products). The trigger causes narrowing of the airways and inflammation and swelling, which can further narrow the airways and block them with mucus. All of this makes it harder for air to move out of and, later, into the lungs. People who have asthma usually know what can trigger an attack and take measures to avoid these triggers.

Recognizing an Asthma Attack

Even when a person takes steps to manage their asthma by avoiding triggers and taking prescribed long-term control medications (Box 5-2), they may still experience asthma attacks occasionally. Signs and symptoms of an asthma attack include:

- Wheezing or coughing.
- Rapid, and/or shallow breathing.
- Trouble breathing.
- Sweating.
- Being unable to talk without stopping for a breath in between every few words or unable to talk at all.
- Limited ability to walk or go upstairs.
- In infants and young children, change in cry or weak cry.
- Feelings of tightness in the chest or being unable to get enough air into the lungs.
- Anxiety and fear.
- Fatigue.

An asthma attack can become life-threatening because it affects the person's ability to breathe. If the person has signs and symptoms of an asthma attack, call 9-1-1 and get equipment immediately or tell someone to do so.

Giving First Aid Care for an Asthma Attack

After calling 9-1-1 and getting equipment, if the person has an **asthma action plan** (a written plan that the person develops with their healthcare provider that details daily management of the condition as well as how to handle an asthma attack), assist the person to follow that plan.

Box 5-2 Asthma Inhalers and Nebulizers

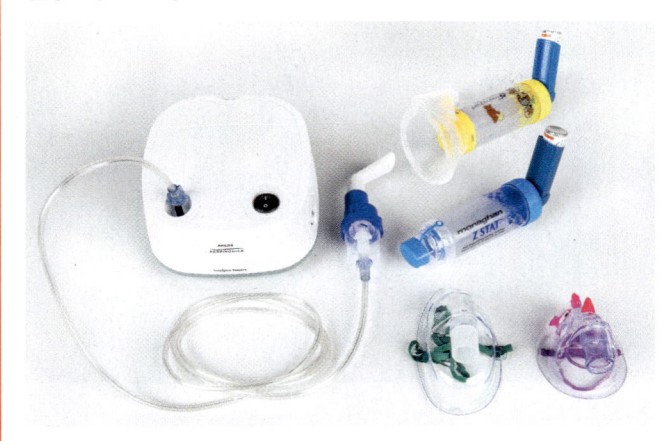

Quick-relief (rescue) medications are taken when the person is experiencing an acute asthma attack. These medications work quickly to relax the muscles that tighten around the airways, opening the airways right away so that the person can breathe more easily. A person who has been diagnosed with asthma may take two forms of medication, quick-relief and long-term control medications.

Long-term control medications are taken regularly, whether or not signs and symptoms of asthma are present. These medications help prevent asthma attacks by reducing inflammation and swelling and making the airways less sensitive to triggers.

Both long-term control medications and quick-relief (rescue) medications may be given through an inhaler and a nebulizer. Long-term control medications can also be given orally. Inhalation allows the medication to reach the airways faster, work quickly and be targeted to where it is needed. Medications are inhaled using a metered dose inhaler (MDI), a dry powder inhaler (DPI) or a small-volume nebulizer.

Metered Dose Inhalers

An MDI delivers a measured dose of medication directly into the person's lungs. The person gently presses down the top of the inhaler. This causes a small amount of pressurized gas to push the medication out quickly.

A spacer (or chamber) should be used to make it easier for the person to coordinate with the inhaler correctly and get the full dose of medication. The medication goes into the spacer, and then the person inhales the medication through the mouthpiece on the spacer. For infants and younger children, a spacer may be used with a face mask instead of a mouthpiece.

Dry Powder Inhalers

A DPI delivers a measured dose of medicine in a dry powder form directly into the person's lungs. Instead of pressing down on the top of the device to dispense the medication, the person breathes in quickly to activate the DPI and dispense the medication. Some people and young children have difficulty using DPIs because they require the user to take in a quick, strong breath.

Small-Volume Nebulizers

Small-volume nebulizers convert liquid medication into a mist, which is delivered over 5 to 15 minutes.

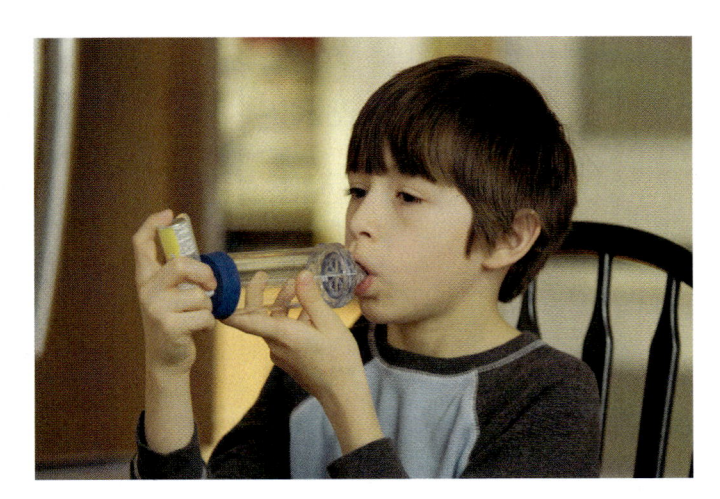

Assisting with Quick-Relief Medications

Encourage or assist the person to use their prescribed quick-relief (rescue) medication, assisting if needed and if asked (see Box 5-2).

Be aware that more than one dose of medication may be needed to stop the asthma attack. The medication may be repeated after 10 to 15 minutes. Stay with the person and monitor their condition until the person is able to breathe normally or EMS personnel arrive and begin their care.

Putting It All Together 5-1 provides step-by-step instructions for responding to a person who is experiencing an asthma attack.

Administering Quick-Relief Medications

You may administer a quick-relief medication that is stocked at your facility, if it is allowable by state laws and regulations and you are trained and authorized to do so. If this is done at your facility, there will be a specific plan in place for you to follow. Under some state laws and regulations you may also administer a medication prescribed to the person.

American Red Cross | First Aid for Sudden Illnesses and Injuries

See Skill Practice Sheets: Administering Quick-Relief Medication Using an Inhaler; Administering Quick-Relief Medication Using a Nebulizer in Appendix D.

Allergic Reactions and Anaphylaxis

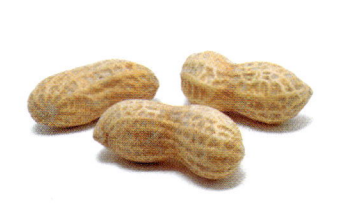

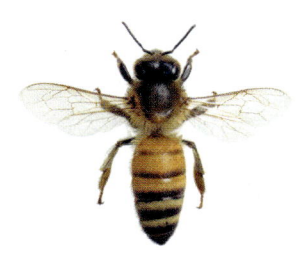

Our immune systems help to keep us healthy by fighting off harmful pathogens that can cause disease. But sometimes our immune systems overreact and try to fight off ordinary things that are not usually harmful, like certain foods, grass or pet dander (tiny flakes of skin that animals shed). A person can have an allergy to almost anything. Common allergens (allergy triggers) include venomous insect stings, certain foods (like peanuts, tree nuts, shellfish, milk, eggs, soy and wheat), animal dander, plant pollen, certain medications (like penicillin and sulfa drugs) and latex.

Recognizing Allergic Reactions and Anaphylaxis

An allergic reaction can range from mild to very severe. A person who is having a mild to moderate allergic reaction may develop a skin rash, a stuffy nose, or red, watery eyes, abdominal cramps or nausea. The skin or area of the body that came in contact with the allergen may swell, turn red and may have hives.

Anaphylaxis is a life-threatening allergic reaction that can cause shock and affect the person's ability to breathe. A person who is having an anaphylactic reaction (severe, life-threatening allergic reaction) may have either signs of an allergic reaction or history of an allergy, and one or more of the following signs and symptoms within seconds or minutes of coming into contact with the allergen:

- Swelling of the face, neck, tongue or lips
- Trouble breathing
- Signs and symptoms of shock (such as excessive thirst; skin that feels cool or moist and looks pale or bluish; an altered level of responsiveness; and a rapid, weak heartbeat)
- A change in responsiveness

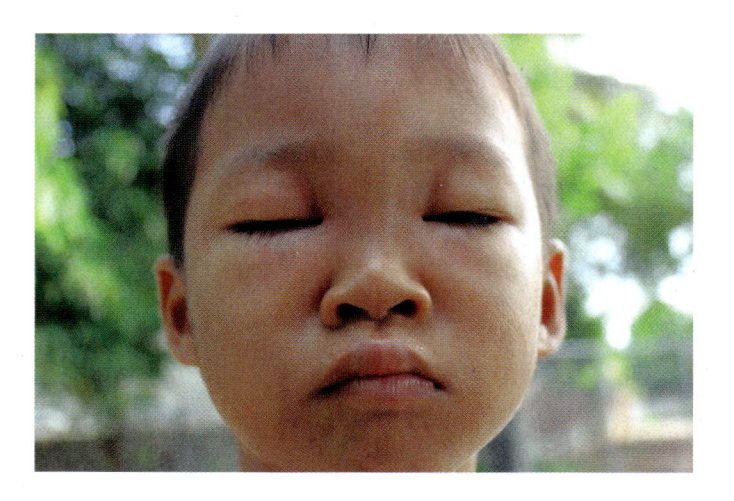

To determine if a person is having a severe, life-threatening allergic reaction (anaphylaxis), look at the situation as well as the person's signs and symptoms (Table 5-1).

If you know that the person has had a severe allergic reaction before, and the person is having trouble breathing or is showing signs and symptoms of shock or anaphylaxis, call 9-1-1 and get equipment immediately or tell someone to do so.

TABLE 5-1 How Do I Know If It Is Anaphylaxis?

SITUATION	LOOK FOR:
You do not know if the person has been exposed to an allergen.	■ Any skin reaction (such as hives, itchiness or flushing) **OR** ■ Swelling of the face, neck, tongue or lips **PLUS** ■ Trouble breathing **OR** ■ Signs and symptoms of shock
You think the person may have been exposed to an allergen.	Any **TWO** of the following: ■ Any skin reaction ■ Swelling of the face, neck, tongue or lips ■ Trouble breathing ■ Signs and symptoms of shock ■ Nausea, vomiting, cramping or diarrhea
You know that the person has been exposed to an allergen.	■ Trouble breathing **OR** ■ Signs and symptoms of shock

88   Chapter 5 | Sudden Illness

Giving First Aid Care for Anaphylaxis

After calling 9-1-1, if the person carries medication for the emergency treatment of anaphylaxis (e.g., epinephrine), offer to assist the person to use the medication.

If you are alone, assist the person with administering the medication and then call 9-1-1 or the designated emergency number. While you wait for help to arrive, make sure the person is sitting in a comfortable position, or have the person lie down if they are showing signs of shock.

Assisting with Epinephrine

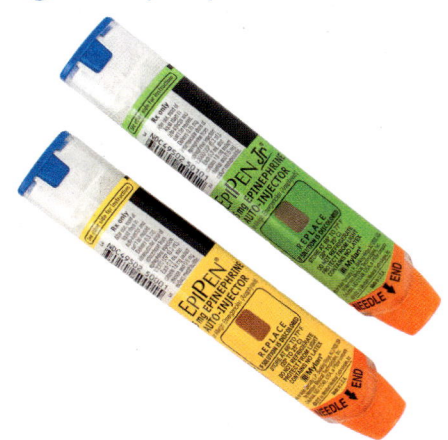

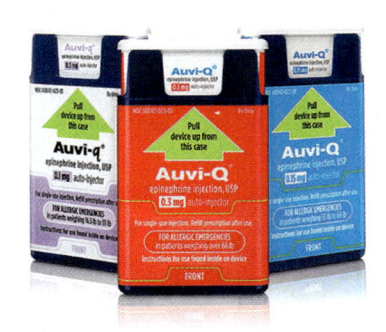

Epinephrine is a drug that slows or stops the effects of anaphylaxis. If a person is known to have an allergy that could lead to anaphylaxis, they may carry an **epinephrine auto-injector** (a syringe system, available by prescription only, that contains a single dose of epinephrine and can administer an injection). Many healthcare providers advise that people with a known history of anaphylaxis carry an anaphylaxis kit containing at least two doses of epinephrine (two auto-injectors) with them at all times. This is because more than one dose may be needed to stop the anaphylactic reaction. Have the person administer a second dose only if emergency responders are delayed and the person is still having signs and symptoms of anaphylaxis 5 to 10 minutes after administering the first dose.

Devices are available containing different doses because the dose of epinephrine is based on weight (0.15 mg for children weighing between 33 and 66 pounds, and 0.3 mg for children and adults weighing more than 66 pounds).

It is important to act fast when a person is having an anaphylactic reaction because difficulty breathing and shock are both life-threatening conditions. If the person is unable to self-administer the medication, you may need to help. You may assist a person with using an epinephrine auto-injector when the person is having an anaphylactic reaction.

Different brands of epinephrine auto-injectors are available, but all work in a similar fashion (and some have audio prompts to guide the user). The device is activated by pushing it against the skin, with the preferred location being the mid-outer thigh. Once activated, the device injects the epinephrine into the thigh muscle. The device must be held in place for the recommended amount of time (about 3 seconds, depending on the device) to deliver the medication. Some medication may still remain in the auto-injector even after the injection is complete. After the person removes the auto-injector, massage the injection site for several seconds (or have the person massage the injection site). Give the container to EMS personnel for proper disposal.

After the person has self-administered epinephrine, stay with them and give care as you have been trained until EMS arrives and begins their care. Have the person rest comfortably, monitor their condition and provide reassurance.

Putting It All Together 5-2 provides step-by-step instructions for responding to a person who is experiencing anaphylaxis.

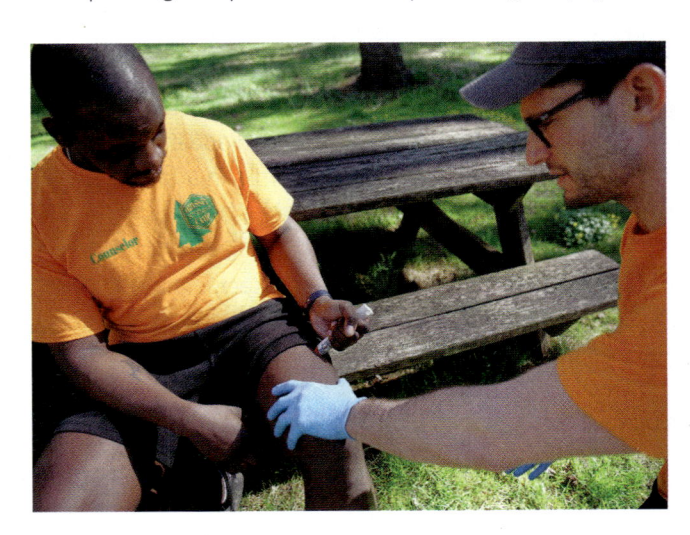

American Red Cross | First Aid for Sudden Illnesses and Injuries

Administering Epinephrine

Where state and local laws allow, some organizations (such as schools, businesses, public venues) keep a stock of epinephrine auto-injectors for designated staff members who have received the proper training to use in an anaphylaxis emergency. If you are using a stock epinephrine auto-injector, follow your organization's emergency action plan and/or protocol for epinephrine auto-injector use. Dispose of the used auto-injector per your facility's protocol. If there is not a specific protocol, give the used auto-injector to EMS. Complete any facility-required paperwork and notifications.

Under some state laws and regulations, you may also administer a person's prescribed medication to them.

See Skill Practice Sheet: Administering Epinephrine Using an Auto-Injector in Appendix D.

Assisting with Antihistamines

The person's healthcare provider may recommend that the person carry an antihistamine in their anaphylaxis kit, in addition to epinephrine. An antihistamine is a medication that counteracts the effects of histamine, a chemical released by the body during an allergic reaction. Antihistamines are supplied as pills, capsules or liquids and are taken by mouth. The person should take the antihistamine according to the medication label and their healthcare provider's instructions. As part of first aid care, you may assist the person with their prescribed antihistamines.

Opioid Overdose

Opioids are drugs that are prescribed to reduce pain for serious injuries or cancer or after surgeries. The effectiveness of opioid drugs has led to their widespread use—but we also have seen misuse and addiction, fueling what is being called the opioid epidemic. In addition, there are illegal derivates of opioids available, such as heroin.

"Drug overdose is the leading cause of accidental death in the United States, surpassing even motor vehicle crashes. Opioids are the number one cause of these deaths, making knowledge of opioid overdose treatment essential for first aid providers."

–Nathan P. Charlton, MD, FACEP, FACMT, FAWM
American Red Cross Scientific Advisory Council

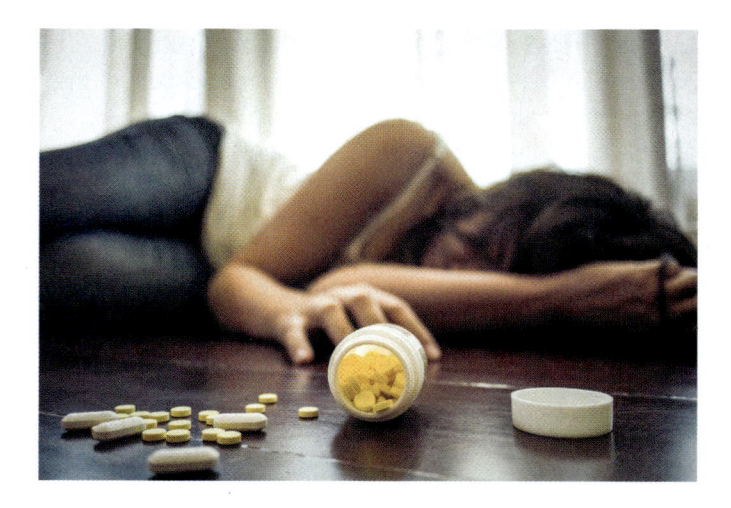

The possible effects of using opioids range from pain relief and euphoria to near-unresponsiveness, stopping breathing and cardiac arrest.

Prescription opioids include:

- Hydrocodone (Vicodin®)
- Oxycodone (OxyContin®, Percocet®)
- Oxymorphone (Opana®)
- Codeine (used alone or in combination with Tylenol® or cough medicine)
- Morphine (Kadian®, Avinza®)
- Fentanyl

Illegal (non-prescription) forms of opioids (e.g., heroin) include drugs with the street names of brown sugar, china white, dope, H, horse, junk, skag, skunk and smack.

Clues that suggest an opioid overdose include prescription pill bottles, pipes, needles, syringes, pill powder or other drug-related items.

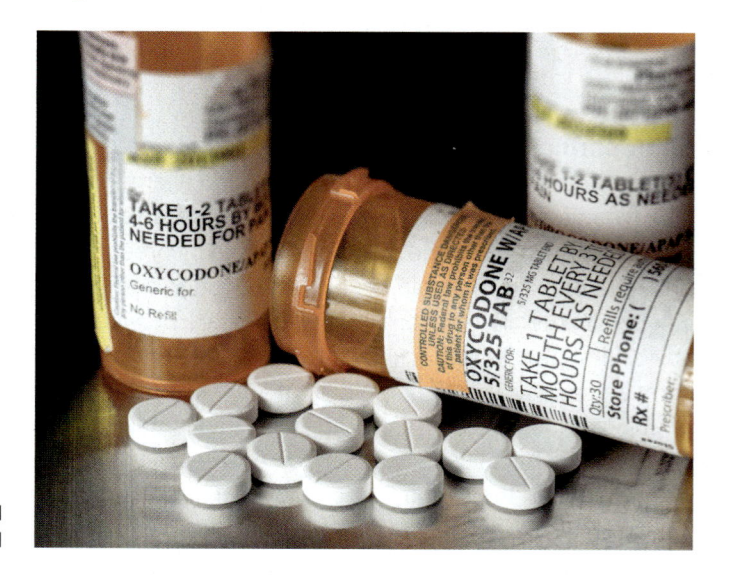

Recognizing an Opioid Overdose

Recognizing an opioid overdose may be difficult. If you aren't sure, it is best to treat the situation like an overdose. You could save a life.

Signs and symptoms of **opioid overdose** include evidence of opioid use and decreased breathing effort; for example, breathing slowly and perhaps only a few times a minute, and gasping or gurgling; unresponsiveness; bluish or grayish colored skin; and cardiac arrest.

If you recognize signs and symptoms of an opioid overdose, call 9-1-1 and get equipment immediately or tell someone to do so.

Giving First Aid Care for an Opioid Overdose

After calling 9-1-1, if the person is unresponsive and not breathing, immediately begin CPR or compression-only CPR, depending on your training. If a family member has been prescribed naloxone for the person, you may assist them with administering naloxone to temporarily reverse the effects of opioids without disrupting or delaying CPR and AED use.

The reason that the appropriate care for a person who is unresponsive and not breathing is CPR is because the person is showing signs and symptoms of cardiac arrest. Cardiac arrest occurs when the heart stops beating or beats too ineffectively to circulate blood to the brain and other vital organs. Thus, it is important to begin CPR right away.

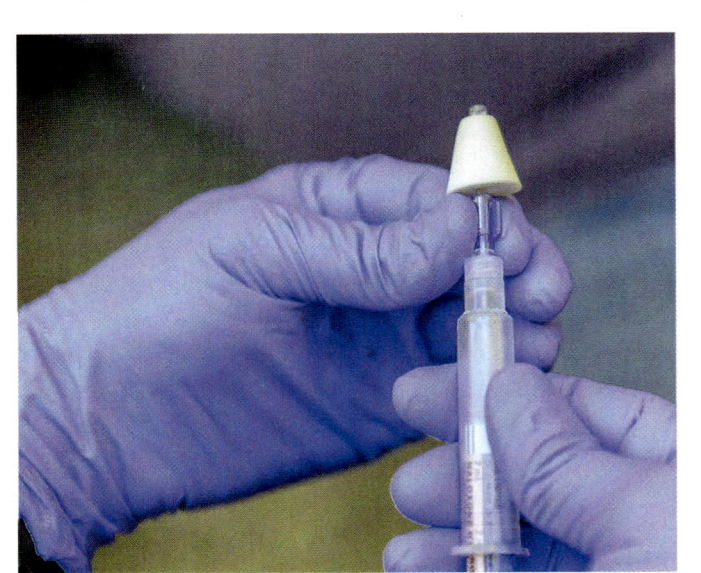

Assisting with Naloxone

If the person is breathing slowly or irregularly and/or is not fully awake or is confused, you may assist a family member with administering naloxone.

Naloxone is a drug that temporarily reverses the effects of opioids (Box 5-3). Naloxone may be given via the nose using a nasal atomizer or nasal spray.

After naloxone is administered, note the time it was administered and look for changes in the person's condition. If they are still having signs and symptoms 2 to 3 minutes after administering the first dose and EMS has not arrived, assist with administering a second dose of naloxone. When you are assisting with administering naloxone via the nose, make sure a new nasal device is used for the second dose. Stay with the person, give care as you have been trained until EMS arrives and begins their care. Have the person rest comfortably, monitor their condition and provide reassurance.

If the person is awake and breathing normally, call 9-1-1 and monitor them until EMS arrives and begins their care.

Administering Naloxone

You may administer naloxone that is stocked at your facility, if it is allowable by state laws and regulations and you are trained and authorized to do so. If this is done at your facility, there will be a specific plan in place for you to follow. Under some state laws and regulations, you may also administer naloxone that is prescribed to the person. If a second responder is with you and they are trained and authorized, they should give naloxone. See Skill Practice Sheets: Administering Naloxone Using a Nasal Spray and Administering Naloxone Using a Nasal Atomizer in Appendix D.

> ### Box 5-3 What Is Naloxone?
>
> Many tools are used to fight the opioid epidemic, including increased awareness and education. However, people still fall victim to accidental death by opioid overdose every day. Fortunately, a medication is available that can save lives by temporarily reversing the effects of opioids. That medication is naloxone, and it's available in generic form or under a brand name like Narcan®.
>
> - Naloxone temporarily reverses the symptoms of an opioid overdose, including change in behavior including unresponsiveness and normalizes breathing.
> - Naloxone can save someone's life until professional medical help arrives.
> - Naloxone does not typically cause serious side effects, even if the person is not overdosing on opioids.
> - Naloxone may be available at your local pharmacy.
>
> ### How Naloxone Works
>
> Naloxone stops the effects of an opioid overdose by blocking the parts of the body that respond to opioids.
>
> Even if given naloxone, a person will also need immediate medical care, as the blocking effects of naloxone often are shorter than the effect of most opioids.
>
> ### Obtaining Naloxone
>
> Depending on where you live, you may need a prescription for naloxone, or it may be available from pharmacies or other distribution locations without a prescription.
>
> Check with your local pharmacy or your state's health department to learn more about availability in your area. 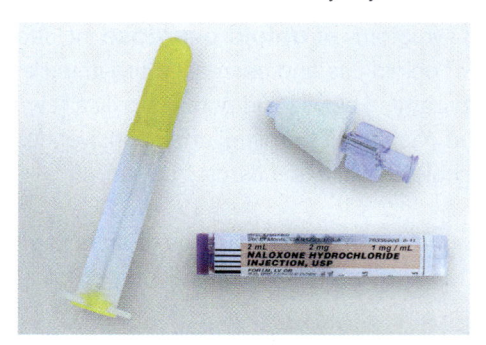
>
> **Nasal atomizer** 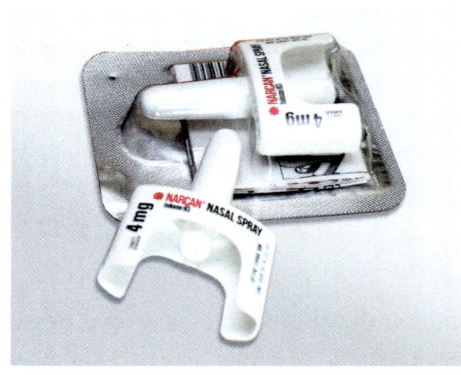
>
> **Nasal spray**

Diabetic Emergencies

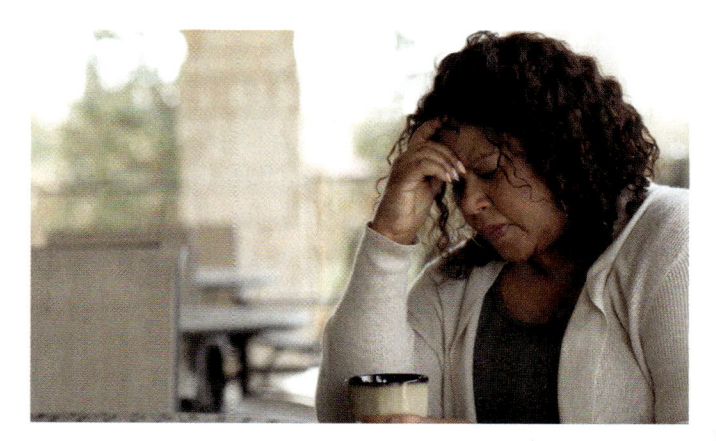

Diabetes is a chronic condition characterized by the body's inability to process glucose (sugar) in the bloodstream. An organ called the pancreas secretes **insulin**, a hormone that causes glucose to be moved from the bloodstream into the cells, where it is used for energy. In a person with diabetes, either the pancreas fails to make enough insulin or the body's cells are unable to respond to insulin. Either situation causes glucose levels in the bloodstream to increase with ingestion of glucose.

A person with diabetes may manage the condition with insulin injections, oral medications, or both. Diet and exercise also play an important role. To keep blood glucose levels within an acceptable range, food intake, exercise and medication must be balanced. A person with diabetes must follow a well-balanced diet with limited sweets and fats. The timing of meals and snacks relative to exercise and medication is important as well.

If food intake, exercise and medication are not in balance, the person may experience a diabetic emergency.

- **Hypoglycemia** (excessively low blood glucose levels) can result if a person misses a meal or snack, eats too little food, exercises more than usual, vomits or takes too much medication.
- **Hyperglycemia** (excessively high blood glucose levels) can result if a person eats too much food, takes too little medication, exercises less than usual or has an infection.

Recognizing Diabetic Emergencies

A person who is having a diabetic emergency will seem generally ill. They may have trouble breathing, experience fast or deep breathing, feel weak or different, experience sweating and have a fast heartbeat. In addition, they may feel dizzy or shaky, have a headache, or have cool, clammy skin. The person's behavior may change; for example, they may become irritable, aggressive or argumentative. If the person is experiencing hyperglycemia, their breath may have a fruity or sweet odor, they may have increased urination, and they may feel dehydrated. Severe hypoglycemia or hyperglycemia can result in confusion, seizures, or unresponsiveness and should be treated as life-threatening.

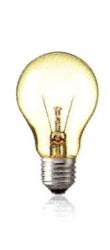

> **THE PROS KNOW.** A person who is experiencing a diabetic emergency may appear to be under the influence of alcohol. For example, the person may slur their words or have difficulty walking. Interviewing the person (or bystanders) using SAM and conducting a focused check may help you identify the true cause of the person's signs and symptoms.

If you recognize signs and symptoms of a diabetic emergency, and the person is unresponsive or not fully awake and alert during your check of the person, call 9-1-1 and get equipment or tell someone to do so immediately. If the person is awake and alert, you can get equipment and give care before calling 9-1-1 but if they don't improve with care, you will need to call 9-1-1 after initial care. If you are unsure whether or not to call 9-1-1 when someone is having a diabetic emergency, the safest approach is always to call 9-1-1 and get equipment and then to give care.

Giving First Aid Care for Diabetic Emergencies

If the person is unresponsive or not fully awake and you are waiting for EMS to arrive, begin their care by placing them in a recovery position, making sure the person's airway is clear of vomit and monitoring the person's breathing until help arrives. If the person is having a seizure, take steps to keep the person safe while you let the seizure run its course.

If the person is alert and able and has their equipment with them, have them check their sugar level and have them tell you if it is low or high. If the blood glucose is low, then giving sugar can be lifesaving. If they don't have their equipment, can't test or can't tell you whether their sugar is low or high, it is good to give some sugar. The volume of sugar you give will be lifesaving if the person's blood glucose is low and will not have a major negative impact if the person's blood glucose is high.

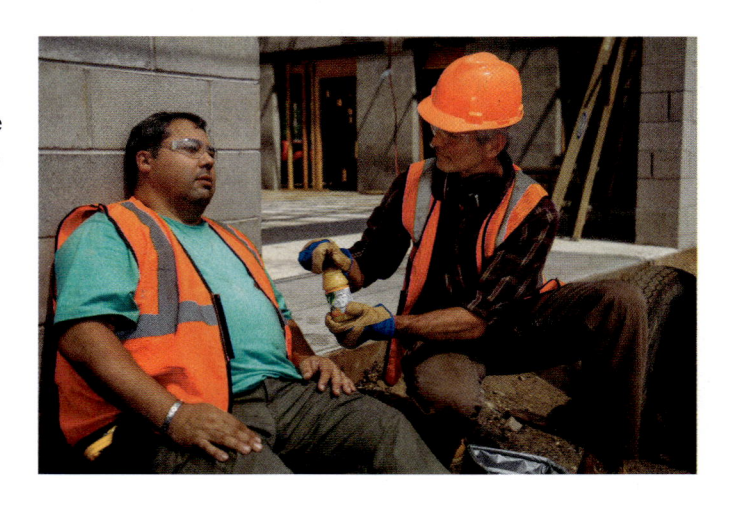

Only offer the person sugar by mouth if the person is awake, able to follow simple commands and able to chew and swallow. Some people may be responsive but not fully awake and therefore not able to safely swallow; in this case, do not attempt to give the person sugar by mouth.

If it is safe for the person to have sugar by mouth, give 15 to 20 grams of sugar. The recommended amount of sugar is 15 grams for children and 20 grams for adults. Check the label on packaged products to determine how much of the package's contents to give.

Acceptable forms of 15 to 20 grams of sugar include:

- Glucose tablets, liquid or gel.
- Orange juice (7 ounces).
- Milk (14 ounces).
- Candies with fructose or sucrose, such as (average):
  - 20 to 25 Skittles.
  - 2 strips of fruit rolls.
  - 10 to 20 jelly beans.

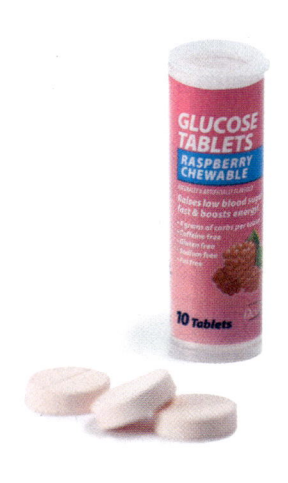

For children who may be uncooperative with swallowing, you can give them a slurry of sugar and water under their tongue that will dissolve.

If possible, after administration of the sugar, have the person check their blood glucose level. If the person's symptoms don't improve within 10 minutes after giving sugar, or if symptoms worsen at any time, call 9-1-1 if you haven't done so already.

If the person improves and you have called 9-1-1, you should call 9-1-1 back and give them an update. If the person becomes more awake, they may decline EMS help upon arrival.

Some people with diabetes may have a prescribed glucagon kit that they carry with them to use in case of a severe hypoglycemic emergency, and you can assist them with this medication. Glucagon is a hormone that stimulates the liver to release glucose into the bloodstream. Those who spend a significant amount of time with the person (e.g., family members, teachers, coaches, co-workers) may receive additional training to learn how to administer a glucagon injection. If the person has someone around who can administer glucagon, you can encourage them to give the medicine if the person meets the indications they have been taught.

Seizures

A **seizure** is the result of abnormal electrical activity in the brain, leading to temporary and involuntary changes in body movement, function, sensation, awareness or behavior. Seizures can have many different causes. Some people have **epilepsy**, a chronic seizure disorder that can often be controlled with medication. Other causes of seizure include fever, infection, poisoning, diabetic emergencies, heat stroke and injuries to the brain tissue.

Recognizing Seizures

There are different types of seizures that may take many forms. Various signs and symptoms of seizures include loss of consciousness, entire body **convulsions** (uncontrolled body movements caused by contraction of the muscles), focal movements of a part of the body, vocalizations and staring.

A person may also experience an **aura** (an unusual sensation or feeling) before the onset of the seizure. If the person recognizes the aura, they may have time to tell someone what is happening and sit down before the seizure occurs.

Although a seizure can be frightening to see, it is easy to care for a person who is having a seizure. Most seizures only last a few minutes, and the person usually recovers fully without any complications. However, because a seizure may become life-threatening, always call 9-1-1 and get equipment or tell someone to do so.

For people with a chronic seizure disorder, they may have given friends, co-workers, school personnel, and so on instructions not to call EMS for every seizure but only under certain conditions, which usually include:

- The seizure lasts more than 5 minutes, or the person has multiple seizures in a row.
- The person was injured as a result of the seizure.
- The person is unresponsive and not breathing or only gasping after the seizure.
- The seizure took place in the water.

However, if you are unsure whether the seizure is life-threatening, always call 9-1-1 and let EMS make the decision about whether further care is needed.

Giving First Aid Care for Seizures

After calling 9-1-1, check the person for responsiveness and breathing as is safe to do so during the seizure and after the seizure.

When a person is having a seizure, do not try to hold the person down or stop the seizure from happening. Just let the seizure run its course and take steps to protect the person from injury. Move furniture or other objects that could cause injury out of the way. A person who is actively seizing should be monitored until the seizing has stopped. Turn them onto their side into a recovery position if it is possible to do so without injury to them or you.

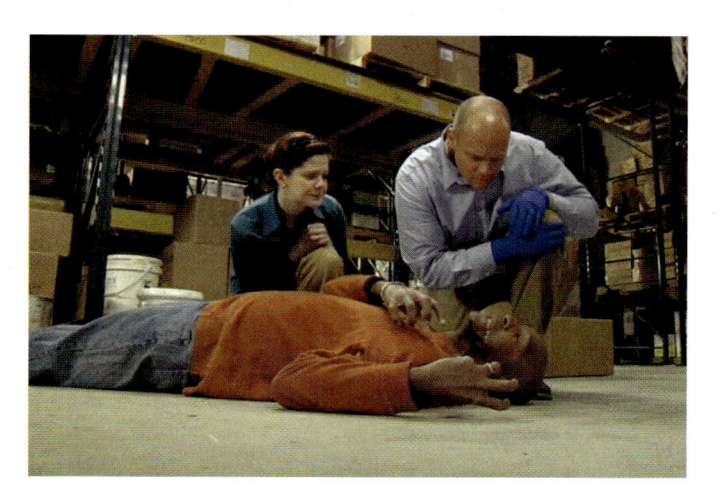

If the person is unresponsive and not breathing or only gasping after the seizure, begin CPR immediately and use an AED as soon as possible, if you are trained in these skills. If the person is unresponsive and breathing or responsive but not yet fully awake after the seizure has stopped, place the person in the recovery position, if you have not already done so, and do a focused check for injuries. Then, stay with the person until they are fully recovered and aware of their surroundings, or until EMS personnel arrive and begin their care. The person may be drowsy and disoriented for as long as 20 minutes after the seizure is over.

> **Myth-Information.** *Put something between the teeth of a person who is having a seizure to prevent the person from biting or swallowing their tongue.* This practice is unsafe and unnecessary. It is impossible to swallow one's own tongue. And although the person may bite down on their tongue, causing it to bleed, this is a minor problem compared with the problems that can be caused by attempting to put an object in the mouth of a person who is having a seizure. You could chip a tooth or knock a tooth loose, putting the person at risk for choking. The person may also bite down with enough force to break the object and then choke on a piece of the object. Additionally, attempting to place an object in the person's mouth puts you at risk for getting bitten.

- Pale, ashen (grayish), cool, moist skin
- Changes in levels of consciousness ranging from unresponsive to confused, restless or irritable
- Nausea or vomiting
- Excessive thirst

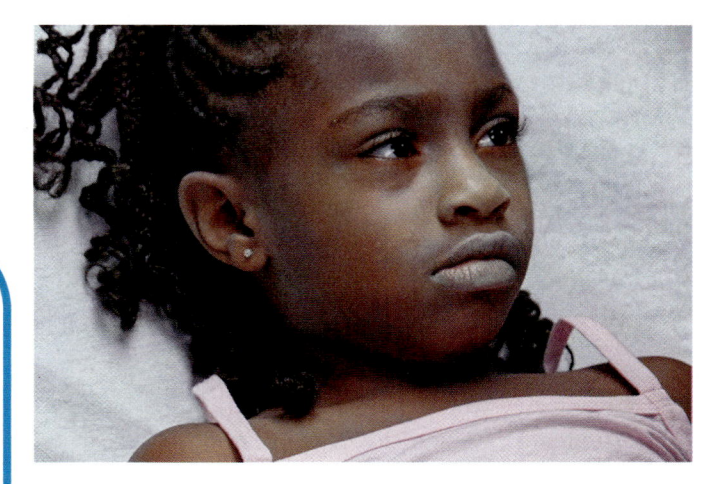

When a person who has been injured or is ill shows signs and symptoms of shock, if not already done, call 9-1-1 and get equipment immediately, or tell someone to do so.

First Aid Care for Shock

Shock cannot be managed effectively by first aid alone, so it is important to get the person emergency medical care as soon as possible. After calling 9-1-1, give care for the person in shock according to your level of training.

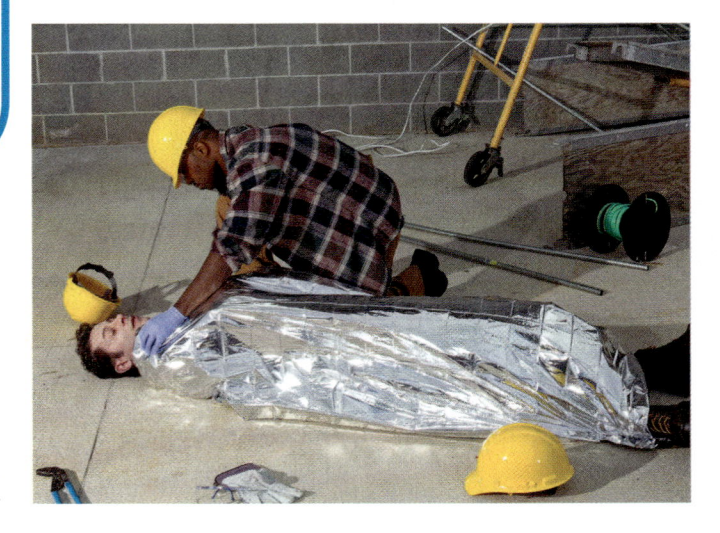

- Give care according to your training *for the condition causing the shock* (e.g., control any external bleeding).
- Have the person lie flat on their back unless they prefer a different position for their comfort and breathing.
- Maintain the person's body temperature. If they get cold, cover them with a blanket to prevent loss of body heat. Or, if they are hot, consider removing a layer of clothing.

Shock

Shock is a progressive, life-threatening condition in which the circulatory system fails to deliver enough oxygen-rich blood to the body's tissues and organs. As a result, organs and body systems begin to fail. Common causes of shock include life-threatening bleeding, infections, dehydration, heart problems and anaphylaxis, but shock can develop quickly after any serious injury or illness. A person who is showing signs and symptoms of shock needs immediate medical attention.

Recognizing Shock

A person who is going into shock may show any of the following signs and symptoms:

- A rapid, weak heartbeat
- Rapid breathing

- Do not give the person anything to eat or drink, even though they may complain of thirst. Eating or drinking increases the person's risk for vomiting and aspiration (inhalation of foreign matter into the lungs). Aspiration can cause serious complications, such as pneumonia.
- Provide reassurance and help the person rest comfortably. Anxiety and pain can intensify the body's stress and speed up the progression of shock.
- Continue to monitor the person's condition and watch for changes in level of consciousness.

Stroke

A **stroke** occurs when blood flow to part of the brain is interrupted by a blood clot or by bleeding from a vessel, resulting in the death of brain cells. Affects throughout the body are possible, including paralysis, loss of speech, problems with memory and trouble with thinking. Strokes can cause permanent damage, but with quick action, sometimes the damage can be stopped or reversed. Although strokes are most common in older adults, a person of any age, even a child, can have a stroke.

Some people experience transient ischemic attacks (TIAs), or "mini-strokes." TIAs cause signs and symptoms similar to those of a stroke, but the signs and symptoms go away after a short period of time. A person who has had a TIA is at very high risk for having a stroke in the near future. In fact, more than 10 percent of people who have a TIA will have a stroke within 3 months, with half of these strokes happening within 48 hours of the TIA. For this reason, whenever a person experiences signs and symptoms of stroke, even if the signs and symptoms seem to go away, the person should seek immediate medical attention.

Recognizing Stroke

The signs and symptoms of stroke can vary from person to person. A person who is having a stroke may suddenly develop one or more of the following signs and symptoms:

- Trouble with speech and language, including slurring of words, being unable to form words or being unable to understand what others are saying
- Drooling or difficulty swallowing
- Drooping of the features on one side of the face (e.g., the eyelid and the corner of the mouth)
- Trouble seeing in one or both eyes
- Weakness, paralysis or numbness of the face, arms or legs, especially on one side of the body
- A sudden, severe headache
- Dizziness or loss of balance
- Confusion
- Loss of consciousness

The FAST mnemonic (Figure 5-1) is one way of remembering the common signs of a stroke.

If you think that a person is having (or has had) a stroke, call 9-1-1 and get equipment immediately, or tell someone to do so.

Giving First Aid Care for Stroke

After calling 9-1-1, note when the signs and symptoms first started (or, if you do not know when the signs and symptoms started, note the last time the person was known to be well). This is important information to give to EMS personnel because some of the medications and procedures used to treat stroke in the hospital are only effective within a certain time frame after the onset of signs and symptoms. Stay with the person and provide reassurance until help arrives. Continue to check for responsiveness and breathing. If the person is responsive but not fully awake, or if the person is drooling or having trouble swallowing, put the person in the recovery position and monitor the person's condition until EMS personnel arrive and begin their care of the person.

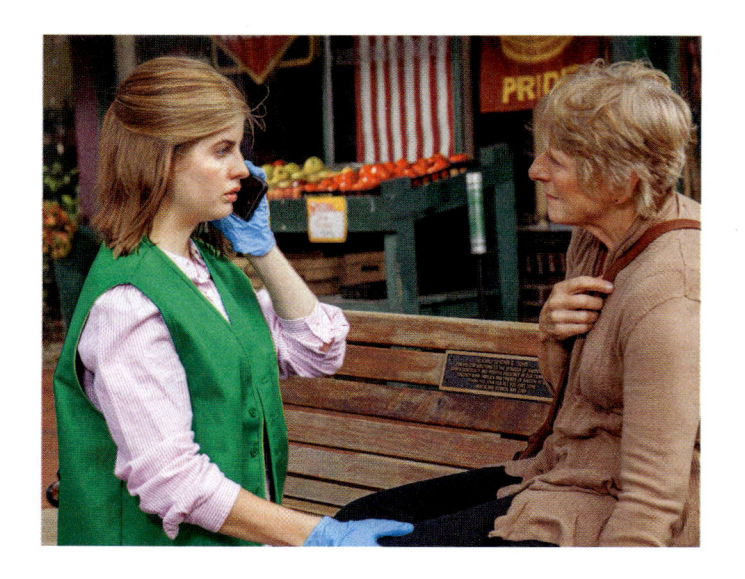

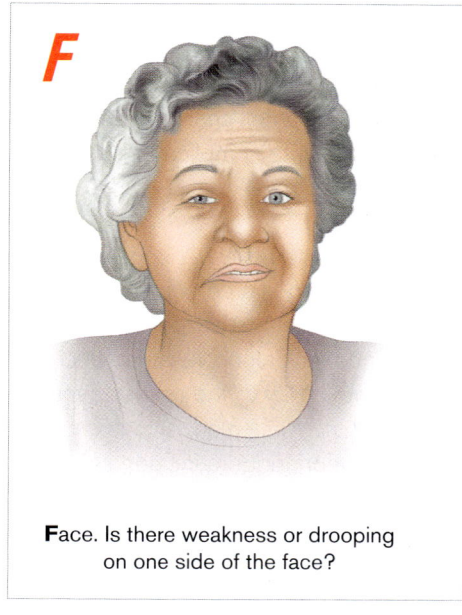

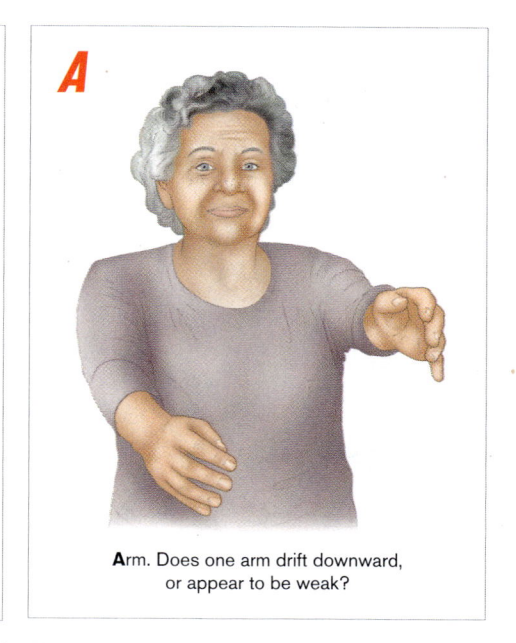

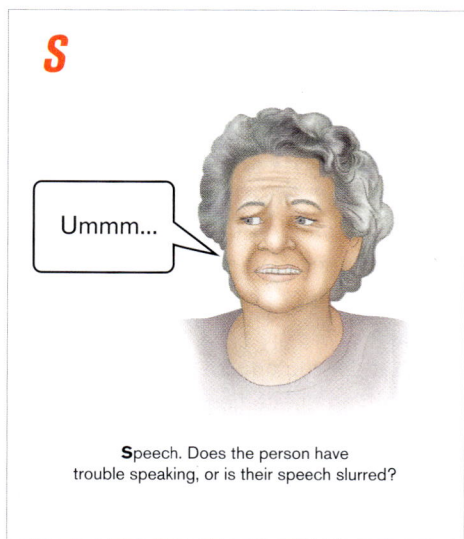

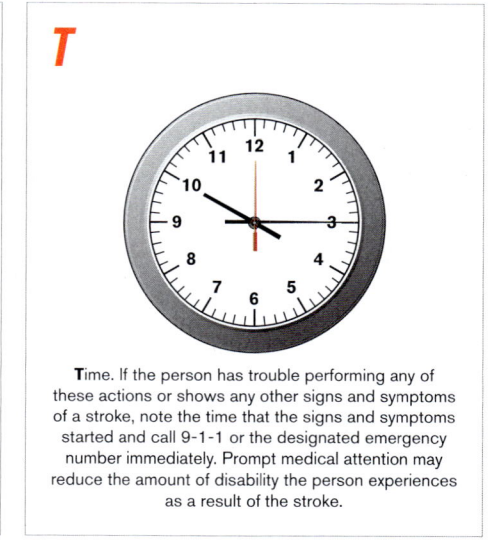

Face. Is there weakness or drooping on one side of the face?

Arm. Does one arm drift downward, or appear to be weak?

Speech. Does the person have trouble speaking, or is their speech slurred?

Time. If the person has trouble performing any of these actions or shows any other signs and symptoms of a stroke, note the time that the signs and symptoms started and call 9-1-1 or the designated emergency number immediately. Prompt medical attention may reduce the amount of disability the person experiences as a result of the stroke.

Figure 5-1. The FAST check for stroke.

Fainting

If a person suddenly loses consciousness and then "comes to" after about a minute, they may simply have fainted. Fainting is caused by a sudden decrease in blood flow to the brain.

Recognizing Fainting

A person who is about to faint often becomes pale, begins to sweat and may feel weak or dizzy. The person may sense that they are about to faint and may attempt to sit down to prevent a fall. In addition, fainting can occur without warning.

Usually the cause of fainting is not serious, but a first aid responder cannot tell and the person may suffer injuries when they faint. So, always call 9-1-1 and get equipment or tell someone to do so because the cause of fainting might be life-threatening. For example, being dehydrated (not having enough fluid in the body), being too hot, being in a crowded room or feeling intense emotion can cause a person to faint.

Giving First Aid Care for Fainting

The person may faint before you even know what is happening, but sometimes it is possible to prevent a fainting spell. If you suspect the person is about to faint and you do not suspect they are having a heart attack or a stroke, have them lie down flat on their back. Then, you can try physical counterpressure maneuvers (PCMs). Lower body PCMs are preferred over upper body or abdominal PCMs. Tell the person to cross their legs while lying down or contract their leg muscles. If their symptoms don't improve within 1 to 2 minutes or if their symptoms reoccur or worsen, call 9-1-1 and get equipment if you haven't already.

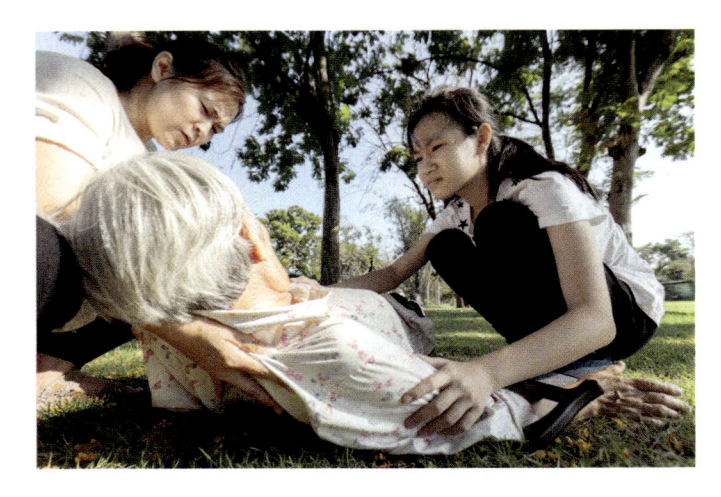

If the person does faint, check them for responsiveness and breathing. If the person does not respond and is not breathing or is only gasping, begin CPR immediately and use an AED as soon as possible, if you are trained in these skills.

If the person is breathing but does not respond, call 9-1-1 if not already done and, if there are no injuries, place them in the recovery position. If the person responds and is breathing, ask SAM questions and do a focused check for injuries that might have happened as a result of the fall. If there are no injuries, place the person in the recovery position so that their head is at the same level as the heart and loosen any tight clothing. This helps blood flow return to the brain and helps the person to quickly recover.

Although the cause of fainting is not usually serious, even if the person refuses EMS care, they should still follow up with their healthcare provider.

Sickle Cell Crisis and Acute Chest Syndrome

Sickle cell disease is a genetic disease characterized by abnormal red cells in the blood. A person with this disease can have complications when the abnormal red blood cells change shape from disc-shaped to sickle-shaped or crescent moon-shaped, which can cause blockages in the small blood vessels.

Some of the complications caused by this disease are chronic, but others are acute and some may even be life-threatening. One of the most common acute complications is called a sickle cell crisis. One of the more severe and life-threatening acute complications is acute chest syndrome (ACS).

A sickle cell crisis is an episode of pain that can occur without warning in a person who has sickle cell disease. It is believed that a crisis occurs when the cells change shape and block blood vessels, which leads to reduced oxygen availability to the tissues served by that vessel and inflammation. While many things can cause a sickle cell crisis, common triggers include cold weather, dehydration, stress or sickness.

ACS is an infection and/or a blockage of blood flow to the chest and lungs. This complication of sickle cell disease can result in lung injury, infection, breathing difficulty, low oxygen, pain to the rest of the body and death. There are many causes of ACS.

Recognizing Sickle Cell Crisis and Acute Chest Syndrome

Signs and symptoms of a sickle cell crisis include pain that starts suddenly and often occurs in the arms or legs, hands or feet, stomach, chest and/or back.

Signs and symptoms of ACS include the combination of breathing difficulties, including lower oxygen levels, cough, wheezing, fast breathing and/or increased work of breathing, possible fever and usually pain in the chest. The person may also have pain in other locations throughout their body. ACS is a life-threatening emergency.

If you recognize the signs and symptoms of sickle cell crisis or ACS in a person, call 9-1-1 and get equipment immediately, or tell someone to do so.

Giving First Aid Care for Sickle Cell Crisis and Acute Chest Syndrome

After calling 9-1-1, care for sickle cell crisis includes having the person rest in a position of comfort and applying a heating pad, if available, to the painful areas as this may reduce the pain. You may also encourage them to drink fluids and assist them with medication that they may take when they experience a sickle cell crisis.

After calling 9-1-1, care for acute chest syndrome includes putting the person in a position of comfort and assisting with any medications they may be prescribed. Continue to monitor them until EMS arrives.

Fever in Young Children and Infants

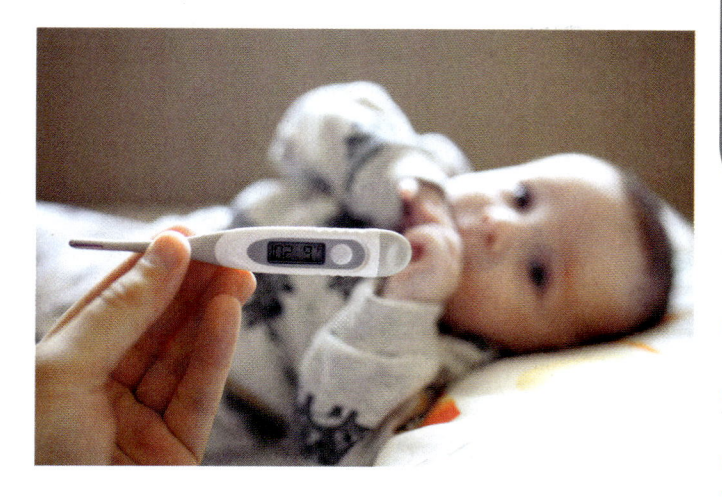

Fever is defined as an elevated body temperature above the normal range of 100.4° F (38° C). Fever is a common sign of illness in young children and infants and is often accompanied by other signs and symptoms of illness, such as a runny nose, cough, nausea, vomiting or sore throat. There also may be headache, muscle aches, chills, loss of appetite, low energy or difficulty sleeping. An infant who has a fever may seem fussy, or they may be quiet and not as active as usual.

General care for fever in a child or infant includes making them as comfortable as possible and encouraging them to rest. Check to ensure that the child or infant is not overdressed or covered with too many blankets. Usually a single layer of clothing and a light blanket is all that is necessary. As long as the child or infant is alert and able to swallow, offer clear liquids such as water and continue to nurse or bottle-feed to prevent dehydration.

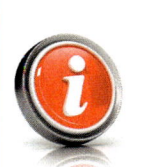

Myth-Information. *Rubbing alcohol helps cool the body and bring down a fever.* Rubbing alcohol (isopropyl alcohol) is dangerous to use to bring down a fever. It is quickly absorbed through the skin and is easily inhaled, placing the infant or child at risk for alcohol poisoning. Moreover, alcohol only cools the skin; it does not lower the internal body temperature.

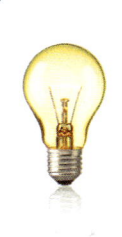

THE PROS KNOW. Never give aspirin to a child or an infant who has a fever or other signs or symptoms of a flu-like or other viral illness. In this situation, taking aspirin can result in Reye's syndrome, an extremely serious and life-threatening condition that causes swelling in the brain and liver.

It is important to contact a healthcare provider if:

- The infant is younger than 3 months and has a fever of 100.4° F (38° C) or greater.
- The child is younger than 2 years and has a fever of 102.5° F (39.2° C) or greater.
- The child or infant has a febrile seizure.
- The fever is associated with change in behavior or activity, neck pain, poor feeding, decreased urination, trouble breathing, abdominal pain, pain with urination, back pain or a rash.

Febrile Seizures

Fevers that suddenly rise can result in febrile seizures. A **febrile seizure** is a convulsion brought on by a fever in a young child or an infant. Febrile seizures are the most common types of seizures in children and in general are not worrisome even though they may be scary to watch. If the child or infant has a seizure, call 9-1-1 and get equipment or tell someone to do so. For children who have had febrile seizures before, parents may be instructed not to routinely call 9-1-1 but only to do so under specific conditions, which usually include:

- The seizure lasts longer than 5 minutes or is repeated.
- The seizure is accompanied by trouble breathing or an injury.
- The child or infant does not become responsive after the seizure.

Vomiting, Diarrhea and Dehydration in Young Children and Infants

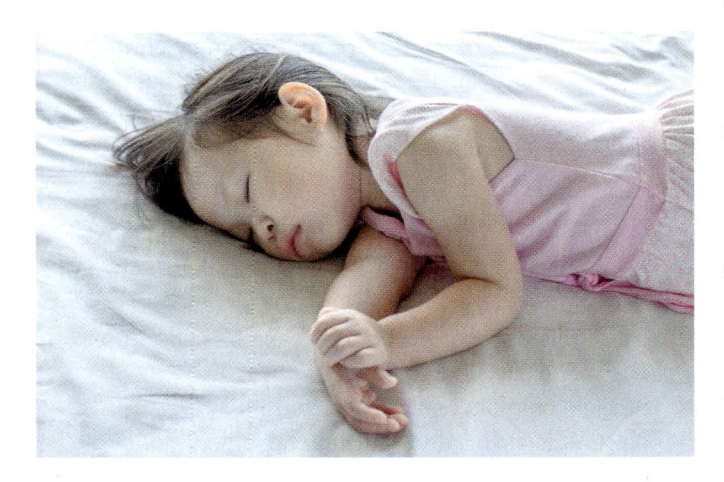

Vomiting, diarrhea, or both are frequently signs and symptoms of infection in children and infants and are most commonly viral. In children, especially younger children and infants, vomiting, diarrhea, or both can lead to **dehydration** (too little fluid in the body) and shock. Young children and infants are at especially high risk for dehydration because they tend to lose more fluid, and at a faster rate, than adults do and often do not have the ability to obtain fluids themselves.

When a child or infant has an illness that causes vomiting, the goal is more frequent but smaller feedings. In addition, the priority is fluids (e.g., water, popsicles or oral rehydration solutions designed specifically for children and infants).

After 12 to 24 hours with no vomiting, gradually reintroduce the child's or infant's normal diet.

To care for diarrhea:

- Maintain the child's or infant's normal well-balanced diet, including a mix of fruits, vegetables, meat, yogurt and complex carbohydrates. Try to limit sugar and artificial sweeteners.
- If the infant will not tolerate his or her normal feedings, or if the child is drinking less fluid than usual, add a commercially available oral rehydration solution designed specifically for children and infants.
- Do not give over-the-counter antidiarrheal medications to young children and infants. In older children, use these medications under the guidance of a healthcare provider.

When a child has vomiting, diarrhea, or both, consult a healthcare provider if:

- The diarrhea or vomiting persists for more than a few days.
- The child or infant is not able to keep fluids down.
- The child has not urinated for more than 6 hours.
- The infant has not had a wet diaper in 3 or more hours.
- The diarrhea is bloody or black.
- The child is unusually sleepy or irritable.
- The child has associated abdominal pain that is sharp or persistent.
- The child cries without tears or has a dry mouth.
- There is a sunken appearance to the child's abdomen, eyes or cheeks (or, in a very young infant, the soft spot at the top of the infant's head).
- The child's skin remains "tented" if pinched and released.

PUTTING IT ALL TOGETHER 5-1

Assisting with an Asthma Inhaler for a Person Experiencing an Asthma Attack

Note: *The instructions for assisting a person with an asthma inhaler found in this Putting It All Together sheet should not be substituted for those given by the manufacturer and the person's healthcare provider. Read and follow all instructions printed on the inhaler prior to assisting the person with administering the medication and consult the person's asthma control plan.*

Check

1. **Check the scene** for safety, **form an initial impression,*** **obtain consent, use PPE** and continue checking the person **(SAM and focused check)**.

   * If you determine the person is unresponsive, responds but is not fully awake, is not breathing, has life-threatening bleeding or another life-threatening condition, immediately go to the call step. Give care immediately for the condition found and continue your check (as appropriate) to obtain more information and determine whether additional care is needed. For a person who is unresponsive and not breathing, start CPR and use an AED immediately.

Call

2. **Call 9-1-1** and get equipment or tell someone to do so.

Care

3. Help the person to **sit up straight**.

4. **Verify the medication** with the person. Make sure the medication is for "quick relief" or "acute attacks" and that it is their medication.
   - Only use if it is for quick relief or acute attacks.

5. **Shake the inhaler** and **remove the mouthpiece cover**.

6. **Attach a spacing device** to the inhaler. A spacing device should be used as it enhances the ability of a person to take the medication.

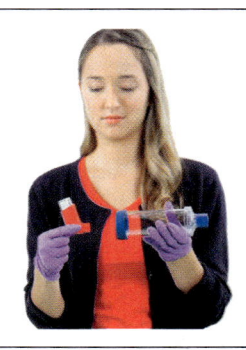

7. Tell the person to **breathe out as much as possible** through the mouth.

(Continued on next page)

PUTTING IT ALL TOGETHER 5-1

Assisting with an Asthma Inhaler for a Person Experiencing an Asthma Attack continued

8. Give the inhaler with the spacer to the person and advise the person to use it as directed by their healthcare provider.

- Have the person **close their lips tightly around the mouthpiece**. Then, have the person push the button on the top of the canister to release the medication into the spacer. Have the person take a slow, deep breath. Then have them hold their breath for 5 to 10 seconds.

   Special Considerations

   - **If the person can't take a slow, deep breath.** Have them take several normal breaths from the spacer.
   - **If the person uses a spacer with mask.** Position the mask over the person's nose and mouth. Have the person push the button on the top of the canister to release the medication into the spacer. Have the person take several normal breaths from the spacer.
   - **If the person does not use a spacer.** Have them place their lips tightly around the mouthpiece of the inhaler. Have the person take a long, slow breath (about 3 to 5 seconds) while pressing down on the top of the canister. Then have the person hold their breath for 5 to 10 seconds.

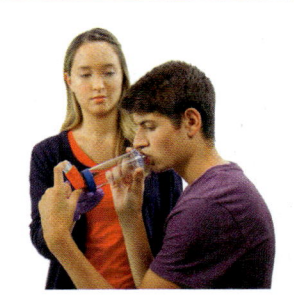

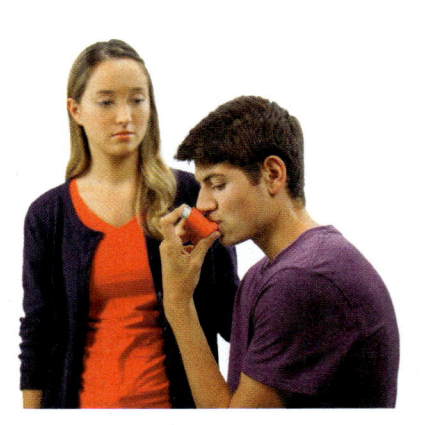

9. Note the time of administration and any change in the person's condition. The person's breathing should improve within 5 to 15 minutes. More than one dose of medication may be needed to stop the asthma attack. The medication may be repeated after 10 to 15 minutes. If the person's breathing does not improve or the person becomes unresponsive, call 9-1-1 if not already done.

Note: *The instructions for assisting a person with an asthma inhaler found in this Putting It All Together sheet should not be substituted for those given by the manufacturer and the person's healthcare provider. Read and follow all instructions printed on the inhaler prior to assisting the person with administering the medication and consult the person's asthma control plan.*

PUTTING IT ALL TOGETHER 5-2

Assisting with an Epinephrine Auto-Injector for a Person Experiencing Anaphylaxis

Note: *The instructions for assisting a person with an epinephrine auto-injector found in this Putting It All Together sheet should not be substituted for those given by the manufacturer and the person's healthcare provider. Read and follow all instructions printed on the auto-injector device prior to assisting the person with administering the medication.*

Check

1. **Check the scene** for safety, **form an initial impression,* obtain consent, use PPE** and continue checking the person **(SAM and focused check).**

   * If you determine the person is unresponsive, responds but is not fully awake, is not breathing, has life-threatening bleeding or another life-threatening condition, immediately go to the call step. Give care immediately for the condition found and continue your check (as appropriate) to obtain more information and determine whether additional care is needed. For a person who is unresponsive and not breathing, start CPR and use an AED immediately.

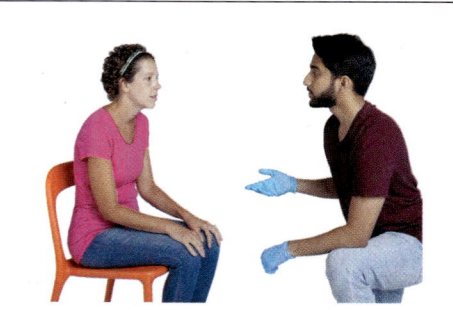

Call

2. **Call 9-1-1** and get equipment or tell someone to do so.

Care

3. **Determine whether the person has already given themselves a dose of the medication.** If they have given themself a first dose, only administer another dose 5 to 10 minutes later if symptoms are still present.

4. **Verify the medication** with the person.

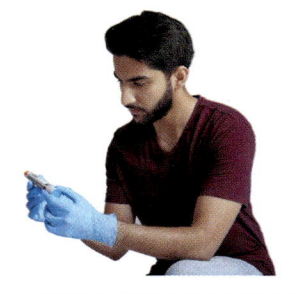

5. **Remove the cap and any safety device** on the auto-injector.

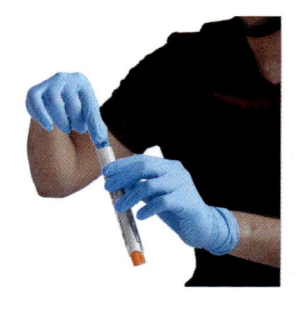

(Continued on next page)

American Red Cross | First Aid for Sudden Illnesses and Injuries 103

PUTTING IT ALL TOGETHER 5-2

Assisting with an Epinephrine Auto-Injector for a Person Experiencing Anaphylaxis continued

6. Have the person **locate the outer middle of one thigh** to use as the injection site.
7. Hand the person their epinephrine auto-injector.
8. Hold the person's leg firmly to limit movement while they use the device to administer the medication.
9. Have the person quickly and firmly push the auto-injector tip straight into their outer thigh at a 90-degree angle. ■ It's OK for them to do this through clothing, if necessary. ■ Have the person **hold the auto-injector firmly in place for 3 seconds** after a click is heard.
10. Have the person **remove the auto-injector from their thigh**.
11. Massage the injection site for 10 seconds (or have the person massage the site).
12. Note the time of administration and any change in their condition. ■ If the person is still having signs and symptoms 5 to 10 minutes after administering the first dose and EMS personnel have not arrived, assist the person with administering a second dose.
13. Give the auto-injector to EMS personnel when they arrive.

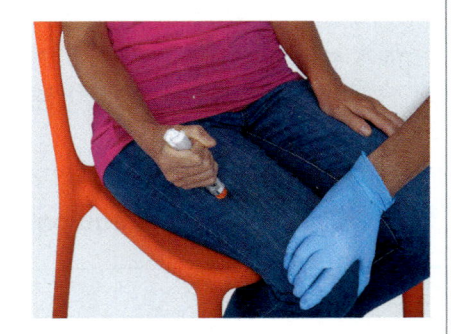

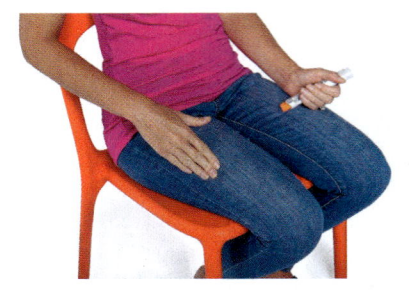

Note: *The instructions for assisting a person with an epinephrine auto-injector found in this Putting It All Together sheet should not be substituted for those given by the manufacturer and the person's healthcare provider. Read and follow all instructions printed on the auto- injector device prior to assisting the person with administering the medication.*

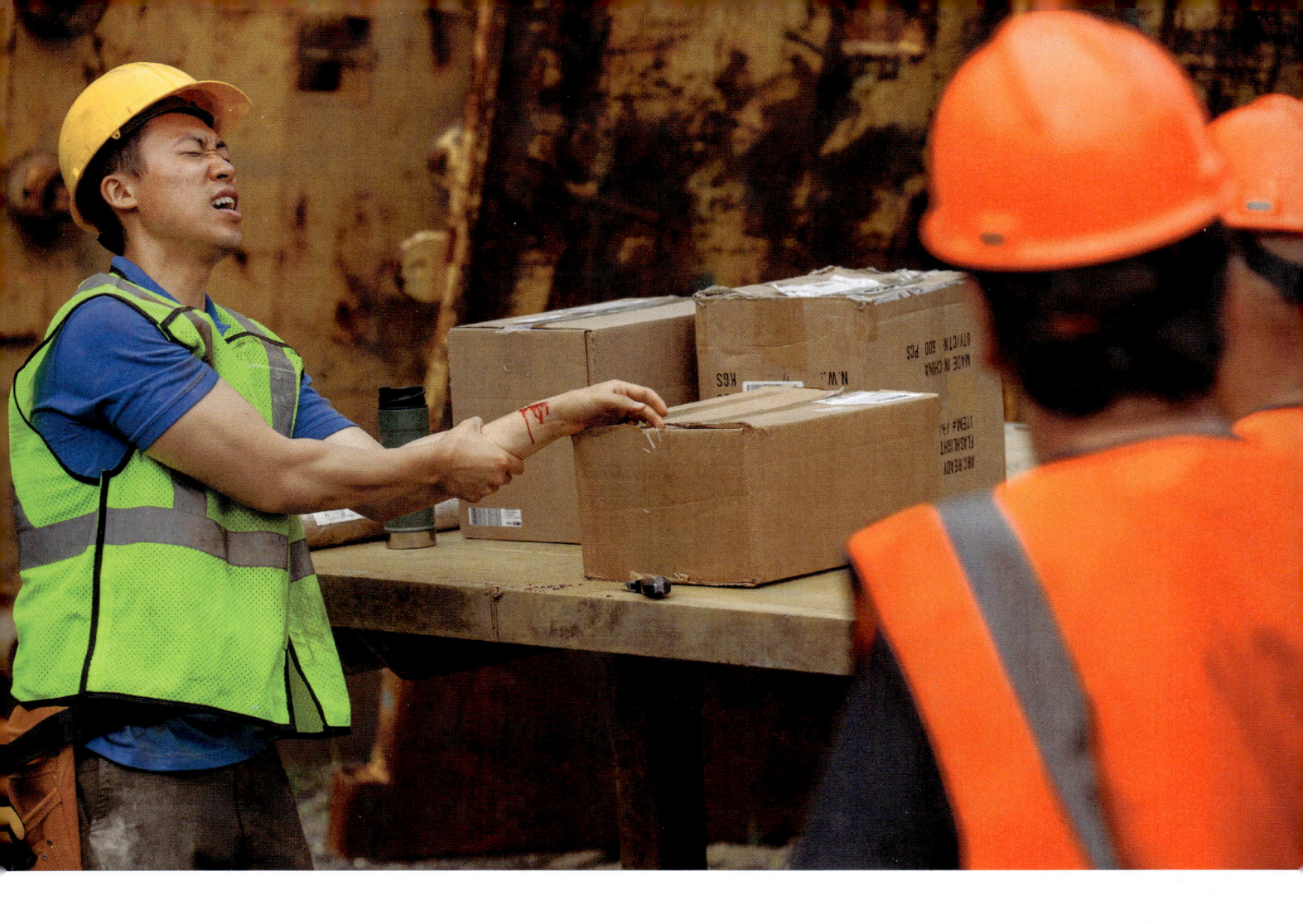

CHAPTER 6
Wounds and Bleeding

A **wound** is an injury that results when the skin or other tissues of the body are damaged. Wounds are generally classified as open or closed. Both open and closed wounds often result in bleeding. Open wounds may cause external bleeding, internal bleeding, or both; closed wounds may cause internal bleeding. External or internal bleeding may be life-threatening (e.g., due to major open wounds or closed wounds) or non-life-threatening (e.g., due to minor open wounds or closed wounds). Recognizing life-threatening bleeding is very important as immediate care is vital.

Open Wounds and External Bleeding

In an **open wound**, the skin's surface is broken, and blood may come through the tear in the skin, resulting in **external bleeding** (bleeding that is visible on the outside of the body).

When giving care for wounds and bleeding, if you have latex-free disposable gloves, put them on. But, if the bleeding is life-threatening and you don't have gloves, begin giving care immediately. The person may have more than one wound. Find the source of any life-threatening bleeding and give care for that wound first.

If available, use other personal protective equipment (PPE) as necessary; for example, if blood is spurting, you may need to wear eye and face protection. Make sure you wash your hands thoroughly with soap and water after giving care, even if you wore gloves.

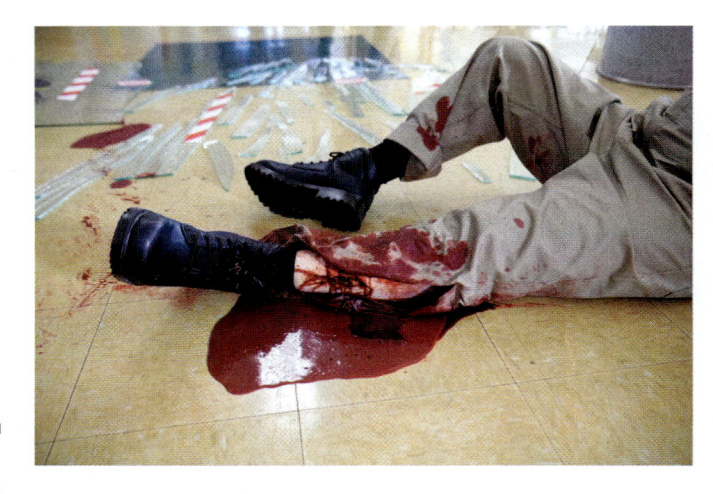

Types of Open Wounds

The four main types of open wounds are abrasions, lacerations, avulsions and puncture wounds (Figure 6-1, A–D) and they may occur together.

- An **abrasion** occurs when something rubs roughly against the skin, causing damage to the skin's surface. You may hear abrasions referred to as "scrapes," "rug

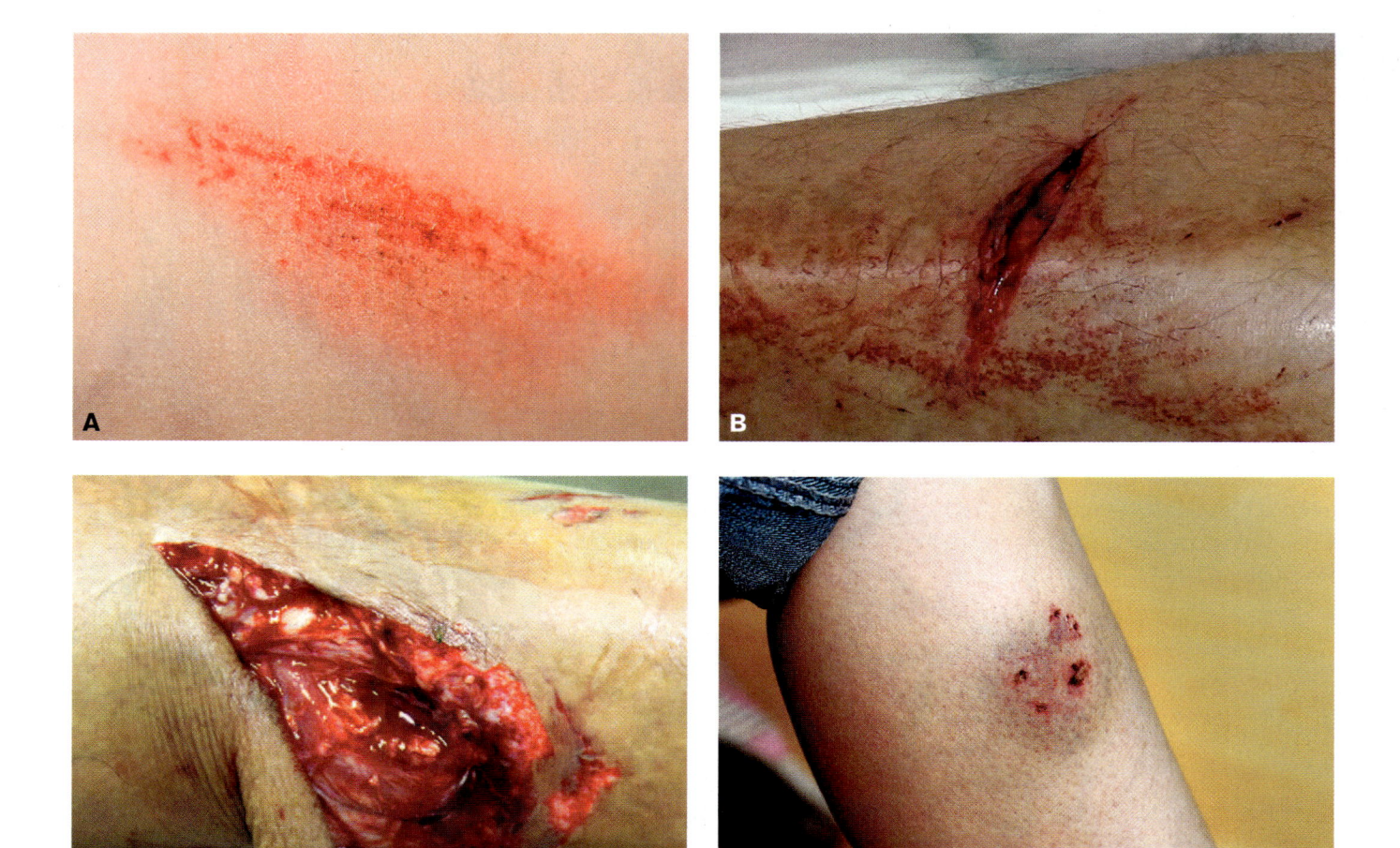

Figure 6-1. Types of open wounds include abrasions (A), lacerations (B), avulsions (C), and puncture wounds (D).

106   Chapter 6 | Wounds and Bleeding

burns," "road rash," or "turf burns." If you have ever had an abrasion, you know how painful these injuries can be! This is because scraping of the outer skin layers exposes sensitive nerve endings. Abrasions are shallow wounds that do not bleed much. However, because of the mechanism of injury (usually a sliding fall), abrasions are often contaminated with dirt and debris.

- **A laceration** is a cut, commonly caused by a sharp object such as broken glass or a knife. A laceration can also occur when blunt force splits the skin. Deep lacerations may extend through layers of fat and muscle, damaging nerves, blood vessels and tendons. Bleeding may be heavy, even life-threatening, or minimal. If deep enough, lacerations can also damage internal organs and structures, causing internal bleeding. These types of wounds also carry a risk for infection because they can penetrate deep into the body's tissues.
- **An avulsion** occurs when a portion of the skin, and sometimes the underlying tissue, is partially or completely torn away. Avulsion wounds may only ooze a little, or they can cause significant, sometimes life-threatening bleeding.
- **A puncture wound** occurs when an object, such as a nail or an animal's tooth, pierces the skin. A gunshot wound is also a puncture wound. Puncture wounds may not bleed much unless a blood vessel has been injured. However, if blood vessels or arteries are damaged, life-threatening external bleeding may be seen. In addition, this type of open wound can cause internal bleeding or puncture internal organs. These types of wounds carry a high risk for infection because the penetrating object can carry pathogens deep into the body's tissues.

Recognizing Life-Threatening Bleeding

Volume and flow are two ways to tell if bleeding is life-threatening. **Volume** is the amount of blood present. Think about a soda can. Bleeding may be life-threatening when the amount of blood present is equal to about half of what a soda can contains. In a small child or an infant, bleeding may be life-threatening when the amount of blood lost is even less. **Flow** is the movement of blood. Blood that is flowing continuously or spurting is a sign of life-threatening bleeding.

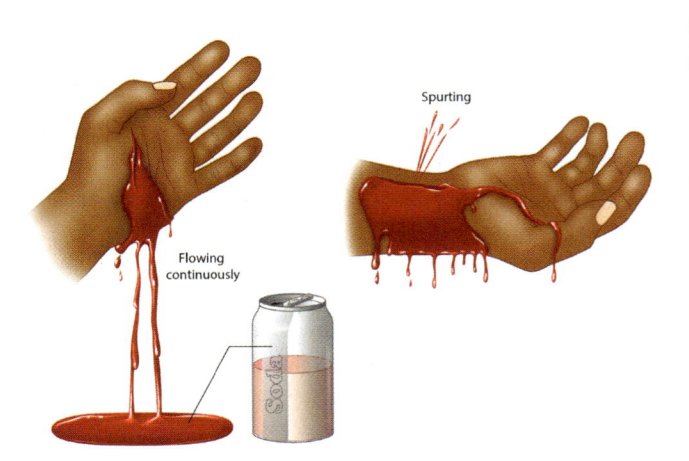

To recognize life-threatening bleeding, look at the amount of blood, volume, and how the blood moves, flow. If you recognize life-threatening bleeding, immediate action is essential. Call 9-1-1 and get a bleeding control kit, first aid kit and an AED immediately or tell someone to do so.

First Aid Care for External Life-Threatening Bleeding

After calling 9-1-1, take steps to control life-threatening bleeding until help arrives. Apply firm, continuous pressure to stop the bleeding. Depending on the situation, the location of the wound and the equipment you have, you may use direct pressure, a tourniquet, or both to control life-threatening bleeding. Mechanical pressure, such as pressure bandages or devices, might be considered in some situations when direct manual pressure is not feasible.

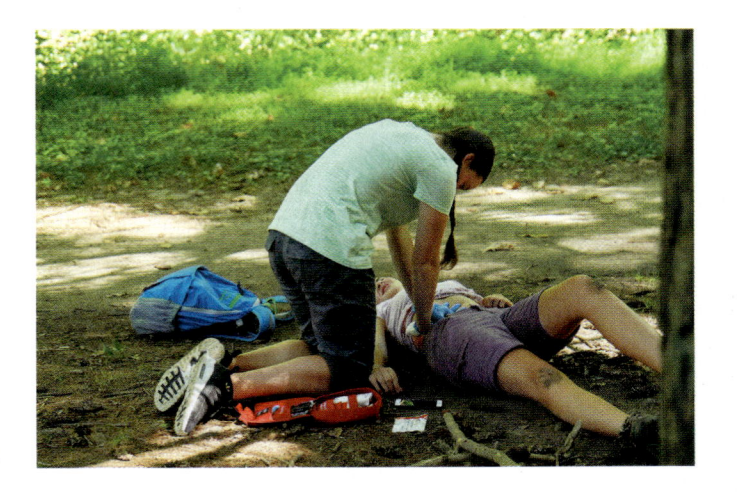

Applying Direct Pressure

Use direct pressure to stop life-threatening bleeding when:

- The wound is on the head, neck, back or trunk.
- The wound is on an arm or a leg and you are waiting for someone to bring a tourniquet, or no tourniquet is available.

You can also use direct pressure to stop non-life-threatening bleeding.

It takes a lot of pressure to stop life-threatening bleeding. To get an idea of how much pressure is needed, think about having your blood pressure taken. To measure your blood pressure, the healthcare provider puts a cuff around your arm and pumps it up. As the cuff fills with air, it puts pressure on your arm, stopping the normal flow of blood. When you are using pressure to control life-threatening bleeding in an emergency situation, you are applying at least as much pressure as a blood pressure cuff, if not more. That's why you need to push *hard*. The amount of pressure might be painful for the injured person. That's OK! You need to use a lot of pressure for the bleeding to stop.

A flat, hard surface underneath the injured body part allows you to press against something, increasing the effectiveness of the direct pressure. First, find the source of the life-threatening bleeding. There may be more than one wound. You need to focus on any wound that is causing life-threatening bleeding first. Next, place a sterile gauze or other clean dressing directly on the wound at the bleeding site (Box 6-1). A dressing is a pad that absorbs blood and can promote clotting. Bleeding control kits and first aid kits often contain special dressings called **hemostatic dressings**.

These dressings contain a substance that promotes clotting and can help to stop bleeding faster. When there is life-threatening bleeding, use a hemostatic dressing if you have one. Otherwise, use a gauze pad or other available material—such as a clean T-shirt—as a dressing.

The technique of applying direct pressure is the same regardless of the type of dressing you use. Place the dressing on the wound and ensure good contact with the source of the bleeding.

Then, put one hand on top of the dressing, put your other hand on top and push down with both hands. You need to apply a lot of pressure to stop life-threatening bleeding, so let the person know that it can be painful. Apply pressure directly on the wound until the bleeding stops.

Box 6-1 Dressings and Bandages

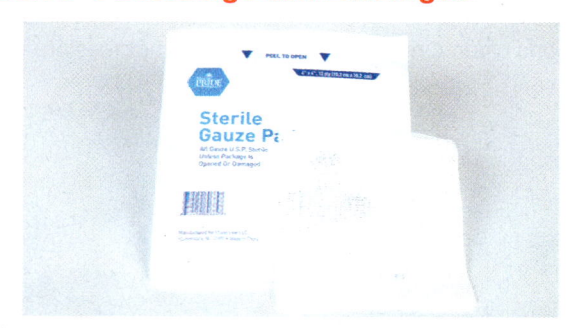

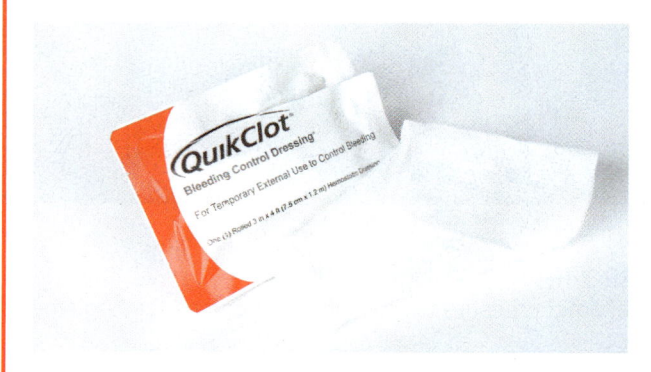

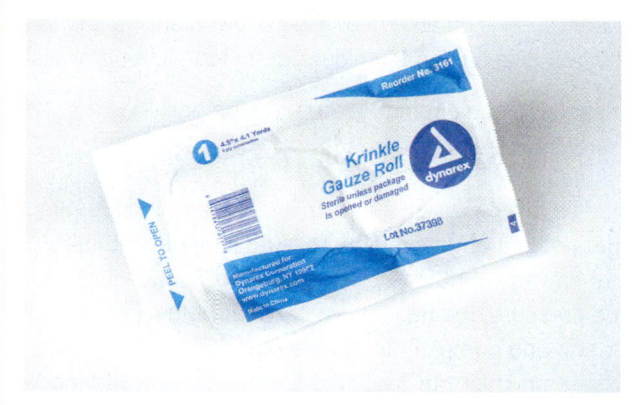

Dressings and bandages are staples of any well-stocked first aid kit or bleeding control kit and have a variety of uses.

Gauze Dressings

A dressing is a pad that is placed directly on a wound to absorb blood and other fluids, promote clotting and prevent infection. To minimize the chance of infection, dressings should be sterile. There are many different types of dressings available. In a first aid situation, gauze pads, which are available in a variety of sizes, are most commonly used as dressings.

Hemostatic Dressings

A hemostatic dressing is a dressing treated with a substance that speeds clot formation. As is the case with tourniquets, hemostatic dressings are used when life-threatening bleeding exists. Typically, hemostatic dressings are used on parts of the body where a tourniquet cannot be applied, such as the neck or torso. A hemostatic dressing can also be used to control bleeding from an open wound on an arm or a leg if a tourniquet is not available or is ineffective. The hemostatic dressing is applied at the site of the bleeding (and inside of the wound in the case of wound packing for those trained in this procedure) and is used along with direct pressure.

Bandages

A bandage is a strip of material used to hold the dressing in place. Roller bandages, made of gauze or a gauze-like material and sometimes with elastic properties, are frequently included in first aid kits and come in a variety of widths and lengths. Wrap the bandage around the injured body part, covering the dressing completely and allowing a margin of several inches on all sides. Then tape the bandage, or, if no tape is available, tie the bandage to secure it in place.

Position your body over the wound so your shoulders are directly over your hands, with your elbows locked. If you have been trained in CPR, you might recognize this position. Push down, using your body weight to increase the pressure. If you need your hands, use your knee to apply pressure.

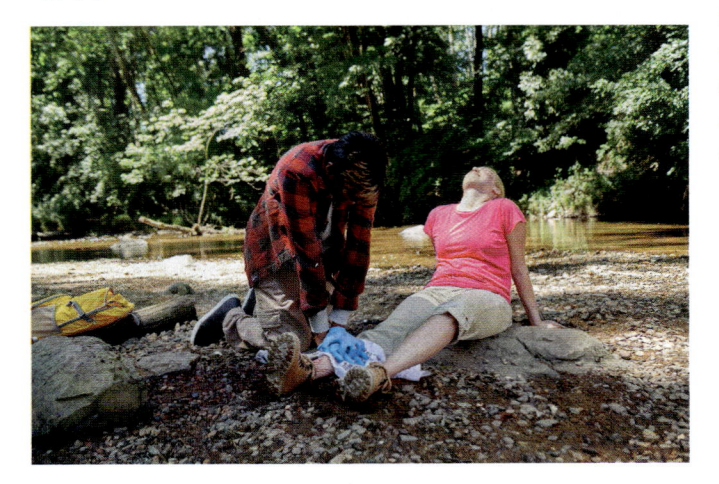

If blood soaks through the original dressing, you don't need to do anything. However, you can place another dressing on top of the first and continue direct pressure (press harder than you did before, if possible). If that dressing becomes soaked, you can remove that one and replace with a new dressing. However, *do not* remove the original dressing that is placed directly on the wound. Also, only add one dressing on top of the original. *Do not* stack multiple dressing as this weakens direct pressure.

When using direct pressure to stop bleeding, remember to press as hard as you can directly on the wound and hold the pressure until:

- The bleeding stops.
- A tourniquet is applied for life-threatening bleeding from an arm or leg.
- Another person relieves you.
- You are too exhausted to continue.
- The situation becomes unsafe.

Applying a Bandage

If the bleeding stops before EMS arrives, first check for circulation beyond the injury. Check the skin on the side of the injury farthest away from the heart (e.g., the hand or foot) for temperature, color and feeling. Ask the person if there is any tingling or numbness. Then, apply a roller bandage over the dressing to maintain pressure on the wound and to hold the dressing in place. To apply a roller bandage, place the end of a bandage on the dressing at a 45-degree angle. Continue wrapping the bandage over the dressing. Make sure the dressing is completely covered and allow a margin of several inches on all sides. Tape to secure the dressing.

If you do not have tape, you can use an alternate "bandage splitting" technique to secure the dressing. Once the dressing is covered, roll out the remaining length of bandage. While holding the bandage, use the index finger of the other hand to split the bandage in half, moving it down and underneath the limb. Bring up the two ends of the bandage and tie them in a bow or a knot (Figure 6-2, A–C).

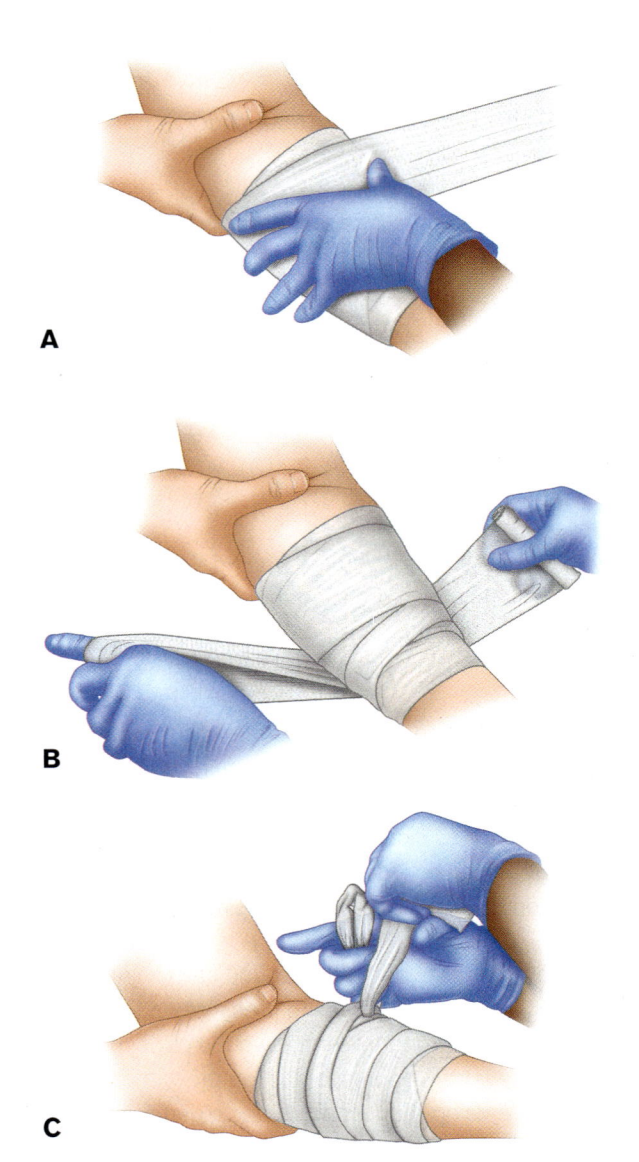

Figure 6-2. To use a "bandage splitting" technique to secure the dressing, once the dressing is covered, roll out the remaining length of the bandage (A). While holding the bandage, use the index finger of the other hand to split the bandage in half, moving it down and underneath the limb (B). Bring the two ends of the bandage up and tie them in a bow or knot (C).

The bandage should be snug but not too tight. Check again for circulation (i.e., temperature, color, feeling) beyond the injury. If there is a change in temperature, color or feeling from your first check (e.g., the skin is cooler or paler than it was before, the area is swollen, or the person complains of a numb or tingly feeling), then the bandage is too tight and needs to be loosened carefully.

After applying a bandage, monitor for re-bleeding by monitoring the person and looking for bleeding through the bandage. If bleeding recurs, do not apply an additional dressing or bandage; instead remove the bandage and leave only the single dressing on the wound in place, and then apply direct manual pressure.

Finally, it is important to give care for shock, if necessary, until help arrives.

Putting It All Together 6-1 describes step-by-step how to use direct pressure to control external bleeding and how to apply a bandage if the bleeding stops.

Wound Packing

Wound packing can help direct pressure and more effectively control life-threatening bleeding from the scalp, neck, shoulder, groin, and back, and from an extremity *if* there is no tourniquet available.

You may pack a wound if you are trained. To pack a wound, use a hemostatic gauze dressing if you have one. If you don't have a hemostatic gauze dressing, you can use a plain gauze pad or other dressing material.

First, open any clothing covering the wound to identify any life-threatening bleeding. Next, try to identify the source of the bleeding within the wound as accurately as you can because the goal is to pack as closely to the source of the bleeding as possible. There may be blood in a large area. If you are unsure about the source of the bleeding, then pack a wider area.

Then, place the dressing into the wound cavity directly onto the bleeding source. While holding pressure on the bleeding source, continue packing the entire wound cavity until it is tightly packed. After you have packed the wound, apply direct pressure using the technique described previously.

Continue applying direct pressure until bleeding has stopped, a tourniquet is available for an extremity, the situation becomes unsafe, or EMS personnel arrive and begin their care of the person.

If bleeding stops before EMS arrives, apply a bandage using the technique described above and monitor and treat for shock.

Applying a Tourniquet

For life-threatening bleeding on an arm or leg, use a tourniquet. While waiting for a tourniquet, or if a tourniquet is not available, use direct pressure and, if trained, wound packing.

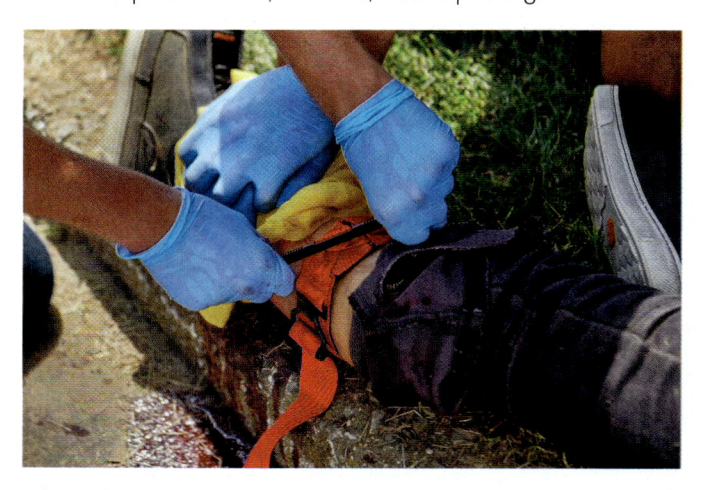

A **tourniquet** is a device placed around an arm or leg that applies pressure to stop blood flow to a wound. There are different types of tourniquets available (Figure 6-3, A–D). All work by applying pressure. A properly applied tourniquet can save a life.

If you find yourself in a situation where you need to apply a tourniquet, a commercially manufactured tourniquet is preferred over an improvised device. If a manufactured tourniquet is not available and direct manual pressure with or without the use of a hemostatic dressing fails to stop life-threatening bleeding, a first aid responder trained in the use of an improvised tourniquet may consider using one.

Follow the manufacturer's instructions for applying the tourniquet. Although tourniquets may have slightly different designs, all are applied in generally the same way. First, place the tourniquet around the wounded extremity about 2 to 3 inches above the wound. The tourniquet should be placed between the wound and the heart. Do not place the tourniquet on top of the wound or a joint.

Tighten the tourniquet according to the manufacturer's instructions until the bleeding stops. Then secure the tourniquet in place as necessary according to the manufacturer's instructions.

> **THE PROS KNOW.** Tourniquets can be extremely painful. If you must apply a tourniquet, make sure the person understands the reason for the tourniquet, and warn the person that it may be painful.

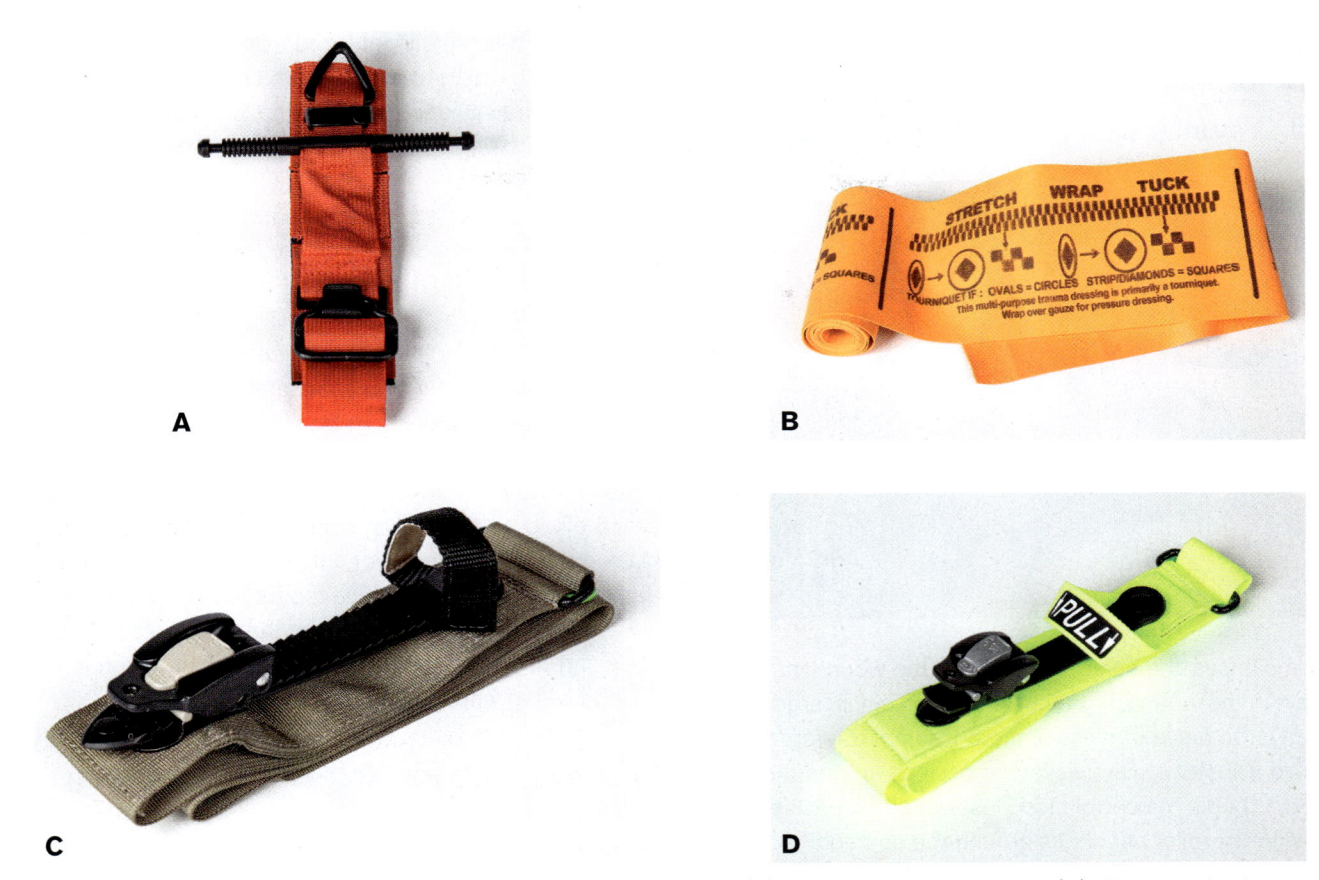

Figure 6-3. Types of tourniquets include windlass rod tourniquet (A), elastic wrap tourniquet (B), TX-3 ratcheting medical tourniquet (C), and TX-1 pediatric ratcheting tourniquet (D).

No matter what type of tourniquet you are using, you can apply a second tourniquet if you've tightened the tourniquet as much as you can, but the bleeding hasn't stopped. Apply the second tourniquet 2 to 3 inches above the first, closer to the heart. As with the first tourniquet, do not apply over a joint. Apply the second tourniquet following the manufacturer's directions.

After you've applied a tourniquet, don't loosen or remove it. That should only be done by a medical professional.

When using a tourniquet for a child, there are special considerations to keep in mind (Box 6-2).

Putting It All Together 6-2 provides step-by-step instructions for applying direct pressure and using a windlass rod tourniquet to control life-threatening bleeding.

See also Appendix D for Skill Practice Sheets that focus on applying other types of tourniquets: Using Direct Pressure and a Ratcheting Tourniquet to Control Life-Threatening Bleeding; Using Direct Pressure and an Elastic Tourniquet to Control Life-Threatening Bleeding.

Box 6-2 Pediatric Considerations for Tourniquet Use

When using a tourniquet on a child it is important to remember that not all tourniquets tighten enough to stop bleeding in small children. If you are using a tourniquet on a small child, make sure the tourniquet you choose will work (see Figure 6-3, D).

Tourniquets are currently not recommended for children under approximately 2 years of age. For these children, direct pressure will likely stop the bleeding.

When placing a tourniquet on a child, make sure you can tighten the strap so that there is *no* room between it and the limb before activating the tightening mechanism. If the tourniquet is not tight enough around the limb, it may be beneficial to move the tourniquet closer on the limb to the body where the extremity is thicker. In addition, if after using the tightening mechanism bleeding is not controlled, place another tourniquet above the first tourniquet higher on the limb.

It is especially important to emphasize to the child and to the parent or guardian that tourniquets can be very painful. Make sure the child and the parent or guardian understand the reason for the tourniquet and warn them that it will likely be very painful, but this means it is applied tight enough to work.

American Red Cross | First Aid for Sudden Illnesses and Injuries

Special Considerations When Giving Care for Major Open Wounds

Open Wounds with Embedded Objects

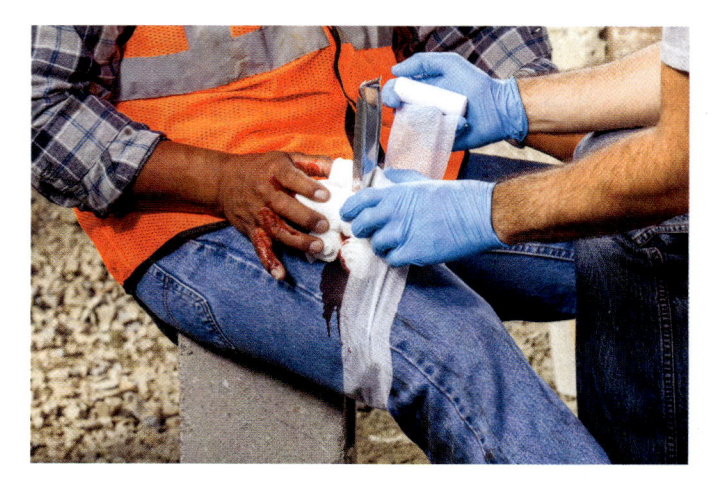

In some cases, the object that caused the wound may remain in the wound. If the embedded object is large (e.g., a large piece of glass or metal), do not attempt to remove it. Instead, place several dressings around the object to begin to control blood loss, and then pack bulk dressings or roller bandages around the embedded object to keep it from moving. Bandage the bulk dressings or roller bandages in place around the object and seek medical care. Remember to monitor the person for signs and symptoms of shock. If this is life-threatening bleeding, apply direct pressure around the embedded object as close to the object as possible. If the embedded object is on an extremity and causing life-threatening bleeding, you can apply a tourniquet above the embedded object.

A small partially embedded object, such as a splinter, can usually be removed using first aid techniques; however, medical care should be sought if the splinter is deep, completely embedded in the skin, or located under the nail or in the eye. To remove a simple shallow splinter, grasp the end of the splinter with clean tweezers and pull it out. Then provide care as you would for any minor open wound.

Traumatic Amputations

Traumatic amputation is the loss of a body part as a result of an injury. Common causes of traumatic amputations include injuries involving power tools, farming or manufacturing equipment; motor-vehicle collisions; explosions and natural disasters. In a traumatic amputation, the body part might be severed cleanly from the body or ripped away as a result of being subjected to violent tearing or twisting forces. Crushing forces can also result in mangled tissue and traumatic amputations. The body part may be completely detached from the body, or it may still be partially attached. Bleeding may be minimal or life-threatening, depending on the location and nature of the injury.

When a person has experienced a traumatic amputation, call 9-1-1 or tell someone to do so. Then control life-threatening bleeding if present.

After life-threatening bleeding is controlled, if present, try to locate any body part that is completely detached from the body because surgeons may be able to reattach it. Wrap the amputated body part in sterile gauze or other clean material. Put the wrapped body part in a plastic bag and seal the bag. Keep the bag containing the body part cool by placing it in a larger bag or container filled with a mixture of ice and water. Do not place the bag containing the body part directly on ice or dry ice. Give the bag containing the body part to EMS personnel so that it can be taken to the hospital along with the person.

First Aid Care for Non-Life-Threatening Bleeding

For non-life-threatening external bleeding, get equipment or tell someone to do so, and take steps to control the bleeding. If the wound is deep or extensive, if the bleeding cannot be stopped with direct pressure, or if the wound carries a high risk for infection (e.g., a puncture or deep laceration wound), medical care will be needed (Box 6-3).

Many open wounds, however, are minor and can be cared for effectively using first aid. To care for a minor open

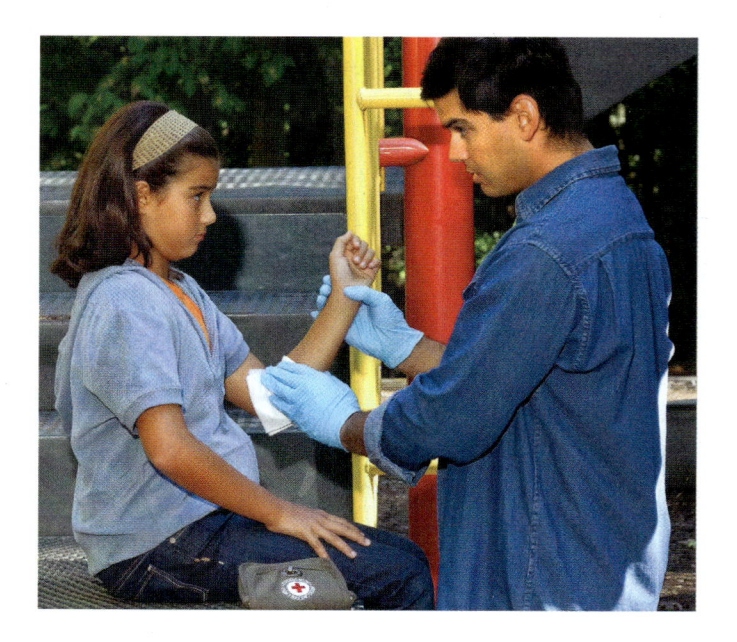

Box 6-3 Does This Wound Need Medical Attention?

Depending on the cause of the wound and the nature of the injury, it may be necessary for the person to see a healthcare provider for treatment.

When a wound is deep or complex, has jagged edges or is dirty, the person should seek care from a healthcare provider because it may require closure and/or antibiotics to prevent an infection of the skin or deeper tissues, including an infection in the bloodstream.

Tetanus Prophylaxis

If the person does not know or cannot remember when they last had a tetanus booster shot, or if it has been more than 5 years since their last tetanus booster shot, they should seek medical care. Tetanus is a severe bacterial infection that can result from a puncture wound or a deep laceration. The bacteria that cause tetanus are commonly found in soil and animal manure. Once introduced into the body via a deep or dirty wound, they produce a powerful toxin that can cause muscle paralysis and death. Signs and symptoms of tetanus infection include muscle spasms and stiffness. The spasms and stiffness begin in the jaw and neck, leading to difficulty swallowing (a classic sign of tetanus). As the infection progresses, the muscle spasms and weakness spread to the abdomen and then to the rest of the body.

Although the effects of the tetanus toxin can be managed through administration of an antitoxin, prevention through immunization is a better strategy. The initial tetanus vaccine series is usually given during childhood, and then immunity is maintained through a booster shot given at least every 10 years. Death rates from tetanus infection are highest among those who were never immunized against tetanus and those who fail to maintain adequate immunization through regular booster shots.

Placement of Stitches

Suturing a wound closed can speed the healing process, reduce the chance for infection and minimize scarring. Wounds should be cleaned and stitched as soon as possible. If you think that a wound needs stitches, it probably does. If in doubt, tell the person to have the wound evaluated by a healthcare provider. In general, the following types of wounds often require stitches:

- Wounds that are deep or longer than ½ inch
- Wounds on parts of the body where scarring could impair appearance or function (e.g., the face, hands or feet)
- Wounds with jagged edges that gape open or wounds with straight edges that don't stay closed
- Wounds that are bleeding heavily and uncontrollably

Treatment of Infection

Proper wound care helps to lower the risk for infection, but sometimes infections develop anyway. An untreated wound infection can cause complications, including delayed wound healing; infection of nearby skin (cellulitis) or bone (osteomyelitis); or infection throughout the body (sepsis, which can be fatal). Tell the person they should see their healthcare provider if they notice signs and symptoms of infection or if the wound does not seem to be healing. Signs and symptoms of an infected wound may include:

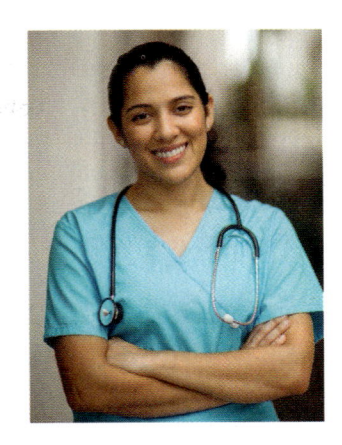

- Increased pain, swelling, redness or warmth in the area of the wound.
- Red streaks extending from the area of the wound.
- Pus (a thick yellow or green fluid) draining from the wound.
- Fever.

The healthcare provider may use advanced wound-care strategies, antibiotics, or both to eliminate the infection and promote wound healing.

Animal and Human Bites

Bites from animals or humans can range from minor scratches and bruises to serious puncture or laceration wounds.

It is important to take the person to a healthcare provider or tell the person to seek medical care for any human or animal bite that breaks the skin because of the high risk for bacterial infection. In these cases, antibiotics may be necessary. In addition, there is a risk of rabies infection from the bite of many wild animals (especially bats) and any stray dog or cat. A rabies vaccine may be necessary. In addition, a tetanus shot may be necessary in these cases.

If the wound is minor (e.g., scratches, bruising or skin was not broken completely through), stop any minor bleeding using direct pressure. Then, clean the wound with soap and water and flush the wound by running it under cool, clean water for at least 5 minutes. Apply an antibiotic ointment and apply ice and/or assist with administering ibuprofen or acetaminophen to help with any pain, bruising or swelling. Tell the person to contact their healthcare provider if they notice signs of infections, such as fever, pus, or redness or red streaks around the wound.

wound, apply direct pressure with a gauze pad to stop the bleeding. It may take several minutes for the bleeding to stop. After the bleeding stops, wash the area with soap and warm water. Rinse under warm running water for about 5 minutes until the wound appears clean and free of dirt and debris, and then dry the area. Cover the area with a sterile gauze pad and a bandage or apply an adhesive bandage. When you are finished providing care, wash your hands with soap and water, even if you wore gloves.

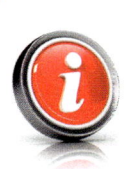

> **Myth-Information.** *Use hydrogen peroxide to clean a wound and prevent infection; the bubbles mean it is working to kill germs.* Although applying hydrogen peroxide to a wound will kill germs, it also can harm the tissue and delay healing. The best way to clean a wound is with soap and warm water.

Life-Threatening Internal Bleeding

Internal bleeding (bleeding that occurs inside the body, into a body cavity or space) can be a consequence of traumatic injury and may be life-threatening. **Blunt trauma**, which is caused by impact with a flat object or surface that does not break the skin, is a common cause of internal bleeding. Mechanisms of injury that can lead to blunt trauma and internal bleeding include falls, being struck by a vehicle or a piece of heavy equipment, being struck by a blunt object (such as a bat) or being thrown into a blunt object (such as a steering wheel). Crushing forces, for example, when a person's body is squeezed between two hard surfaces, can also cause blunt trauma, leading to internal bleeding. **Penetrating trauma**, which occurs when the body is pierced by an object (such as a knife or bullet) or impaled on an object (such as a branch or piece of metal) can also lead to internal bleeding.

Internal bleeding may not be immediately obvious because the blood is contained within the body (e.g., within the abdomen, chest or skull). Often, when a person has sustained an injury that could cause internal bleeding, they will have other, more obvious injuries as well or other signs such as bruising of the skin overlying the injury or significant pain at the site, nausea or vomiting. However, internal bleeding can also occur as a result of seemingly minor trauma, and it may reveal itself hours or days after the initial injury. When the mechanism of injury is one that could lead to internal bleeding (such as blunt or penetrating trauma), be alert to signs and symptoms that may indicate internal bleeding. If there is any thought that internal bleeding may be present, treat it as a life-threatening emergency.

Signs and Symptoms of Internal Bleeding

As a result of the blood loss, the person may show signs and symptoms of shock, such as excessive thirst; skin that feels cool or moist and looks pale or bluish; an altered level of consciousness; a rapid, weak heartbeat; nausea or vomiting. The person may cough, vomit or urinate blood. You may also notice that the area of the body where the blood is collecting (such as the abdomen) is tender, swollen or rigid, and there may be bruising over the area. If internal bleeding is occurring in an injured limb, the limb may be blue or extremely pale, swollen and rigid.

First Aid Care for Internal Bleeding

If a person is showing signs and symptoms of internal bleeding, call 9-1-1 and get equipment or tell someone to do so. If necessary, give first aid care for shock until EMS personnel arrive.

Minor Closed Wounds

When a person has a minor **closed wound**, the surface of the skin is intact, but the superficial underlying tissues are injured. A **bruise (contusion)** is a very common type of minor closed wound, usually caused by trauma that doesn't break the skin. Bruises occur when the small blood vessels under the surface of the skin are damaged and blood leaks into the surrounding tissues.

Signs and Symptoms of Minor Closed Wounds

The area around minor closed wounds may appear red or purple, and there may be swelling. The bruised area may be painful.

First Aid Care for Minor Closed Wounds

Get equipment or tell someone to do so. Then, apply a cold pack to the bruised area, which can help to reduce pain and swelling. To make a cold pack, fill a sealable plastic bag with a mixture of ice and water. Before applying the cold pack to the person's skin, wrap it in a thin, dry towel to protect the skin from injury. Hold the cold pack in place for no more than 20 minutes, and then wait at least 20 minutes before applying the cold pack again. If the person is not able to tolerate a 20-minute application, apply the cold pack for periods of 10 minutes on and off.

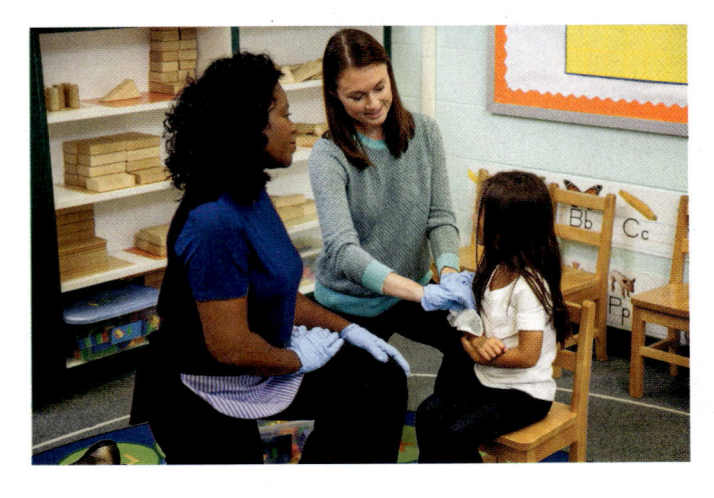

PUTTING IT ALL TOGETHER 6-1

Using Direct Pressure to Control Life-Threatening Bleeding

Check 1. **Check** the scene for safety, form an initial impression, obtain consent and use PPE.

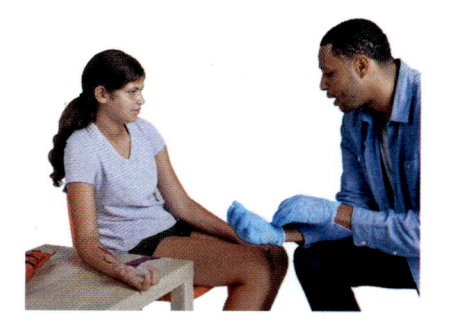

Call 2. **Call 9-1-1** and get equipment (bleeding control kit and first aid kit) or tell someone to do so.

Care 3. **Find the source of the bleeding.**
- There may be one wound or more than one wound.
- Care for life-threatening bleeding first.

4. **Tell the person to expect pain.**
- The amount of pressure you need to apply may be painful for the person, but it is necessary to control the bleeding.

5. **Choose a dressing.**
- If the bleeding is life-threatening, use a hemostatic dressing if you have one.
- Otherwise, use a gauze pad or other available material (such as a clean T-shirt) as a dressing.

6. **Place the dressing on the wound.**
- Ensure good contact with the bleeding surfaces of the wound.

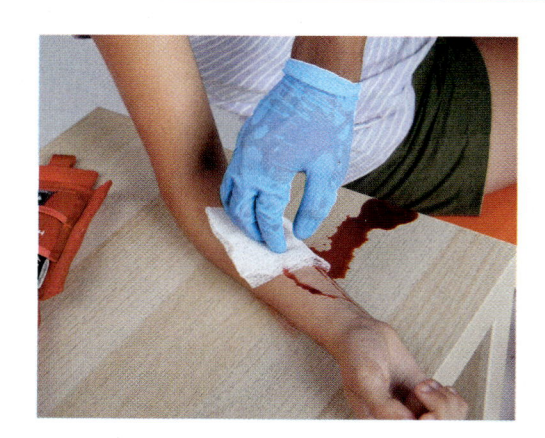

PUTTING IT ALL TOGETHER 6-1

7. Apply steady, firm pressure directly over the wound until the bleeding stops.
- Put one hand on top of the dressing and put your other hand on top.
- Position your shoulders over your hands and lock your elbows.
- Push down as hard as you can.
- If you need your hands, use your knee to apply pressure.
- Remember that direct pressure is most effective when the injured body part is on a firm, flat surface.
- If blood soaks through the original gauze pad, you do not need to do anything, but you can put another gauze pad on top. Replace the new gauze pad as necessary if blood soaks through the pads.

Note: Do not remove the original gauze pad and **do not** stack multiple gauze pads.

8. Hold direct pressure until:
- The bleeding stops.
- A tourniquet is applied (for life-threatening bleeding from an arm or leg) and the bleeding has stopped.
- Another person relieves you.
- You are too exhausted to continue.
- The situation becomes unsafe.

9. Apply a roller bandage (only if the bleeding stops before EMS arrives).
- Check for circulation beyond the injury before applying bandage.
- Apply the bandage over the dressing and secure it firmly to keep pressure on the wound.
  - Place the end of a bandage on the dressing at a 45-degree angle.
  - Continue wrapping the bandage over the dressing.
  - Tape to secure the dressing.
- Check again for circulation beyond the injury. If there is any change, the bandage may be too tight; carefully loosen the bandage.

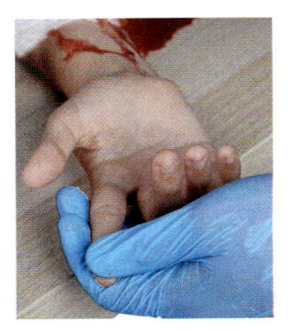

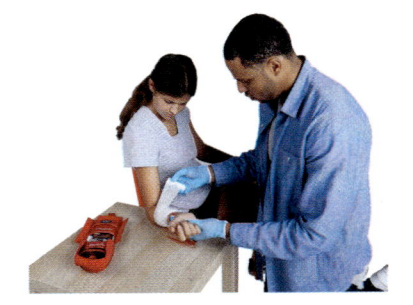

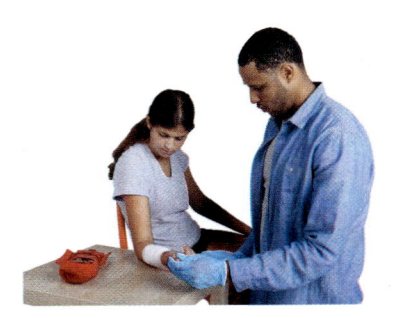

(Continued on next page)

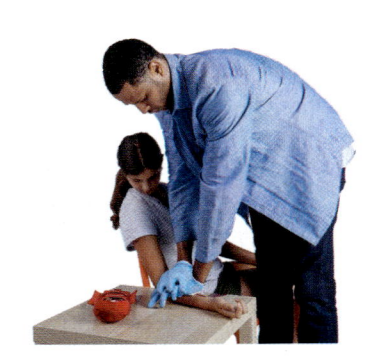

American Red Cross | First Aid for Sudden Illnesses and Injuries

PUTTING IT ALL TOGETHER 6-1

Using Direct Pressure to Control Life-Threatening Bleeding continued

10. Monitor for re-bleeding.
- Monitor the person and look for bleeding through the bandage.
- If bleeding recurs:
  - Do not apply an additional dressing or bandage.
  - Remove the bandage and leave only the single dressing on the wound in place.
  - Apply direct manual pressure.

11. After giving care, remove your gloves and wash hands.

PUTTING IT ALL TOGETHER 6-2

Using Direct Pressure and a Windlass Rod Tourniquet to Control Life-Threatening Bleeding

Check 1. **Check the scene** for safety, **form an initial impression, obtain consent and use PPE.**

Call 2. **Call 9-1-1** and get equipment (bleeding control kit, first kit and AED) or tell someone to do so.

Care 3. **Find the source of the bleeding.**
- There may be one wound or more than one wound.
- Care for life-threatening bleeding first.

4. **Tell the person to expect pain.**
- The amount of pressure you need to apply may be painful for the person, but it is necessary to control the bleeding.

5. **Choose a dressing.**
- If the bleeding is life-threatening, use a hemostatic dressing if you have one.
- Otherwise, use a gauze pad or other available material (such as a clean T-shirt) as a dressing.

6. **Place the dressing on the wound.**
- Ensure good contact with the bleeding surfaces of the wound.

7. **Apply direct pressure** to the wound until the tourniquet is available.
- Place the dressing (a hemostatic dressing, if available) over the wound.
- Push down with both hands and apply steady, firm pressure over the wound until the bleeding stops:
  - Position your body over the wound so your shoulders are directly over your hands with your elbows locked.
  - Push down with all of your body weight.

Note: *If you need your hands, use your knee to apply pressure.*

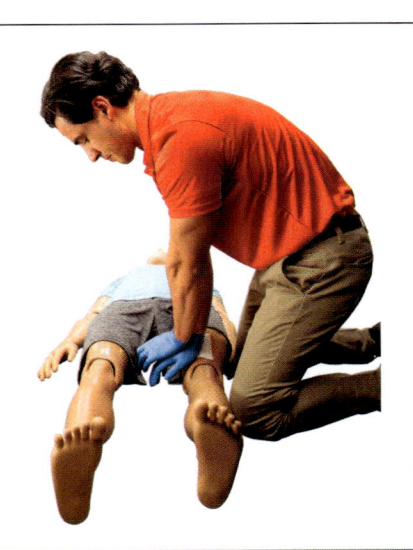

(Continued on next page)

American Red Cross | First Aid for Sudden Illnesses and Injuries

PUTTING IT ALL TOGETHER 6-2

Using Direct Pressure and a Windlass Rod Tourniquet to Control Life-Threatening Bleeding continued

8. Once a tourniquet is available, have a bystander continue applying direct pressure while you apply the tourniquet.
- If you are alone, use your knee to apply pressure while you apply the tourniquet.

9. Place the tourniquet around the limb, approximately 2 to 3 inches above the wound.
- Do not place the tourniquet on top of the wound or a joint.
- If the wound is over a joint, apply the tourniquet 2 to 3 inches above the joint.

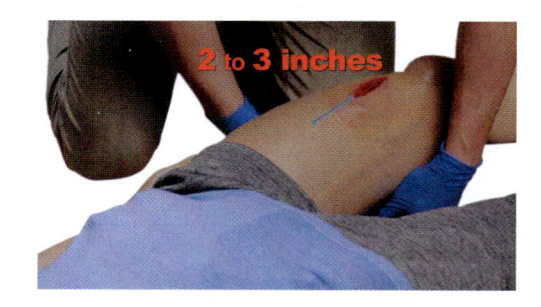

10. Attach the buckle or pass the end of the strap through the buckle and then think, PULL–TWIST–CLIP.

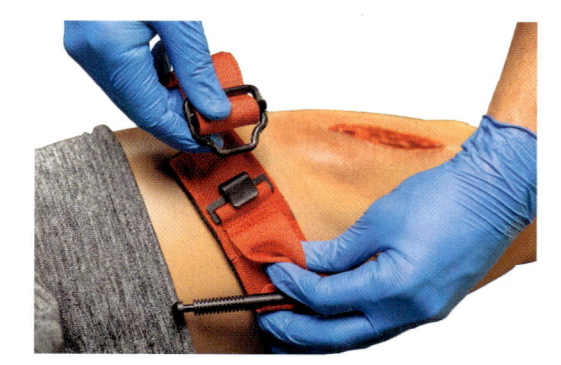

11. PULL the free end of the strap until the tourniquet is as tight as you can get it around the limb.
- Make sure there is no room between the tourniquet and the limb before activating the tightening mechanism.
- If the tourniquet is not tight enough around the extremity, it may be beneficial to move the tourniquet closer on the limb to where the extremity is thicker.

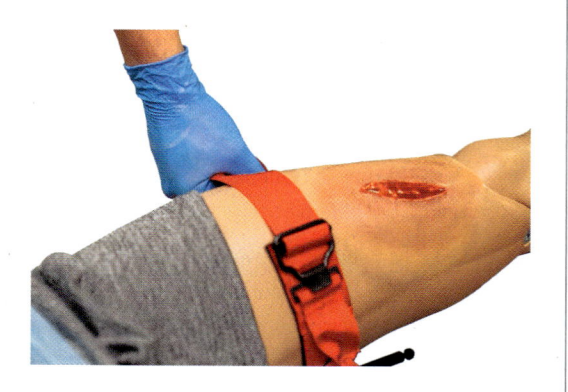

120 Chapter 6 | Wounds and Bleeding

PUTTING IT ALL TOGETHER 6-2

12. TWIST the rod until the bleeding stops, or until you can't twist it anymore.

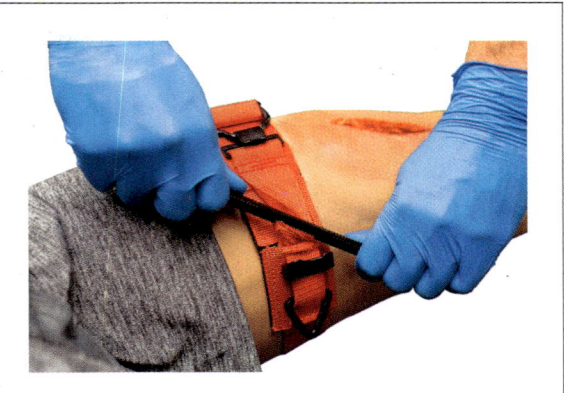

13. CLIP the rod in place to prevent it from untwisting.

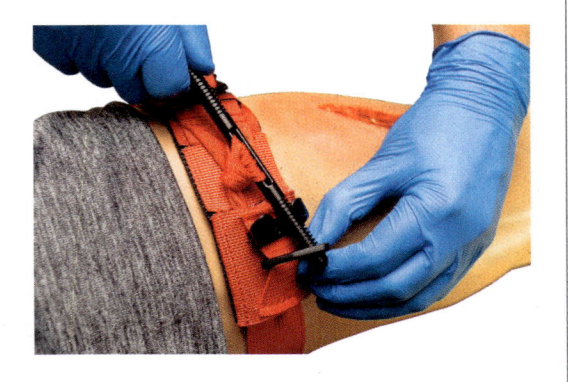

Note: *These steps are a guide to using a windlass rod tourniquet. Instructions for using ratcheting and elastic tourniquets can be found in Appendix D: Skill Practice Sheets for Skill Boosts. Always follow the instructions of the particular tourniquet to which you have access.*

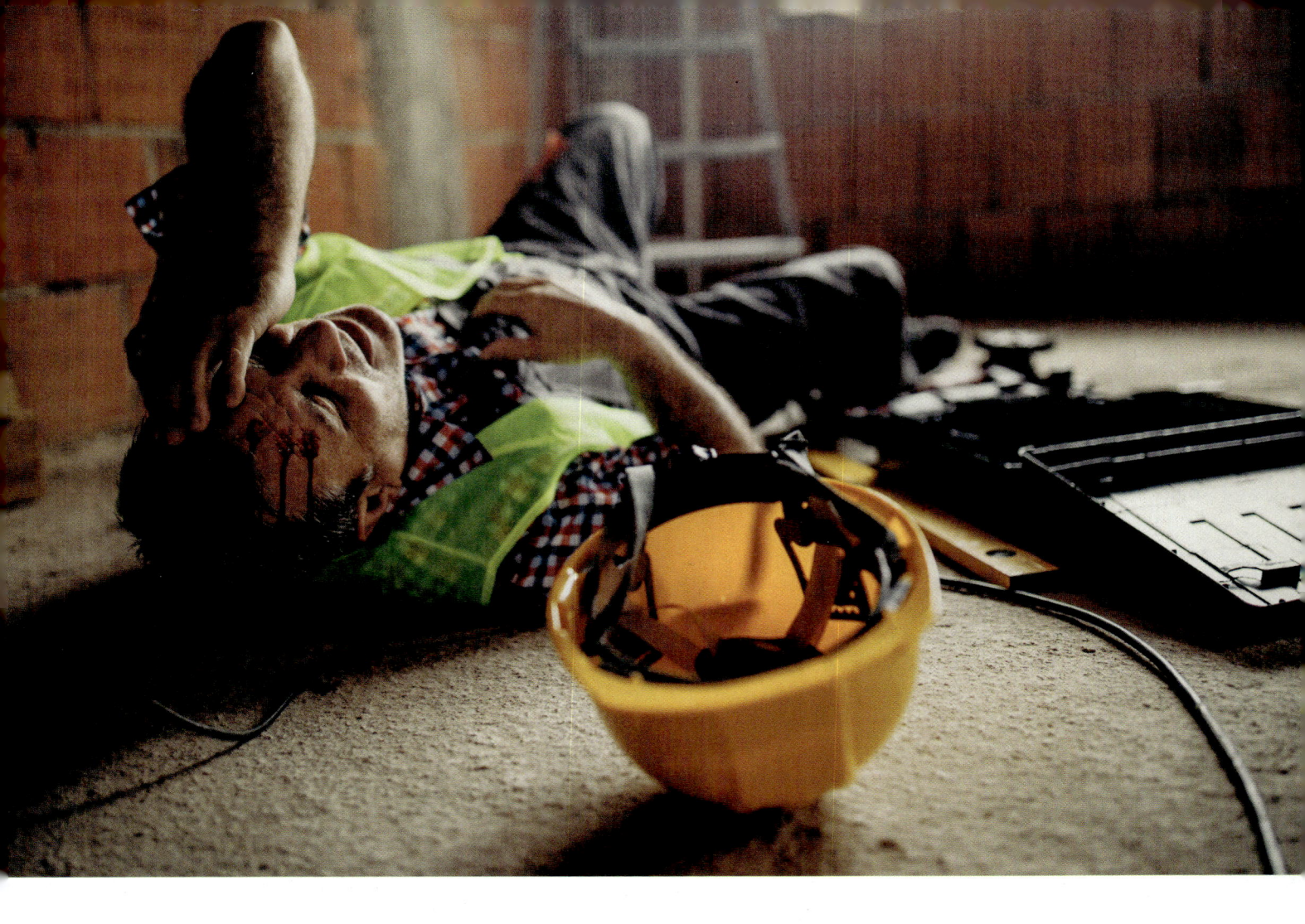

CHAPTER 7
Injuries and Environmental Emergencies

The risk for injury and environmental emergencies is always present as we go about our daily activities and interact with the world around us. Taking appropriate safety precautions significantly reduces that risk, but injuries do happen and it is not possible to eliminate all environmental hazards, especially when work or play brings us outdoors.

Recognizing the signs and symptoms of injuries and environmental emergencies will allow you to make quick decisions and give appropriate first aid care that can speed recovery and even save the person's life.

General Approach to Injuries and Environmental Emergencies

Follow the emergency action steps, CHECK—CALL—CARE, as you have learned to do for any emergency situation.

First you will check the scene for safety, obtain consent and form an initial impression. Then, check the person for responsiveness, breathing, life-threatening bleeding and other life-threatening conditions.

> **ALERT!**
>
> If you see life-threatening bleeding at any time during your initial impression or check of the person, control the bleeding using any available resources.

If you encounter fire, chemicals, exposed electrical wires or other hazards, do not enter the scene. Instead immediately call 9-1-1 or tell someone to do so and follow your facility protocol.

Note: *If, during the initial impression, you determine that the person appears to be experiencing a life-threatening emergency, immediately go to the call step and give general care for the condition found. Then, continue your check (as appropriate) to determine if additional care is needed.*

If the person is responsive and experiencing a non-life-threatening emergency, continue the check by asking them (or bystanders, if necessary) questions using SAM (**S**igns and symptoms, **A**llergies, **M**edications and medical conditions) to gain a better understanding of the situation. Then do a focused check, focusing in on the area of concern (see Chapter 1).

Call 9-1-1 and get equipment or tell someone to do so if the person is unresponsive, is not breathing normally, is experiencing life-threatening bleeding or has a condition that is potentially life-threatening. If you don't need to call 9-1-1, get equipment or tell someone to do so.

Then give care. Follow the same general guidelines as you would for any emergency.

- Give care consistent with your knowledge and training as needed.
- Ask SAM questions and do a focused check if not already done.
- Offer to *assist* the person with their own medication, if needed.
  - You can *administer* medications if it is allowable by state laws and regulations and you are trained and authorized to do so. Additional training on medication administration is available through the American Red Cross, if you need it.
- Position the person:
  - Help the responsive person rest in the most comfortable position.
  - For head, neck and spinal injuries, you will need to keep the person in the position they are found in unless you need to perform CPR.
  - Place an unresponsive person who is breathing or a person who responds but is not fully awake in the recovery position except for head, neck and spinal injuries.
- Keep the person from getting chilled or overheated.
- Reassure the person by telling the person that you will help and that EMS personnel have been called (if appropriate).
- Continue to watch for changes in the person's condition, including breathing and level of responsiveness.

INJURIES

Open and closed wounds and bleeding were covered in Chapter 6. This chapter will focus on burns; head, neck and spinal injuries; muscle, bone and joint injuries; and injuries to specific parts of the body (e.g., nose and mouth, abdomen).

Burns

A **burn** is a type of wound; a traumatic injury to the skin (and sometimes the underlying tissues as well) that can be caused by contact with heat, chemicals, radiation or electricity (Figure 7-1, A–D).

If you enter a scene and see that a person is being burned, it is important to stop the burning. Once you have determined that the scene is safe for you to enter, remove the source of the injury if it is safe for you to do so. Depending on the cause of the burn, this may involve removing the person from the source or removing the source from the person. Then, check the person.

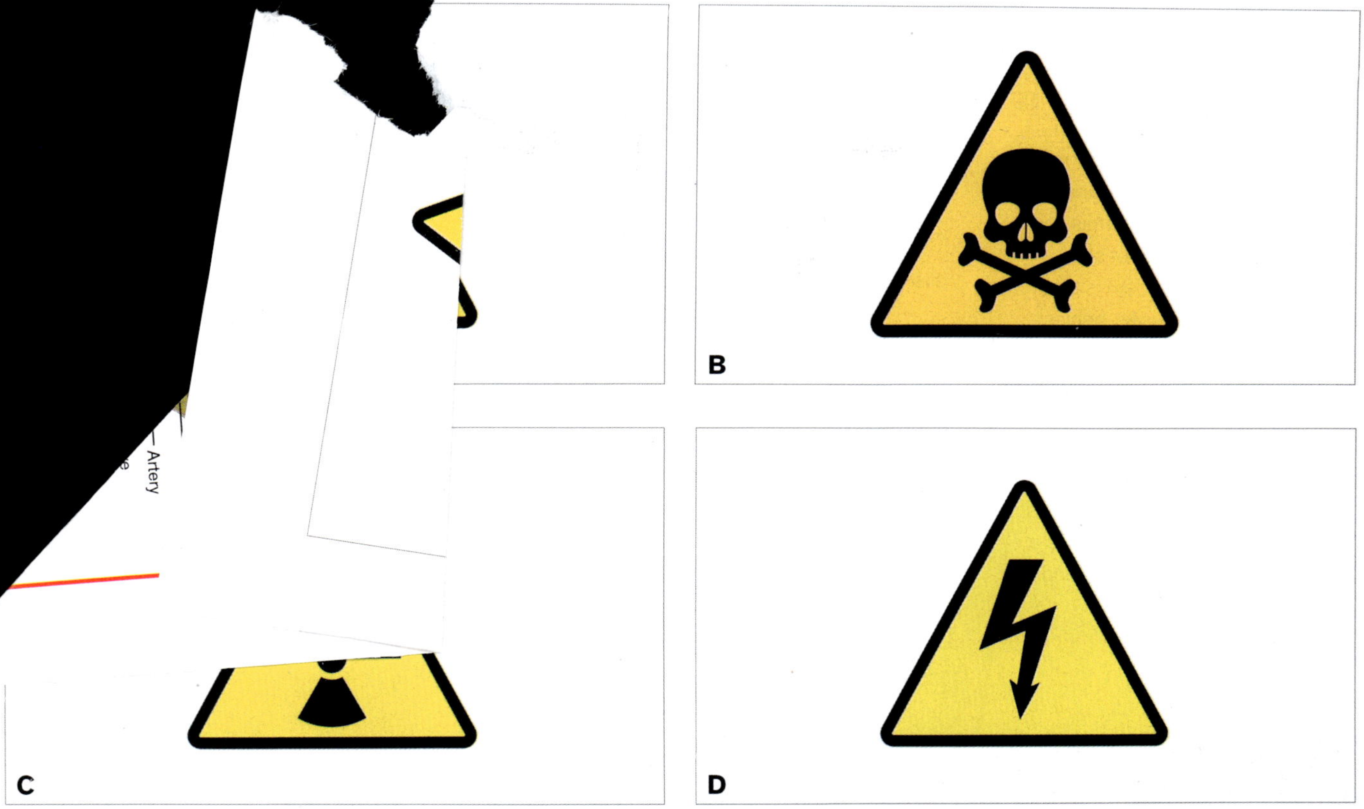

Figure 7-1. Causes of burns include extreme heat (A), chemicals (B), radiation (C) and electricity (D).

Recognizing Signs, Symptoms and Severity of Burns

Burned areas can appear red, brown, black (charred) or white. The burned area may be extremely painful or almost painless (if the burn is deep enough to destroy the nerve endings). There may be swelling, blisters or both. The blisters may break and ooze a clear fluid.

Burns range in severity from minor to life-threatening. A life-threatening burn is potentially disfiguring or disabling and it requires immediate medical attention. In addition to life-threatening burns, other burns may need immediate medical attention. Burns requiring immediate medical attention include:

- Burns that extend through deeper layers of skin or the fat, muscle or bone underneath (Box 7-1).
- Burns that cover more than one body part or a large percentage of the person's total body surface area.
- Burns that affect areas that could impair a person's function or their ability to breath, such as burns on the face, hands, feet, joints or groin.
- Inhalation burns. Burns can occur when someone inhales hot gasses.
- Burns caused by electricity, chemicals, radiation or an explosion.
- Burns in people with medical conditions or other injuries.
- Burns in a young child, an infant or an older adult.
- Circumferential burns (that is, burns that go all the way around a limb, the chest, the neck or another body part).

If you think that a person has a burn that requires immediate medical attention, call 9-1-1 and get equipment immediately, or tell someone to do so. If you are not sure if a burn is severe enough to require immediate medical attention, be safe and call 9-1-1. If you do not need to call 9-1-1, get equipment or tell someone to do so.

Giving First Aid Care for Burns

First aid care for burns focuses on cooling. First, remove any clothing or jewelry at the burn site. Then, cool the burn and relieve pain using clean, cool, running water for at least 10 minutes and ideally 20 minutes. Use water that you could drink. If clean, cool running water is not available, you can use clean, lukewarm water or apply a cool or cold compress instead. If cooling was not started immediately after the burn, you can consider starting the cooling process up to 3 hours after the injury.

American Red Cross | First Aid for Sudden Illnesses and Injuries

Box 7-1 Classifying the Depth of the Burn

Burns can be classified according to depth. Superficial burns only involve the epidermis (the top layer of skin). Partial-thickness burns involve the epidermis and the dermis (the layer of skin underneath the epidermis that contains blood vessels, nerves, hair follicles and glands). Full-thickness burns involve both layers of skin and may extend into the subcutaneous tissue, muscle or bone underneath. Any burn that is more than superficial requires medical care, and many burns are potentially life-threatening and require EMS.

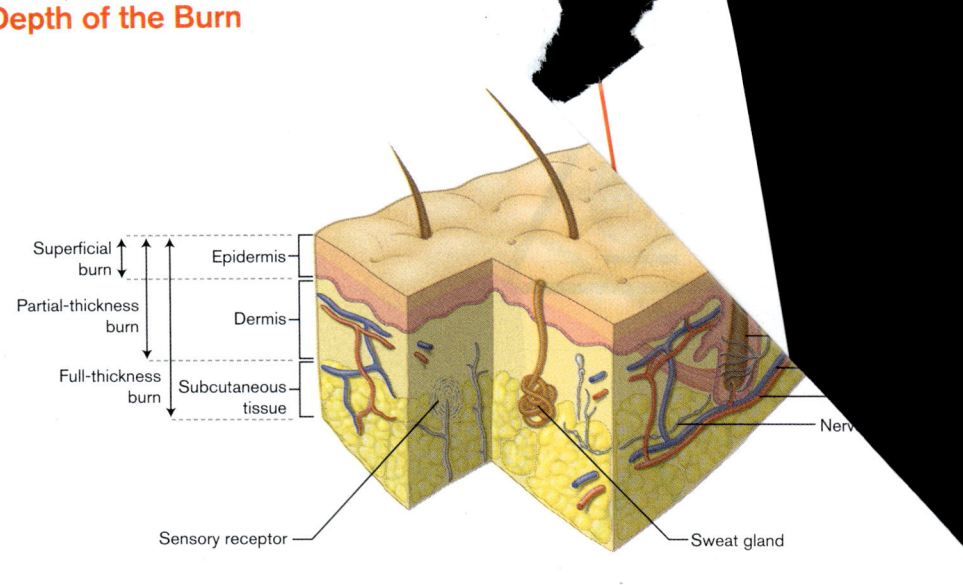

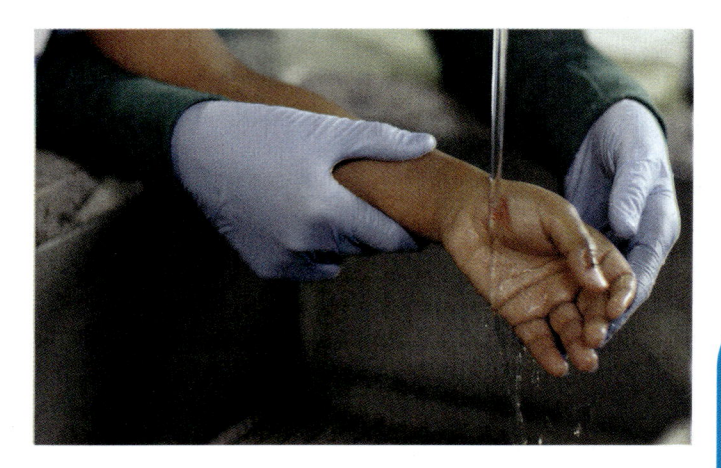

Burns of all types, especially if they cover a large percentage of the body, can cause a person to go into shock, so monitor the person closely. When caring for a burn, do not remove pieces of clothing that are stuck to the burned area, do not attempt to clean a severe burn, and do not break any blisters.

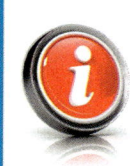

Myth-Information. *Soothe a burn with butter.* Not a good idea! Putting butter, mayonnaise, petroleum jelly or any other greasy substance on a burn is not effective for relieving pain or promoting healing. In fact, applying a greasy substance to the burn can seal in the heat and make the burn worse.

Never use ice, ice water or a freezing compress to cool a burn because doing so can cause more damage to the skin. Cooling a burn over a large area of the body can bring on hypothermia (a body temperature below normal), so be alert to signs and symptoms of this condition. In addition, avoid cooling beyond 40 minutes due to the risk of hypothermia. Hypothermia is discussed later in this chapter.

Leave the burn uncovered; EMS personnel will give care when they arrive. However, if EMS is delayed or you are in a remote location, cover the burn loosely with a sterile dressing. If a sterile dressing is not available, a clean dressing or even plastic wrap may be used to cover the burn. It is important to make sure that whatever you use to cover the wound is sterile or at least clean, because burns leave the person highly susceptible to infection.

Chemical Burns

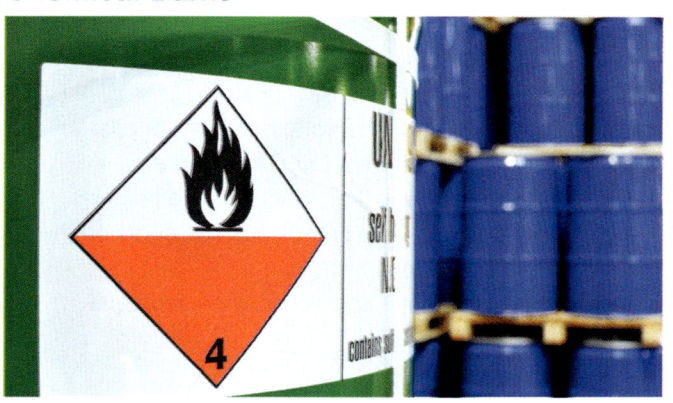

The general care for a chemical burn is the same as for any other type of burn: stop and cool. However, there are some special considerations for the "stop" step. Because the chemical will continue to burn as long as it is on the skin, you must remove the chemical from the skin as quickly as possible. Carefully remove, or help the person to remove, any clothing that was contaminated with the chemical if you are trained, wearing personal protective equipment and it is safe to do so.

- **Dry chemicals.** If the burn was caused by a dry chemical, such as lime, brush off the powder or granules with gloved hands or a cloth, being careful not to get any of the chemical on your skin or on a different area of the person's skin. Then flush the area thoroughly with large amounts of cool, clean, running water for at least 15 minutes or until EMS personnel arrive and begin their care of the person.
- **Liquid chemicals.** If the burn resulted from a liquid chemical coming into contact with the skin, flush the affected area with large amounts of cool, clean, running water for at least 15 minutes or until EMS personnel arrive and begin their care of the person.

If the chemical is in the person's eye, flush the eye with water until EMS personnel arrive and begin their care of the person. Tilt the person's head so that the affected eye is lower than the unaffected eye as you flush.

Electrical Burns

As always, check the scene for safety before entering. Make sure 9-1-1 has been called, and if possible, turn off the power at its source. Do not approach or touch the person until you are sure they are no longer in contact with the electrical current. Once you have determined that it is safe to approach the person, give care as needed until help arrives.

First aid for electrical burns also follows the general principle of "stop and cool," but as with chemical burns, there are some special care considerations when electricity is the cause of the burn. Because the electrical current that caused the burns can also affect the heart's rhythm or the person's ability to breathe (causing the person to go into cardiac arrest), be prepared to give CPR and use an AED if you are trained in these skills.

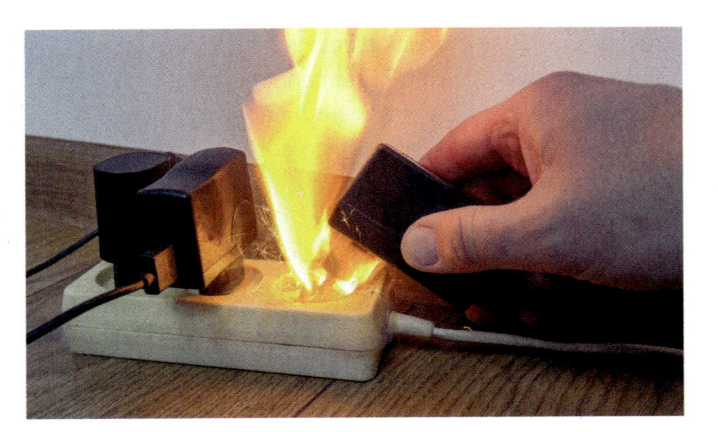

Anyone who has experienced an electrical burn should be evaluated by a healthcare provider because the person's injuries may be more extensive than they appear. Although the person may only have a small burn wound where the electrical current entered or left the body, there may be significant internal injuries caused by the current passing through the body.

Head, Neck and Spinal Injuries

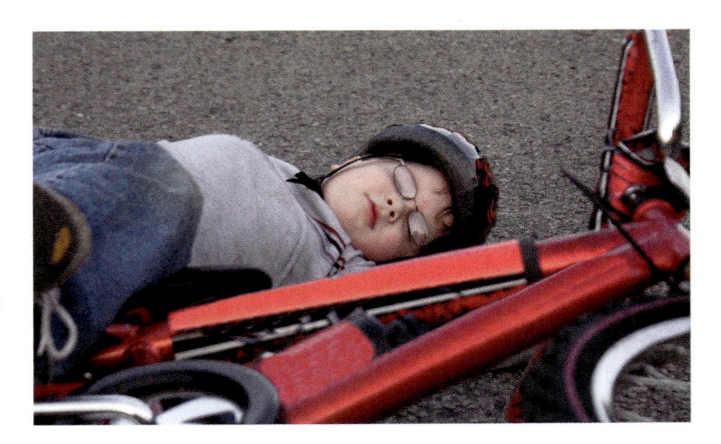

Traumatic accidents (such as falling from a height, getting hit by or being thrown from a vehicle, or sustaining a blow to the head) can cause head, neck or spinal injuries. Head, neck or spinal injuries are serious because they may involve the spinal cord or the brain. Depending on the nature and severity of the injury, the person may be left with a permanent disability (e.g., traumatic brain injury, paralysis). Head, neck or spinal injuries can be fatal so all should be treated as potentially life-threatening.

- **Spinal cord injuries** can result from trauma that causes one or more vertebrae (the bones that surround and protect the spinal cord) to break. The sharp bone fragments can press into the soft tissue of the spinal cord, damaging it. Damage can also occur if the injury causes the soft tissue of the spinal cord to swell, compressing it against the hard bone that surrounds it. Finally, in children, the bones of the spine can move, damage the spinal cord, and then return to the original position. Depending on the location and severity of the spinal cord injury, the person may develop **paralysis** (the loss of movement, sensation or both) in body parts below the level of the injury. **Paraplegia** is paralysis that

affects both legs and the lower trunk. **Quadriplegia** is paralysis that affects both arms, the trunk and both legs.
- **Brain injuries** can occur as a result of a blow to the head, a penetrating injury to the head (such as a bullet wound), or exposure to acceleration-deceleration forces that cause the head to snap forward and then back. A blow to the head can lead to a **concussion** (a traumatic brain injury that alters the way the brain functions; Box 7-2), a **brain contusion** (bruising of the brain tissue) or a **brain hematoma** (bleeding into the space between the brain and the skull). Acceleration-deceleration forces, such as can occur with a motor vehicle collision or a fall from a height, can lead to **diffuse axonal injury** (tearing of nerves throughout the brain tissue).

Causes of Head, Neck and Spinal Injuries

Many different types of accidents can lead to head, neck or spinal injuries. You should especially consider the possibility of a head, neck or spinal injury if the person:

- Was hit by a vehicle, thrown from a moving vehicle, or was the occupant of a vehicle involved in a motor vehicle collision.
- Was injured as a result of entering shallow water headfirst.
- Was injured as a result of a fall from a height greater than the person's own height.
- Was participating in a sport and sustained a blow to the head or collided with another player, the ground or a piece of equipment.

Recognizing Head, Neck and Spinal Injuries

The signs and symptoms of a head, neck or spinal injury depend on the nature and location of the injury, but could include:

- Mechanism of injury, which means the method by which the injury occurred.
- A change in behavior or mental status, for example, unresponsiveness, confusion, stumbling, repeatedly asking the same questions, memory loss, nausea or vomiting, or speech problems.
- Head, neck or back pain or a visible injury.
- A partial or complete loss of sensation or movement in part of the body.
- Seizures.
- Crying, especially if inconsolable.
- Inability to do activities that the person could previously do, such as walking.
- Unusual bumps, bruises or depressions on the head, neck or back.
- Heavy external bleeding of the head, neck or back.
- Bruising of the head, especially around the eyes and behind the ears.
- Blood or other fluids in the ears or nose.
- Confusion or disorientation.
- Impaired breathing or vision.
- Nausea or vomiting.
- Partial or complete loss of movement or feeling of any body part.
- Loss of balance.
- Severe pain or pressure in the head, neck or back (reported by the person or indicated by the person holding their head, neck or back).
- Back pain, weakness, tingling or loss of sensation in the hands, fingers, feet or toes.
- Persistent headache.
- A broken or damaged safety helmet.

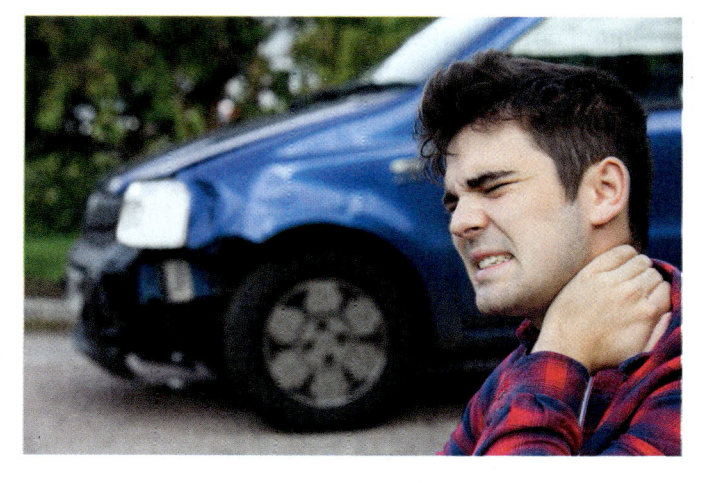

If you suspect a head, neck or spinal injury, call 9-1-1 and get equipment immediately, or tell someone to do so. Evaluation by medical personnel is needed to determine the severity of a head, neck or spinal injury and you should always assume that an injury involving the head, neck or spine is serious and provide care accordingly.

Giving First Aid Care for Head, Neck and Spinal Injuries

After calling 9-1-1, first aid care for a person with a suspected head, neck or spinal injury involves having the person remain in the position in which they were found, unless you need to give CPR or cannot control bleeding in the position in which they were found. For example, if a child is strapped into a car seat, do not remove them from it unless you need to give CPR.

If the person is wearing a helmet, do not remove it unless removing the helmet is necessary to give CPR. In addition, it is important to maintain the person's body temperature and, based on your level of training, care for any other injuries that may be present.

128 Chapter 7 | Injuries and Environmental Emergencies

Box 7-2 Concussions

A concussion is a traumatic brain injury that alters the way the brain functions. Concussions often occur as sports-related injuries, but they can occur whenever a person experiences a bump, blow or jolt to the head or body that results in rapid movement of the brain within the head. A person who has had one concussion is at increased risk for complications from subsequent concussions.

A concussion can result from even a seemingly minor bump, blow or jolt and may be tricky to recognize. Many people who experience a concussion do not lose consciousness, or they may only lose consciousness very briefly. Your best clues that a person may have a concussion are often changes in the person's behavior or other signs noted after the person has experienced a bump, blow or jolt. For example, the person may seem confused, dazed or stunned; lose the ability to remember or follow simple instructions; or ask repeatedly what happened. The person may complain of a headache, feel nauseated, vomit, have blurred or double vision, complain of dizziness, or be especially sensitive to light or noise. Many people who have experienced a concussion say that the concussion caused them to feel sluggish, groggy or just "not right."

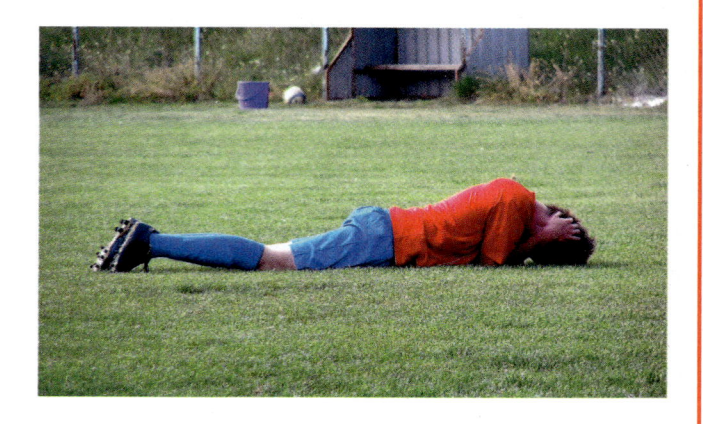

Signs and symptoms of a concussion usually are apparent soon after the injury, although some can appear hours or days later. For example, the person may sleep more or less than usual. Children may show changes in playing or eating habits. The effects of the concussion can last for several days or weeks or longer.

Signs and Symptoms of Concussion

THINKING AND REMEMBERING	PHYSICAL	EMOTIONAL	BEHAVIORAL
■ Difficulty thinking clearly ■ Difficulty remembering events that occurred just prior to the incident and just after the incident ■ Difficulty remembering new information ■ Difficulty concentrating ■ Feeling mentally "foggy" ■ Difficulty processing information	■ Headache ■ Blurred and/or double vision ■ Nausea or vomiting ■ Dizziness ■ Seizures ■ Sensitivity to noise or light ■ Balance problems ■ Feeling sluggish (lack of energy)	■ Irritability ■ Sadness ■ Heightened emotions ■ Nervousness or anxiety	■ Changes in sleeping habits (sleeping more or less than usual, difficulty falling asleep) ■ Changes in playing and eating habits (in children) ■ Loss of consciousness ■ Confusion ■ Inability to do activities that the person could previously do

If you think that a person has sustained a concussion, advise the person to stop the activity they were engaged in when the incident occurred and call 9-1-1 and get equipment, or tell someone to do so.

First aid care for concussion is the same as for all types of injuries to the body. While you are waiting for EMS personnel to arrive, have the person rest without moving and give care for any other injuries that may be present based on your level of training.

If, for any reason EMS was not called, the person should follow up with a healthcare provider as soon as possible for a full evaluation. A healthcare provider is best able to evaluate the severity of the injury and make recommendations about when the person can return to normal activities. And, while rare, permanent brain injury and death are potential consequences of failing to identify and respond to a concussion in a timely manner.

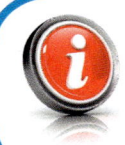

> **Myth-Information.** *A person with a concussion who falls asleep could die.* It is generally considered safe for a person with a concussion to go to sleep. However, this should be after evaluation by a healthcare provider. The person's healthcare provider may recommend that you wake the person periodically to make sure that their condition has not worsened.

> **THE PROS KNOW.** If you suspect that a person has a head, neck or spinal injury, approach the person from the front so that they can see you without turning their head. Tell the person to respond verbally to your questions, rather than nodding or shaking their head.

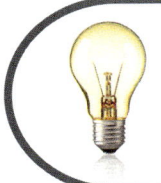

Muscle, Bone and Joint Injuries

Injuries to the muscles, bones and joints include sprains, strains, dislocations and fractures. You will likely not be able to tell the difference between these injuries, except in the cases of very deformed fractures and dislocations. Just remember two key points: treat all injuries as potential fractures, and decide if a call to 9-1-1 is needed based on signs and symptoms.

- A **strain** occurs when a tendon or muscle is stretched, torn or damaged. Tendons attach muscles to bones. Strains often are caused by lifting something heavy or working a muscle too hard. They usually involve the muscles in the neck, back, thigh or the back of the lower leg but can occur anywhere. Some strains can reoccur, especially in the neck and back.
- A **sprain** occurs when a ligament is stretched, torn or damaged. Ligaments connect bones to bones at the joints. Sprains most commonly affect the ankle, knee, wrist and finger joints but can occur anywhere.
- A **dislocation** occurs when a bone within a joint moves out of its normal position in the joint. This type of injury is usually caused by a violent force, allowing the bones to move out of place.
- A **fracture** is a complete break, a chip or a crack in a bone. Fractures can be open (the end of the broken bone breaks through the skin) or closed (the broken bone does not break through the skin).

Recognizing Muscle, Bone and Joint Injuries

Muscle, bone and joint injuries can be extremely painful. Sometimes the injury will be very obvious—for example, you may see the ends of a broken bone protruding through the skin, or the injured body part might appear bent or crooked (deformed). If a joint is dislocated, you may see an abnormal bump, ridge or hollow formed by the displaced end of the bone. Other times, signs and symptoms of injury may be more subtle, such as swelling or bruising. Usually, the person will try to avoid using the injured body part because using it causes pain. In some cases, the person may be unable to move the injured body part. The person might also report feeling or hearing "popping" or "snapping" at the time of the injury, "grating" when moving the injured part, or changes in circulation and feeling, like numbness and tingling, at and below the injured area.

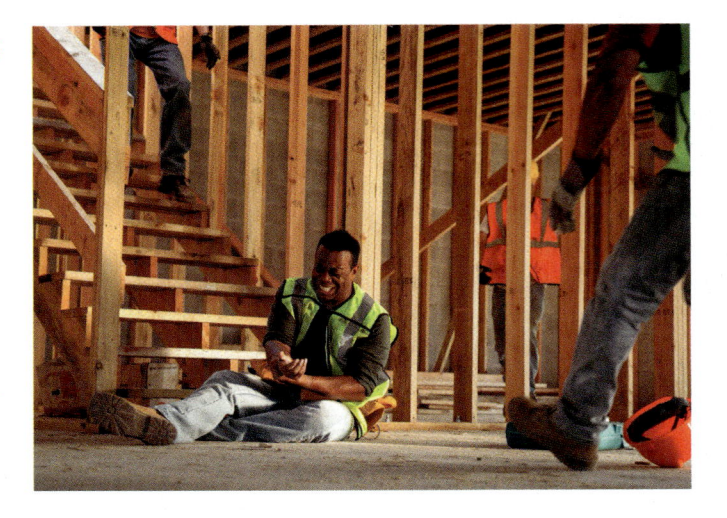

It is not *always* necessary to call 9-1-1 for a muscle, bone or joint injury.

However, you should call 9-1-1 and get equipment if:

- A broken bone is protruding through the skin.
- There is bleeding with the fracture.
- There is moderate or severe swelling and bruising.
- The person cannot move or use the injured body part.
- The injured body part is bent, crooked or looks deformed.
- The person heard or felt the injured area pop or snap at the time of the injury.
- The person hears a grating sound when attempting to move the injured body part.
- The injured area or area below the site of injury is cold, or there is numbness or tingling.
- The injury involves the head, neck or spine, pelvis or upper leg.
- The person is showing signs or symptoms of shock, including difficulty breathing.
- The cause of the injury makes you think that the injury may be severe or that the person may have multiple injuries (e.g., a fall from a height or getting hit by a vehicle).

130 Chapter 7 | Injuries and Environmental Emergencies

- It is not possible to safely or comfortably move the person.
- You are unsure if it is serious or not.

If you do not need to call 9-1-1, you should get equipment or tell someone to do so. In addition, medical care is always still needed. The person should either be taken to the hospital or a medical provider should be contacted for further instruction.

Giving First Aid Care for Muscle, Bone and Joint Injuries

Give care according to the condition found and your level of training. General care for all types of muscle, bone and joint injuries is the same; specific care differs according to severity and location of the injury.

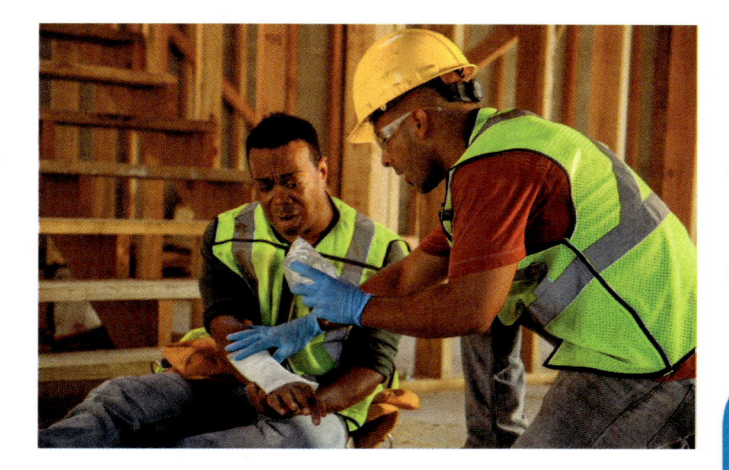

If the injury is severe and you have called 9-1-1 and are waiting for EMS personnel to arrive, have the person rest without moving or straightening the body part. Don't splint the injured body part unless you must move the person.

If the wound is closed and the person can tolerate it, apply a cold pack wrapped in a thin, dry towel to the area to reduce swelling and pain.

Apply cold for no more than 20 minutes at a time and wait at least 20 minutes before applying cold again. To apply cold, fill a sealable plastic bag with a mixture of ice and water. As an alternative you can you use a commercial ice pack.

For muscle, bone and joint injuries that do not require a 9-1-1 call, have the person limit use of the injured body part. Then, either call their healthcare provider or take the person to a healthcare provider. If you call a healthcare provider, follow their guidance. If you take the person to a healthcare provider, first splint the injured body part and then apply a cold pack wrapped in a thin, dry towel for no more than 20 minutes at a time and wait at least 20 minutes before applying cold again.

If the person has an ankle sprain or strain, you can apply a compression wrap to promote comfort if you are trained in their use. First, check for circulation and sensation beyond the injured area. Before applying the compression wrap, apply a cold pack to the area to reduce pain and swelling. After 20 minutes, dry the injured area and apply the compression wrap. To apply the compression wrap, follow these simple steps:

- Wrap the compression wrap around the foot two times to anchor it; with each wrap, unroll the wrap and pull it slightly to maintain light pressure.
- Continue wrapping above the ankle joint in a spiral pattern, around the ankle joint and below the ankle joint to form a figure 8.
  - With each wrap, overlap the previous layer by one-half the width of the compression wrap.
  - It is important to note that more tension should be applied toward the toes and less toward the calf.
  - Make sure to leave the toes and heel uncovered.
- As you near the end of the compression wrap, wrap twice around the limb above the ankle joint and secure the ends of the wrap with tape.
- Recheck for circulation and sensation beyond the injured area.

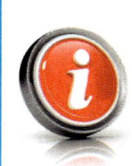

> **Myth-Information.** *Apply heat to a muscle, bone or joint injury to speed healing.* Although applying heat is commonly used to relieve pain associated with chronic muscle, bone and joint conditions such as arthritis, it is not the best treatment for an acute muscle, bone or joint injury.

Splinting

If you need to move or transport the person to receive medical care, you must **splint** the injured body part to limit motion.

Types of Splints

There are different types of splints available. Two of the most common are rigid splints and soft splints. A common type of rigid splint is the padded board. Other rigid splints include the SAM splint, C-splint and cardboard splints.

An example of a soft splint is a sling and binder. If the person has a shoulder injury, you can use a sling and binder to limit motion and provide support. A sling and binder can also be used to secure the shoulder for an upper arm injury or support a splinted lower arm to make it easier to move.

There are some splints that start soft and become rigid. One example is a vacuum splint. Once it is in place, the air is sucked out, creating a vacuum inside and making the splint rigid. Another example is an air splint, which, when placed around the area, is inflated to become more rigid.

You can also make a splint using soft materials (such as blankets, towels or pillows) or rigid materials (such as a folded magazine or a board). You can even use an adjacent part of the body as a splint; for example, you can splint an injured finger to the uninjured finger next to it. This is called an anatomic splint.

Triangular bandages are handy to keep in your first aid kit in case you need to make a splint. A triangular bandage can be used to make a sling (a special kind of splint that is used to hold an injured arm against the chest) and to make ties to hold other kinds of splints in place. A "cravat fold" is used to turn a triangular bandage into a tie (Figure 7-2).

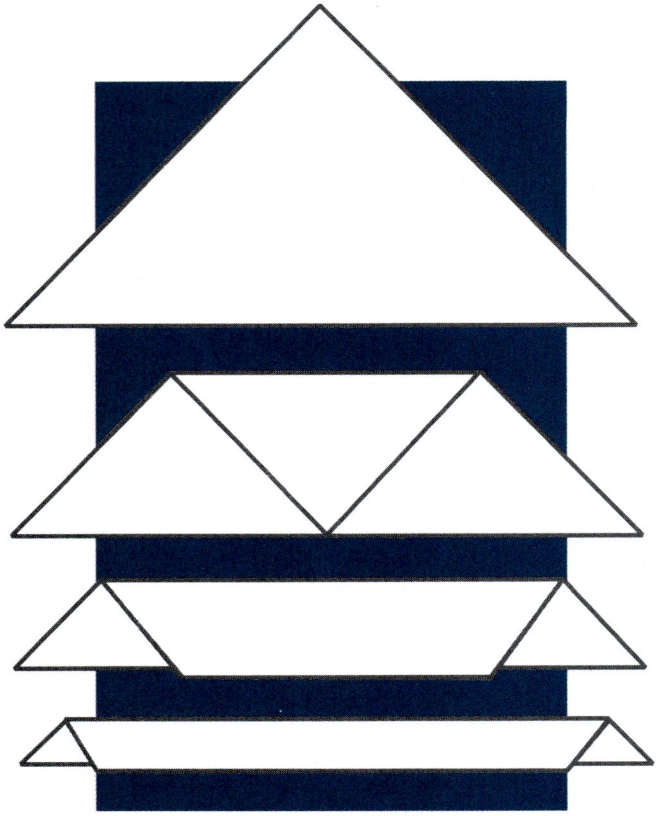

Figure 7-2. A triangular bandage can be folded into a tie using a cravat fold.

General Splinting Principles

You should always splint the body part in the position in which you found it. Never try to straighten or move the body part. If a *joint* is injured, include the bones above and below the joint in the splint and if a *bone* is injured, include the joints above and below the bone in the splint. If you are *not sure* what is injured, include both the bones and the joints above and below the injured area in the splint.

Make sure the splint is long enough to include the joints above and below the injured bone or the bones above and below the injured joint.

Never allow the person to bear weight on an injured lower extremity. Pad splints with gauze to make them more comfortable and help them conform to the shape of the injured body part. Secure the splint in place as per manufacturer's instructions. Some splints have securing devices. For items such as padded boards or improvised splints, you can use folded triangular bandages, roller bandages or other wide strips of cloth.

After splinting, you should elevate the splinted body part, if possible. Finally, check for circulation and sensation beyond the site of injury before and after splinting to make sure that the splint is not too tight. If circulation or sensation changes after splinting, loosen the bandages or other securing mechanism.

See Skill Practice Sheets: Applying a Rigid Splint; Applying a Sling and Binder; Applying a Vacuum Splint in Appendix D.

Nose and Mouth Injuries

Facial trauma can range from minor injuries (cuts and abrasions, bruises, bloody noses and knocked-out teeth) to more severe injuries, such as a fracture of one or more of the facial bones. A person with a facial injury may also have a head, neck or spinal injury, such as a concussion. For these types of injuries, get equipment or tell someone to do so. In some cases, you may need to call 9-1-1.

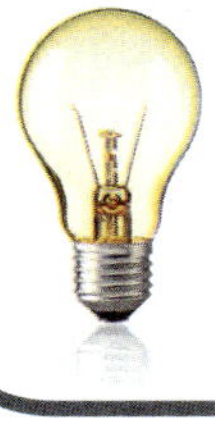

> **THE PROS KNOW.** Although open wounds on the face and scalp can bleed profusely, the bleeding is usually controlled with direct pressure and time.

Nose Injuries

Falling or getting hit in the nose can result in a nosebleed. Other, nontraumatic causes of nosebleeds include breathing dry air and changes in altitude. Certain medical conditions (such as hypertension, or high blood pressure) and the use of certain medications (such as blood thinners) can make a person more susceptible to nosebleeds.

In most cases, you can stop a nosebleed by having the person pinch their nostrils together while sitting with their head slightly forward. Sitting with the head slightly forward helps to keep blood from pooling in the back of the throat, which can lead to choking or, if the blood is swallowed, vomiting. Keep the nostrils pinched shut for at least 5 minutes before checking to see if the bleeding has stopped. If the bleeding has not stopped after 5 minutes, keep pinching the nostrils shut for another 5 minutes. If the bleeding is severe or gushing, call 9-1-1 or the designated emergency number.

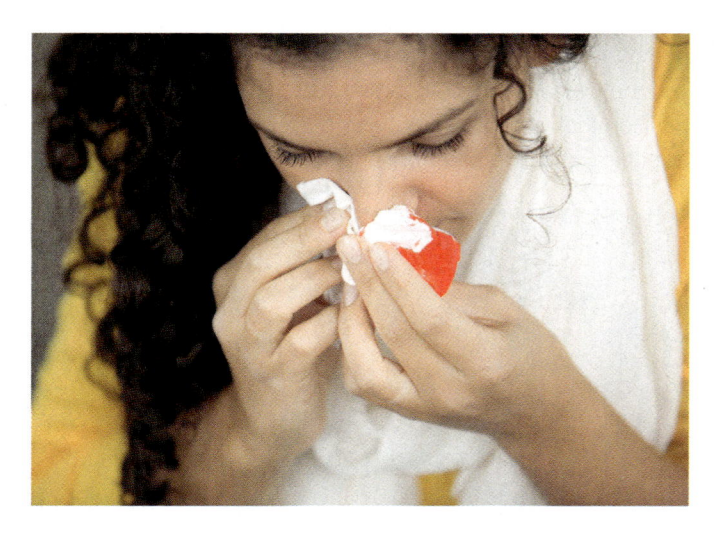

Mouth Injuries

Injuries to the mouth may cause breathing problems if blood or loose teeth block the airway, so make sure the person is able to breathe. If the person is bleeding from the mouth and you do not suspect a serious head, neck or spinal injury, place the person in a seated position leaning slightly forward. This will allow any blood to drain from the mouth. If this position is not possible, place the person on their side in the recovery position. Have the person hold a gauze pad at the site of the bleeding and apply direct pressure to stop the bleeding. (If the person is responsive, having the person apply direct pressure to a wound inside their own mouth is easier and safer than doing it for the person.) With any injury to the face, one needs to consider the possibility of neck or spine injury due to the force.

Lip and Tongue Injuries

For injuries that penetrate the lip, place a rolled gauze pad between the lip and the gum. You can place another gauze pad on the outer surface of the lip. If the tongue is bleeding, apply a gauze pad and direct pressure. Applying a cold pack wrapped in a dry towel to the lips or tongue can help to reduce swelling and ease pain.

Dental Injuries

If a tooth is knocked out, control the bleeding by placing a rolled gauze pad into the space left by the missing tooth and have the person gently bite down to maintain pressure. Try to locate and save the tooth, because a dentist or other healthcare provider may be able to reimplant it.

Be careful to pick up the tooth only by the crown (the part of the tooth that is normally visible above the gum line) rather than by the root. Place the tooth in Hank's Balanced Salt Solution (e.g., Save-A-Tooth®) or in an oral rehydration salt solution, or wrap it in cling film to improve the likelihood of successful reimplantation. If these are not available, place the tooth in cow's milk or saliva. Never place the tooth in tap water.

The person should seek dental or emergency care as soon as possible after the injury. The sooner the tooth is reimplanted, the better the chance that it will survive. Ideally, reimplantation should take place within 30 minutes.

Chest Injuries

The chest cavity contains the heart, the major blood vessels that enter and leave the heart, the lungs, the trachea and most of the esophagus. These vital organs are protected by a bony cage formed by the ribs and breastbone (sternum). Chest injuries may involve the organs and major blood vessels housed in the chest cavity, the bones that form the chest cavity, or both.

Traumatic chest injuries are frequently caused by **blunt trauma**. Penetrating trauma (e.g., a stab or gunshot wound) is also a common cause of traumatic chest injuries. Internal bleeding is likely when a person has sustained significant trauma to the chest.

- **Rib fractures** are a common chest injury associated with blunt trauma. Although painful, a simple broken rib is rarely life-threatening. Broken ribs are less common in children than in adults because children's ribs are more flexible and tend to bend rather than break. However, the forces that can cause a broken rib in adults can severely

bruise the lung tissue of children, which can be a life-threatening injury.
- **Flail chest** occurs when multiple ribs are broken in more than one place, usually as a result of severe blunt trauma. This interferes with the mechanics of breathing because the injured area is not able to expand properly. (Expansion of the chest is what draws air into the lungs.) Flail chest can be life-threatening and is also frequently associated with a **lung contusion** (bruising of the lung tissue).
- **Sucking chest wounds** can occur as a result of penetrating trauma. The puncture wound can allow air to enter the space between the lung and the chest wall. The abnormal collection of air in this space puts pressure on the lung, causing it to collapse (a condition called **pneumothorax**). In addition to putting the person at risk for pneumothorax, the object that caused the puncture wound can injure the organs or vessels contained within the chest cavity and cause varying degrees of internal or external bleeding.

Recognizing Chest Injuries

A person with a broken rib may take small, shallow breaths because normal or deep breathing is uncomfortable or painful. The person usually will attempt to ease the pain by supporting the injured area with a hand or arm.

Signs and symptoms of a more serious chest injury (such as multiple broken ribs, internal bleeding, a lung contusion or a sucking chest wound) could include:

- Difficulty breathing.
- Breathing fast.
- Fast heart rate.
- Flushed, pale, ashen or bluish skin.
- Severe pain at the site of the injury.
- Bruising at the site of a blunt injury, such as that caused by a seat belt.
- Deformity of the chest wall.
- Unusual movement of the chest wall when the person breathes, which may include movement of only one side of the chest or **paradoxical breathing** (when the person inhales, the injured area draws in while the rest of the chest expands, and when the person exhales, the injured area expands while the rest of the chest draws in).
- Coughing up blood, which may be bright red or dark like coffee grounds.
- A "sucking" sound coming from the wound with each breath the person takes (caused by air entering the chest cavity through an open chest wound).
- Signs and symptoms of shock, such as excessive thirst; skin that feels cool or moist and looks pale or bluish; an altered level of consciousness; and a rapid, weak heartbeat.

Call 9-1-1 and get equipment immediately, or tell someone to do so, if the person is showing signs and symptoms of a serious chest injury or if you think that the person might also have a spinal injury.

Giving First Aid Care for Chest Injuries

First aid care for a chest injury depends on the type of injury. See Chapter 6 for first aid care for life-threatening external and internal bleeding.

Rib Fracture

Give the person a pillow or folded blanket to hold against the injured area to provide support and make breathing more comfortable. The person should be evaluated by a healthcare provider, so call 9-1-1 and get equipment or tell someone to do so if it is not possible to safely or comfortably move the person to a vehicle for transport to a healthcare facility. While you are waiting for help to arrive, have the person rest in a position that will make breathing easier, monitor the person's breathing and give care for shock, if necessary.

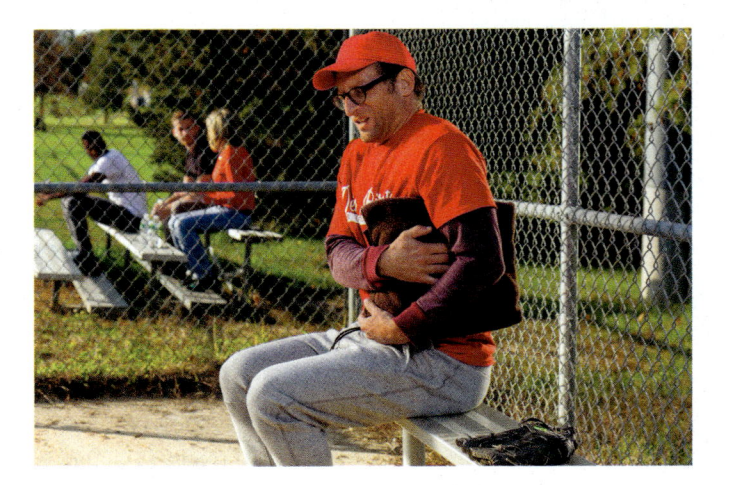

Sucking Chest Wound

The care for a sucking chest wound is slightly different from the care for other types of open wounds. After calling 9-1-1, if external bleeding is present, apply direct pressure to the wound to control the bleeding, but remove each dressing as it becomes saturated with blood and replace it with a clean one as needed. If there is no external bleeding, do not cover the wound. It is important to avoid sealing an open chest wound because doing so could lead to additional life-threatening complications. While you are waiting for help to arrive, monitor the person's breathing and care for shock, if necessary.

Abdominal Injuries

As with chest injuries, abdominal injuries can result from blunt or penetrating trauma and may be accompanied by internal bleeding. It is especially difficult to determine if a person has an abdominal injury if the person is unresponsive and has no visible signs and symptoms of injury. Always suspect an abdominal injury in a person who has multiple injuries. Conversely, if a person has an abdominal injury, be sure to check the person for other injuries because abdominal injuries are often accompanied by injuries to the chest, pelvis or head.

Recognizing Abdominal Injuries

Signs and symptoms of a serious abdominal injury could include:

- Severe pain.
- Organs protruding from the abdomen.
- A tender, swollen or rigid abdomen.
- Bruising over the abdomen.
- Nausea.
- Vomiting (sometimes blood).
- Signs and symptoms of shock, such as excessive thirst; skin that feels cool or moist and looks pale or bluish; an altered level of consciousness; and a rapid, weak heartbeat.

Call 9-1-1 and get equipment immediately, or tell someone to do so, for any serious abdominal injury.

Giving First Aid Care for Abdominal Injuries

After calling 9-1-1, carefully position the person on their back with their knees bent, unless the person has other injuries or that position causes the person pain. While you are waiting for help to arrive, monitor the person's condition and give care for shock, if necessary.

Abdominal organs may protrude through an open wound. If organs are protruding through the wound, do not push them back in and do not apply direct pressure to try and stop minor bleeding. After putting on latex-free disposable gloves, remove clothing from around the wound. Moisten sterile dressings with clean, warm tap water or saline and apply them loosely over the wound. Then cover the dressings loosely with plastic wrap or aluminum foil, if available.

Pelvic Injuries

The pelvis is a ring-shaped group of bones that provides support for the trunk; connects the trunk to the legs; and protects the bladder, the rectum, several major arteries and the reproductive organs. The hip joint is formed by the acetabulum (a cup-shaped indentation on the pelvis) and the upper part of the femur (the thigh bone).

Blunt trauma to the pelvic region can result in pelvic fractures and damage to the internal organs, blood vessels and nerves that are normally protected by the pelvic bones. Usually pelvic fractures result from high-energy impacts (e.g., a motor vehicle collision), but in older adults with osteoporosis (a disease in which loss of bone tissue causes the bones to become fragile and prone to breaking), minor trauma or a fall can result in breaking the pelvis or the upper part of the femur where it forms the hip joint with the pelvis. Pelvic injuries are serious and may be life-threatening because of the risk of damage to major arteries or internal organs. Fractures of bones in this area may cause severe internal bleeding and are associated with an increased risk for death in older adults.

Recognizing Pelvic Injuries

Signs and symptoms of a pelvic injury may include the following:

- Severe pain at the site of the injury
- Bruising, swelling or both at the site of the injury
- Instability of the pelvic bones
- Blood-tinged urine
- Loss of sensation in the legs or an inability to move the legs
- Signs and symptoms of shock, such as excessive thirst; skin that feels cool or moist and looks pale or bluish; an altered level of consciousness; and a rapid, weak heartbeat

Always call 9-1-1 and get equipment immediately, or tell someone to do so, if you suspect a pelvic injury.

Giving First Aid Care for Pelvic Injuries

After calling 9-1-1, avoid moving the person unnecessarily because movement can make the pelvic injury worse, and the person may also have injuries to the lower spine. If possible, try to keep the person lying flat, and give care for shock if necessary.

ENVIRONMENTAL EMERGENCIES

Common environmental emergencies include heat-related illnesses, cold-related illness and injuries, poison exposure, bites and stings, exposure to rash-causing plants and lightning strike injuries.

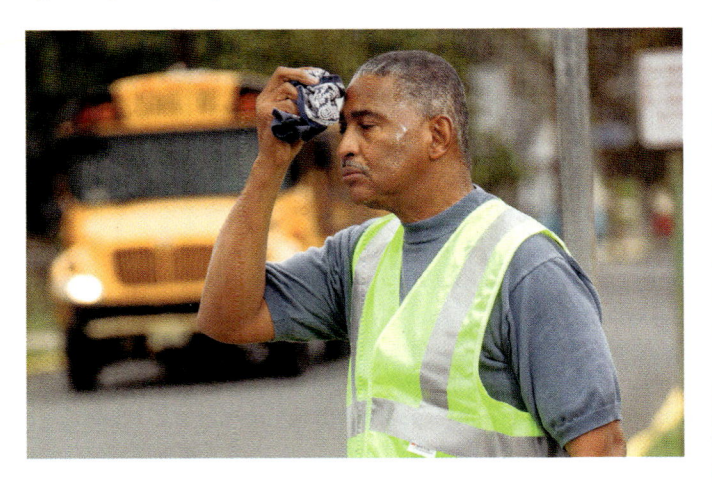

Heat-Related Illnesses

Heat-related illnesses are caused by overexposure to heat and the loss of fluids and electrolytes. While being outdoors is a risk factor for developing a heat-related illness, these illnesses can also affect people who are indoors. People who live or work in buildings that are inadequately cooled or ventilated are at risk, as are those who perform indoor jobs in hot environments (e.g., kitchen and laundry workers, factory workers). People who habitually work or exercise in hot environments tend to become more tolerant of the heat over time but may still be at risk for developing heat-related illnesses, especially when environmental temperatures are very high (e.g., greater than 100° F or 38° C).

Although extremely high environmental temperatures increase the risk for heat-related illnesses, these illnesses can also occur at more moderate environmental temperatures. For example, a person who is doing strenuous work and is clothed in heavy protective clothing may be at risk for experiencing a heat-related illness at a lower environmental temperature. Similarly, a person who is unaccustomed to doing strenuous labor or exercising in the heat may develop a heat-related illness at lower environmental temperatures. Other factors, such as humid air, inadequate fluid intake and personal characteristics (e.g., the presence of certain medical conditions, taking certain medications and the person's age, especially older adults and young children and infants) can increase the risk for heat-related illness.

The three types of heat-related illnesses (in order from least to most severe) are heat cramps, heat exhaustion and heat stroke.

Heat Cramps

Heat cramps are painful muscle spasms, usually in the legs, arms and abdomen, caused by loss of fluids and electrolytes as a result of sweating. These cramps are possibly more common in hot and humid conditions, but they are not directly related to a rise in body temperature.

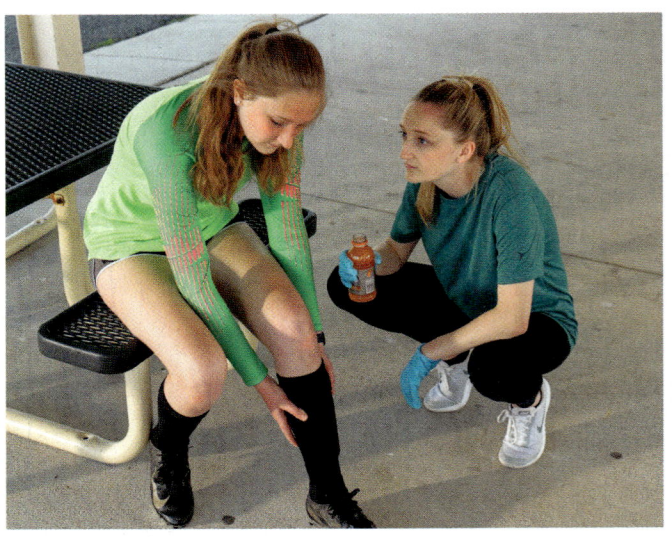

To care for heat cramps, have the person stop the activity associated with the cramping and rest. The person should sip a drink containing electrolytes and carbohydrates (such as a commercial sports drink, coconut water or milk). If a drink containing electrolytes and carbohydrates is not available, have the person drink water. Lightly stretch the muscle and gently massage the area to relieve the cramps. When the cramps stop, the person usually can resume their activity as long as there are no other signs or symptoms of illness. Encourage the person to keep drinking plenty of fluids and watch the person carefully for additional signs or symptoms of heat-related illness.

> **Myth-Information.** *When a person has heat cramps, you should give the person salt tablets to replenish lost sodium.* Salt tablets are not an effective treatment for heat cramps. Consuming a concentrated form of salt can promote loss of fluid from the body, which will make the person's condition worse, not better.

Heat Exhaustion

Heat exhaustion occurs when fluids lost through sweating are not replaced and other cooling mechanisms become compromised. The body's primary mechanism of cooling itself is through sweating. As sweat evaporates from the body, it takes body heat with it, cooling the body. If a person does not take in enough fluids, the body does not have what it needs to make adequate amounts of sweat. Humid environments and environments without good air circulation can make it difficult for the sweat to evaporate. Under these conditions, a person may develop heat exhaustion. Heat exhaustion is often accompanied by dehydration, as the body's excessive production of sweat in an attempt to cool itself depletes fluid levels in the body.

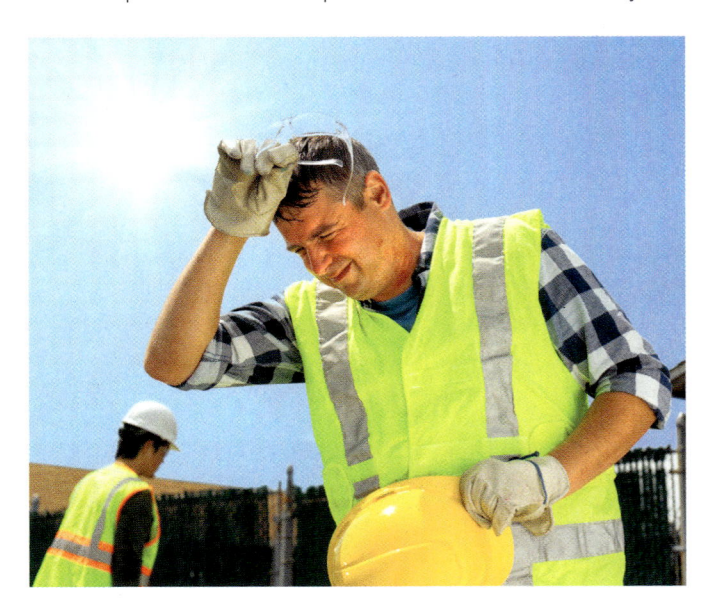

Recognizing Heat Exhaustion

Signs and symptoms of heat exhaustion include fatigue, nausea and/or vomiting, loss of appetite, dehydration, heat cramps, dizziness with fainting possible, and elevated heart and respiratory rate. The person's skin may be cool and clammy, and pale, ashen (gray) or slightly flushed. The person may be weak and not able to stand or walk but will have a normal level of responsiveness.

Giving First Aid Care for Heat Exhaustion

Move the person to a cooler environment with circulating air. Loosen or remove as much clothing as possible and apply cool, wet cloths to the person's skin or spray the person with cool water. Fanning the person may also help by increasing evaporative cooling. If the person is responsive and able to swallow, have the person drink a cool electrolyte- and carbohydrate-containing fluid (such as a commercial sports drink, coconut water or milk). Give water if none of these are available. Do not let the person drink too quickly. Encourage the person to rest in a comfortable position and watch carefully for changes in their condition. Call 9-1-1 and get equipment or tell someone to do so if the person's condition does not improve. The person should wait for several hours after they are no longer having signs and symptoms to resume activity.

If the person is unable to take fluids by mouth, has a change in level of consciousness or vomits, call 9-1-1 and get equipment, or tell someone to do so, because these are indications that the person's condition is getting worse. Stop giving fluids and place the person in the recovery position. Keep the person lying down and continue to take steps to lower the person's body temperature. Monitor the person for signs and symptoms of breathing problems and shock.

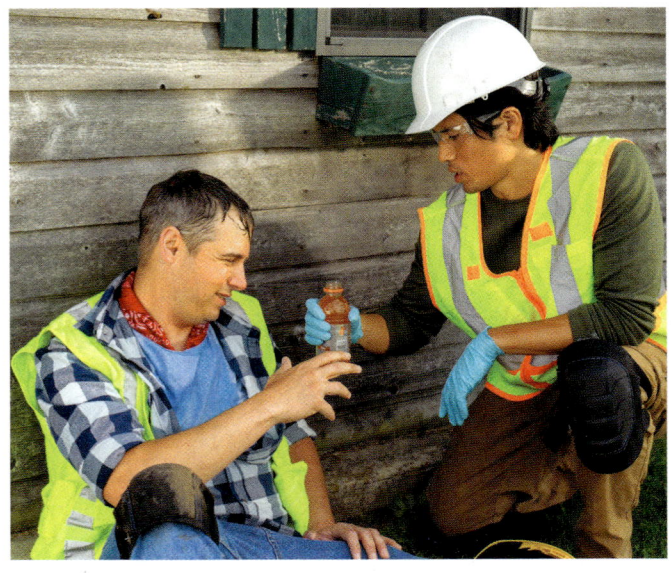

Heat Stroke

Heat stroke is the least common but most severe heat-related illness. It occurs when the body's cooling system becomes completely overwhelmed and stops working. Heat stroke is a life-threatening emergency.

Recognizing Heat Stroke

A person with heat stroke may have moist, pale or flushed skin. They may also experience an absence of sweating or some degree of sweating, unresponsiveness, confusion, seizure, headache, nausea, dizziness, weakness and exhaustion.

The person may vomit. The person's breathing may be rapid and shallow, and their heartbeat may be rapid and weak.

If you suspect a person is experiencing heat stroke, call 9-1-1 and get equipment immediately, or tell someone to do so.

Giving First Aid Care for Heat Stroke

After calling 9-1-1, take steps to rapidly cool the person's body. The preferred way of doing this is to immerse the person up to their neck in cold water, if you can do this safely. If you can't immerse the person in cold water, apply cold, wet cloths or towels to the person's skin. Then apply ice packs over the towels and fan the person. You can also have them take a cold shower. If you are not able to measure and monitor the person's temperature, apply rapid cooling methods for 20 minutes or until the person's condition improves or EMS personnel arrive and begin their care of the person. Finally, it is important to watch for changes in the person's condition and to give care as needed for other conditions that you find.

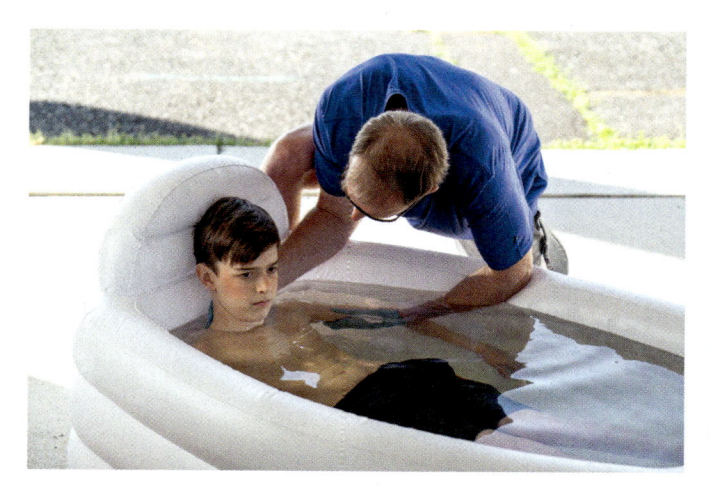

Cold-Related Illnesses and Injuries

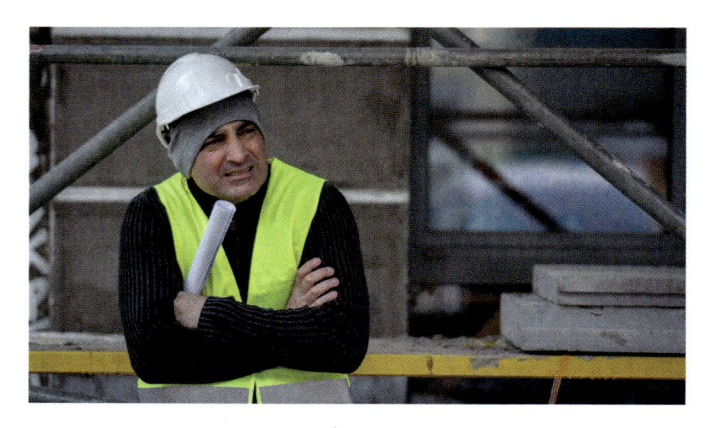

Exposure illnesses and injuries result from exposure to cold air temperatures and/or cold water. In cold temperatures, the body uses shivering to contract the muscles generating heat from energy usage in an attempt to warm the body.

However, prolonged exposure to cold can overwhelm the body's thermoregulatory mechanisms, leading to life-threatening illness. People who are at increased risk for experiencing a first aid emergency due to exposure to cold include:

- Those who work or exercise outdoors.
- Older adults and young children and infants.
- Those with medical conditions.
- Those who take certain medications.

Preventing cold-related illnesses and injuries is key (Box 7-3).

Hypothermia

Hypothermia is a potentially life-threatening, cold-related emergency that occurs when the body loses heat faster than it can produce heat, causing the core body temperature to fall below 95° F (35° C).

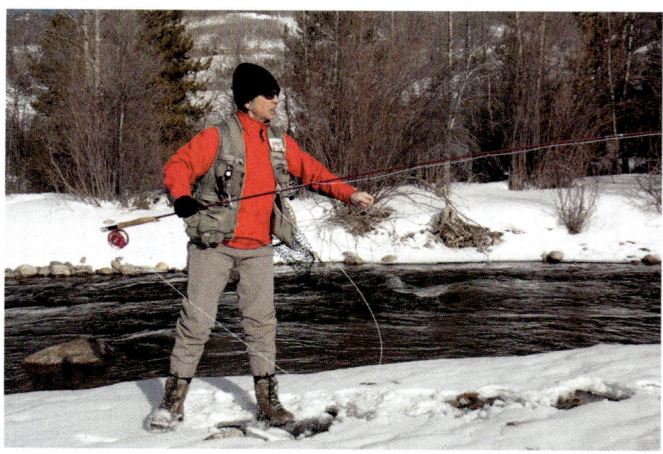

Box 7-3 Dressing for Cold Weather

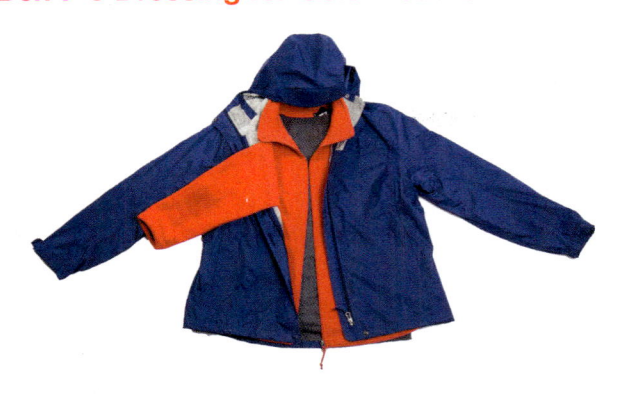

Dressing in layers can help to protect you from illness as a result of exposure to cold external temperatures. The first layer, called the base layer, is next to your skin. The base layer helps to regulate your body temperature by wicking perspiration away from your skin. This is important because if perspiration gets trapped inside your clothes, you can become chilled rapidly, which can lead to hypothermia. The fabrics that are best at wicking sweat away from the skin are silk, merino wool and certain synthetics. Cotton is not a good choice because it traps moisture, rather than wicking it away. The job of the middle layer is insulation. This layer keeps you warm; it helps you retain heat by trapping air close to your body. Natural fibers, such as wool and goose down, are excellent insulators. So is synthetic fleece. Vests, jackets and tights are examples of clothing that can be worn for insulation.

The shell or outer layer protects you from wind, rain or snow. For cold weather, the shell layer should be both waterproof and "breathable." This will keep wind and water from getting inside of the other two layers while allowing perspiration to evaporate. The shell also should be roomy enough to fit easily over the other layers without restricting your movement. In addition to layering your clothes, wear the following to stay warm in cold weather:

- A hat
- A scarf or knit mask that covers your face and mouth
- Sleeves that are snug at the wrist
- Mittens (they are warmer than gloves)
- Water-resistant boots

Typically, the person experiences exposure to cold air temperatures, cold water or both. Hypothermia can also occur when the weather is not cold. Examples of how this can occur include prolonged exposure to a wet or windy environment, wet clothes or sweating.

Recognizing Hypothermia

The person with hypothermia may be shivering, pale and cold to the touch. But as the hypothermia worsens, the person may lose the ability to shiver, which is the mechanism that allows them to create heat. This is a sign that the person's condition is worsening and the person needs immediate medical care.

The person may also be disoriented, indifferent or confused. You may notice that the person has a "glassy" stare. In advanced cases of hypothermia, the person may become unresponsive, and their breathing may slow or stop. There may be slow heart rate, abnormal rhythm, or the heart can stop. The body may feel stiff because the muscles became rigid.

Call 9-1-1 and get equipment immediately, or tell someone to do so, for any case of hypothermia, which is a life-threatening emergency.

Giving First Aid Care for Hypothermia

After calling 9-1-1, if the person is unresponsive and not breathing or only gasping, give CPR and use an automated external defibrillator (AED) if you are trained in these skills.

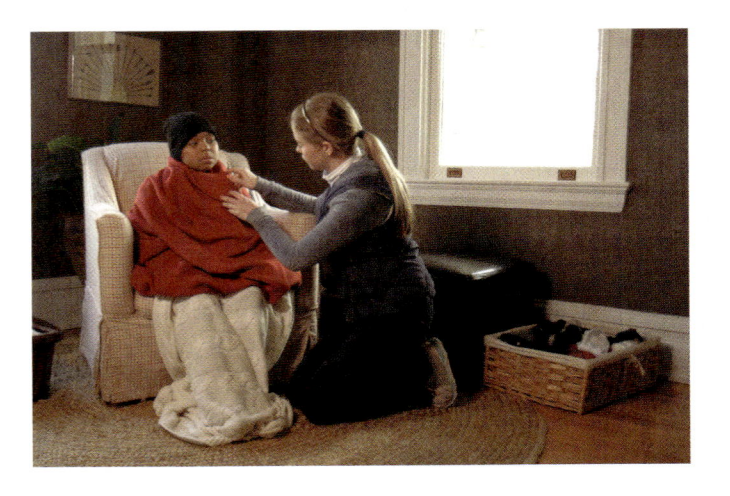

First aid care for the person with hypothermia consists of moving them to a warmer place and warming them slowly. Raising the body temperature must be accomplished gradually. Rapid rewarming, for example, by immersing the person in a hot bath or shower, can lead to dangerous heart rhythms and should be avoided. To gradually rewarm the person, remove any wet clothing, dry the person, and help the person to put on dry clothing (including a hat, gloves and socks). Then wrap the person in dry blankets and plastic sheeting, if available, to hold in body heat. Make sure you cover their head.

If you are far from medical care, position the person near a heat source or apply heating pads or hot water bottles filled with warm water to the body. If you have positioned the person near a heat source, carefully monitor the heat source to avoid burning the person. If you are using heating pads or hot water bottles, wrap them in thin, dry cloths to protect the person's skin. If the person is alert and able to swallow, you can give the person small sips of a warm, non-caffeinated liquid such as broth or warm water. In addition, reassure the person, continue warming them and monitor for changes in condition (including changes in breathing or level of responsiveness and the development of shock) until EMS personnel arrive and begin their care of the person.

> **Myth-Information.** *Giving a person with hypothermia an alcoholic drink can help the person to warm up.* Never give alcohol to a person who has hypothermia. Although alcohol may temporarily make the person feel warmer, it actually increases loss of body heat. You should also avoid giving a person who has hypothermia beverages containing caffeine, because caffeine promotes fluid loss and can lead to dehydration.

Frostbite

Frostbite is an injury caused by freezing of the skin and underlying tissues as a result of prolonged exposure to freezing or subfreezing temperatures. Frostbite can cause the loss of fingers, hands, arms, toes, feet and legs.

Recognizing Frostbite

The frostbitten area is numb, and the skin is cold to the touch and appears waxy. The skin may be white, yellow, blue or red. In severe cases, there may be blisters and the skin may turn black.

If the frostbite is severe or the person is also showing signs and symptoms of hypothermia, call 9-1-1 and get equipment, or tell someone to do so.

Giving First Aid Care for Frostbite

Give care for hypothermia, if necessary. If the frostbite has caused blisters, do not break them. Monitor the person's condition, and if you see that the person is going into shock, give care accordingly.

If the frostbite is mild, you may be able to care for it using first aid. When providing first aid care for frostbite, handle the affected area gently. Never rub the frostbitten area, because this can cause additional damage to the tissue. Remove wet clothing and jewelry (if possible) from the affected area and care for hypothermia, if necessary.

Do not attempt to rewarm the frostbitten area if there is a chance that the body part could refreeze before the person receives medical attention. Once the rewarming process is started, the tissue cannot be allowed to refreeze because refreezing can lead to tissue necrosis (death). Skin-to-skin contact, for example, cupping the affected area in your hands, may be sufficient to rewarm the frostbitten body part if the frostbite is mild. Alternatively, you can rewarm the affected body part by soaking it in warm water until normal color and warmth returns (about 20 to 30 minutes). The water temperature should not be more than 100° F to 105° F (38° C to 40.5° C). If you do not have a thermometer, test the water with your hand. It should feel warm (about body temperature), not hot. After rewarming, loosely bandage the area with a dry, sterile bandage. If the fingers or toes were affected, place cotton or gauze between them before bandaging the area (Figure 7-3, A–B).

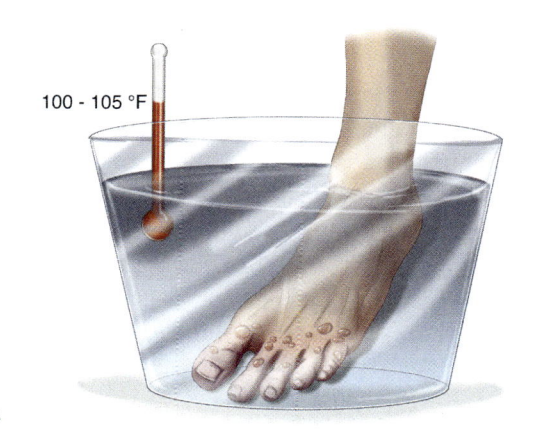

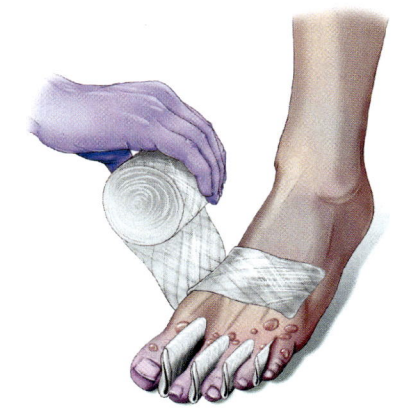

Figure 7-3. To care for frostbite, rewarm the body part by immersing it in warm water (A) and then loosely bandage it (B).

Poison Exposure

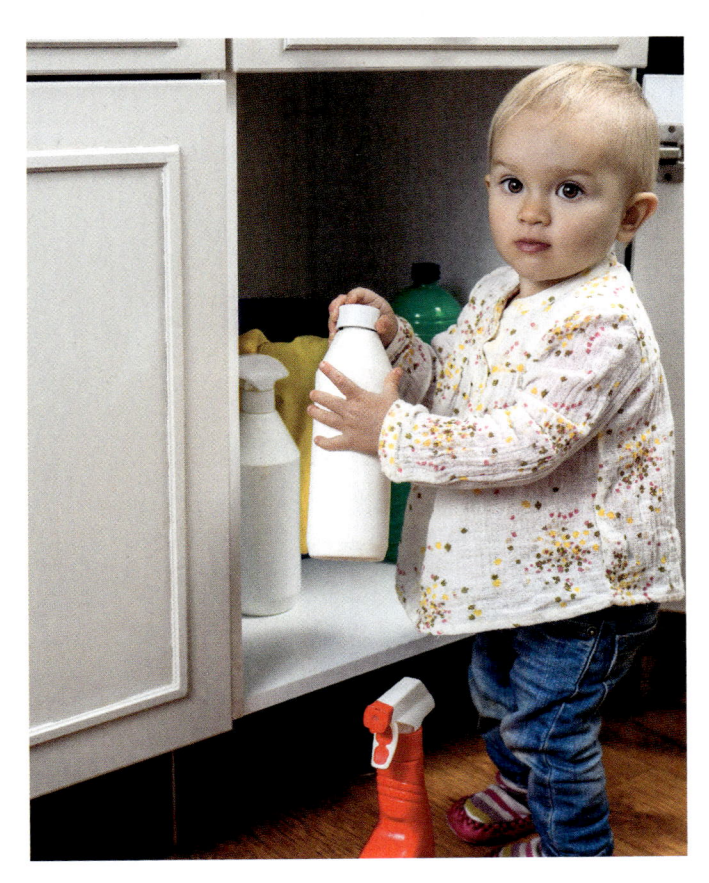

A poison is any substance that causes injury, illness or death if it enters the body. Poisons can be ingested (swallowed), inhaled, absorbed through the skin or eyes, or injected (via a sting or bite). Practically anything can be a poison if it is not meant to be taken into the body. Even some substances that are meant to be taken into the body, such as medications, can be poisonous if they are taken by the wrong person, or if the person takes too much. Combining certain substances can also result in poisoning.

Poisoning can happen anywhere, but most poisonings take place in the home. Children younger than 5 years, especially toddlers, are at the highest risk for poisoning. Children may be attracted to pretty liquids in bottles, sweet-smelling powders, berries on plants that look like they are edible, medications or vitamins that look like candy or detergent pods that look like sweets. Additionally, very young children explore their world by touching and tasting things around them, so even substances that do not look or smell attractive are poison exposure hazards among this age group. Older adults who have medical conditions that cause confusion (such as dementia) or who have impaired vision are also at high risk for unintentional poison exposure. Box 7-4 lists common household poisons, and Box 7-5 describes strategies for reducing the risk for unintentional poison exposure at home.

Box 7-4 Household Poisons

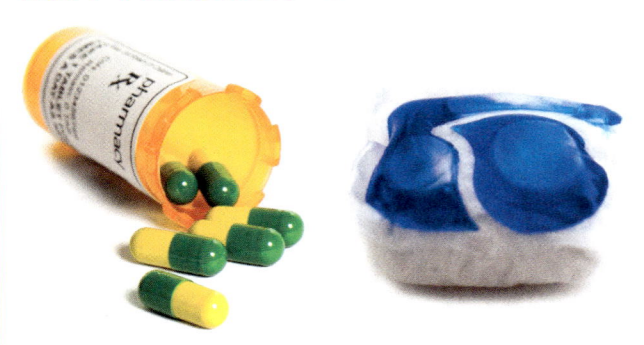

Many everyday household items can be poisonous if they are used incorrectly. Young children and older adults with medical conditions that are associated with confusion (e.g., dementia) or who have impaired vision are at particularly high risk for unintentional poisoning. Common causes of unintentional poisonings at home include:

- Alcohol (found in many products, including hand sanitizer, mouthwash, perfume, cologne, aftershave and vanilla extract).
- Medications (over-the-counter and prescription) and vitamins.
- Cleaning products (detergent "pods" are especially attractive to children).
- Glues and paints.
- Insect and weed killers.
- Car maintenance products (e.g., antifreeze, windshield washer fluid).
- Plants (both houseplants and outdoor plants).
- Oils, lubricants and polishes.
- Personal care products.
- Tobacco.
- Heavy metals, such as lead (often found in old, peeling paint).

Box 7-5 Lowering the Risk for Unintentional Poisoning

If your household contains members who are at high risk for unintentional poisoning, there are simple steps you can take to help keep them safe.

- Keep all medications and household products well out of reach of children or confused older adults, preferably up, away and out of sight.
- Store potentially poisonous substances in locked cabinets.
- Be aware that purses and bags may contain potential poisons (such as medications or hand sanitizer). Avoid putting bags or purses down where they are within reach of curious children or confused older adults.
- Closely supervise children and confused older adults, especially in areas where potential poisons are commonly stored (such as kitchens, bathrooms and garages).
- Keep medications and products in their original containers with their original labels in place.
- Use poison symbols to identify potentially poisonous substances and teach children the meaning of the symbols.
- Be aware that a child or confused older adult may try to consume products that feature fruit on the label (e.g., cleaning products), so take care when storing these.
- Never call a medicine "candy" to entice a child to take it, even if the medicine has a pleasant candy-like flavor.
- Use child-resistant safety caps on containers of medication and other potentially dangerous products, but do not assume that children cannot open them; there is no such thing as "childproof."
- Dispose of medications and other potentially poisonous substances properly. Check with your local government for procedures for the safe disposal of unused and expired medications and other hazardous materials.

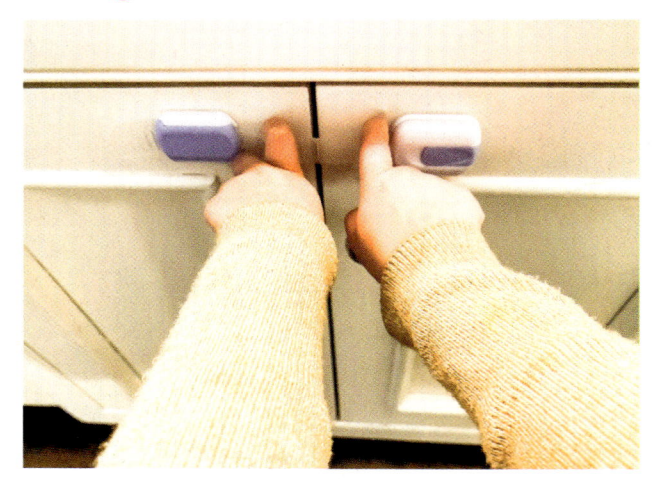

Common causes of death as a result of poison exposure include drug overdose (of over-the-counter, prescription and illicit or "street" drugs), alcohol poisoning and carbon monoxide poisoning (Box 7-6). A specific type of drug overdose, opioid overdose is covered in Chapter 5: Sudden Illness.

Recognizing Poison Exposure

Signs and symptoms of poison exposure vary depending on the type and amount of poison taken into the body and the way it enters the body. The person may experience:

- Abdominal pain, nausea, vomiting or diarrhea.
- Abnormal skin color or sweating.

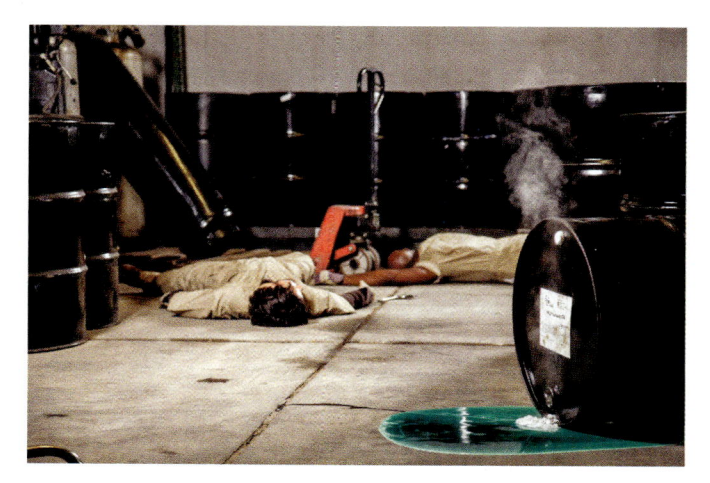

They may also experience life-threatening conditions such as:

- Trouble breathing, breathing too fast or breathing too slow and shallow breathing.
- Fast or slow heart rate.
- Unresponsiveness, changes in level of responsiveness, seizures, headache, dizziness or weakness.

Your check of the scene, initial impression and check of the person will often yield clues that point to poisoning as the cause of the person's illness. For example, you may note an open or spilled container, an unusual odor, burns around the person's mouth, a strange odor on the person's breath or other people in the area who are also ill.

If you think that a person has been poisoned, try to find out:

- The type of poison.
- The quantity taken.
- When it was taken.
- How much the person weighs.

This information can help poison control, 9-1-1, and you and others to give the most appropriate care.

If the person who has been exposed to a poison shows signs and symptoms of a life-threatening condition (e.g., unresponsiveness, changes in level of responsiveness, seizures, headache, dizziness or weakness, fast or slow

142   Chapter 7 | Injuries and Environmental Emergencies

Box 7-6 Lethal Poisons

There are many different types of poisoning, but three in particular warrant special mention because they are common and can be fatal: drug overdose, alcohol poisoning and carbon monoxide poisoning.

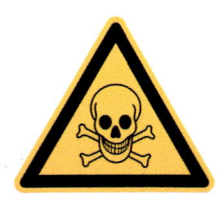

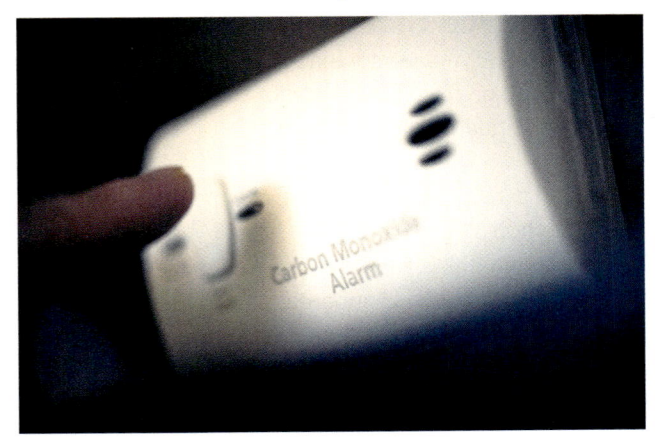

Drug Overdose

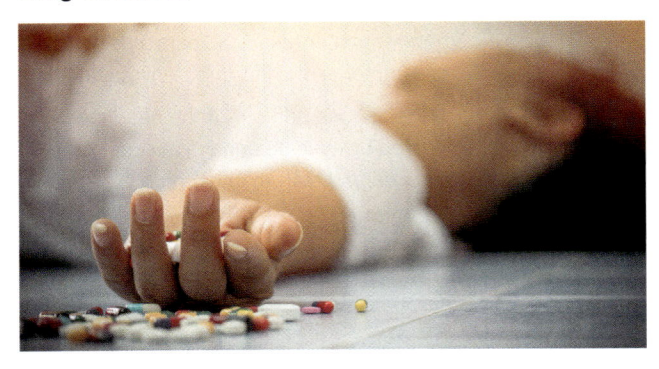

Drugs (whether over-the-counter, prescription or illicit) are frequently a cause of death as a result of poisoning. Drug overdose may be accidental or intentional. Signs and symptoms will vary depending on the drug but may include loss of responsiveness, changes in behavior, changes in breathing and heart rate, and nausea or vomiting. If you suspect a drug overdose, call 9-1-1 or the designated emergency number if the person:

- Is unresponsive or seems to be losing consciousness.
- Is having difficulty breathing.
- Has persistent pain or pressure in the chest or abdomen.
- Is vomiting blood or passing blood.
- Has a seizure, severe headache or slurred speech.
- Is aggressive or uncooperative.
- Is showing signs of shock.

While you are waiting for EMS personnel to arrive, try to find out from others at the scene what substance or substances the person may have taken. Keep the person covered to minimize shock.

Opioid drugs, such as heroin and oxycodone, are a common cause of drug overdose in the United States. Recognizing and giving first aid care for opioid overdose is covered in depth in Chapter 5: Sudden Illness.

Alcohol Poisoning

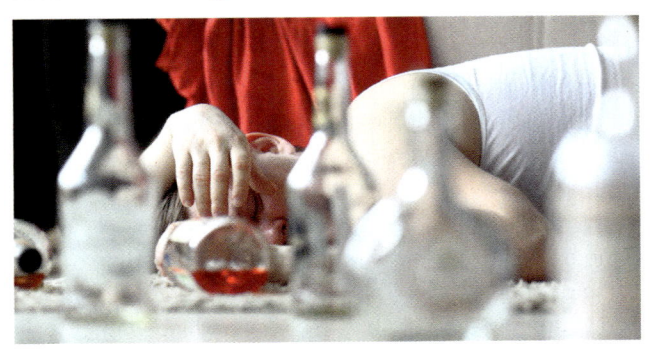

Alcohol poisoning is caused by drinking large quantities of alcohol in a short period of time (binge drinking). The National Institute on Alcohol Abuse and Alcoholism defines binge drinking as a pattern of drinking that brings a person's blood alcohol concentration (BAC) to 0.08 percent or more. This typically happens when a man consumes 5 or more drinks over a period of about 2 hours, or when a woman consumes 4 or more drinks over the same amount of time. Alcohol is a depressant that affects the central nervous system. Very high levels of alcohol in the bloodstream can affect the brain's ability to control breathing, heart rate and body temperature, resulting in death. Signs and symptoms of alcohol poisoning include loss of consciousness, slow or irregular breathing, vomiting, seizures and hypothermia. If you suspect alcohol poisoning, call 9-1-1 and get equipment, or tell someone to do so immediately. Place the person in the recovery position and take steps to keep the airway clear as needed until EMS personnel arrive and begin their care of the person.

Carbon Monoxide Poisoning

Carbon monoxide is a gas that is produced whenever a fuel such as gas, oil, kerosene, diesel, wood or charcoal is burned. When equipment that burns these fuels is ventilated properly, carbon monoxide is not a problem. But if the equipment or ventilation system is faulty, or if equipment that is only supposed to be run outdoors is run inside an enclosed area, toxic levels of carbon monoxide can build up quickly, leading to carbon monoxide poisoning. Carbon monoxide poisoning is often called a "silent killer" because the gas has no smell and you cannot see it. Signs and symptoms of carbon monoxide poisoning include drowsiness, confusion, headache, dizziness, weakness, and nausea or vomiting. A person with signs or symptoms of carbon monoxide poisoning needs fresh air and medical attention immediately. Remove the person from the area if you can do so without endangering yourself and call 9-1-1 or the designated emergency number.

> **Box 7-7 Poison Control Centers**
>
> There are 55 regional poison control centers in the United States. By dialing the national Poison Help hotline (1-800-222-1222), you will be put in touch with the poison control center that serves your area. The call is toll free, and the phone number works from anywhere in the United States. The poison control centers are staffed by medical professionals who have access to information about most types of poisoning. They can tell you what care to give if you think or know that someone has been poisoned.
>
> Callers are often able to get the help they need from the poison control center without having to call 9-1-1 when the person is not showing signs of a life-threatening condition. This helps to reduce the workload of EMS personnel and also reduces the number of emergency room visits. Of course, in some cases, the poison control center staff member may tell you to call 9-1-1, and, remember, you should always call 9-1-1 or the designated emergency number first if the person is showing signs or symptoms of a life-threatening condition.
>
> Be prepared: Keep the telephone number of the national Poison Help hotline posted by every telephone in your home or office! The service is free and staff members are available 24 hours a day, 7 days a week.

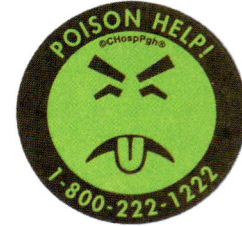

heart rate, difficulty breathing) or if multiple people are affected, call 9-1-1 and get equipment immediately or tell someone to do so.

Giving First Aid Care for Poison Exposure

After calling 9-1-1, if a person has been exposed to poison, remove the person from the source of the poison if you can do so without endangering yourself.

If the person is responsive and alert, call the national Poison Help hotline at 1-800-222-1222. When you dial this number, your call is routed to the regional poison control center that serves your area, based on the area code and exchange of the phone number you are calling from (Box 7-7). The poison control center staff member will tell you what care to give.

Do not give the person anything to eat or drink unless the poison control center staff member tells you to do so. Also, if you do not know what the poison was, and the person vomits, save a sample for analysis.

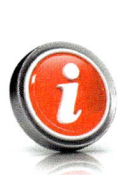

> **Myth-Information.** *If a person has been poisoned, you should make the person vomit to get rid of the poison.* Inducing vomiting in a person who has been poisoned often causes additional harm and is not recommended. Sometimes the person may vomit on their own, but you should never give the person anything to make them vomit unless you are specifically instructed to do so by the poison center staff member.

Bites and Stings

Bites and stings can range in severity from mildly irritating to life-threatening. When a person is bitten or stung, proper first aid care can help to limit complications and speed healing and may even be lifesaving.

Animal Bites

Any animal that has teeth, whether domesticated (e.g., pets or livestock) or wild, can be the source of a bite wound. When the animal is unknown to the person (e.g., a stray or wild animal), rabies may be a concern (Box 7-8).

Recognizing Animal Bites

Animal bites may result in bruising, breaks in the skin or both. Open wounds, such as avulsion wounds and lacerations, may be accompanied by a great deal of bleeding. Puncture wounds typically do not bleed as much.

Always call 9-1-1 and get equipment, or tell someone to do so, if the wound is bleeding heavily and/or the person was bitten by a wild or stray animal or if you suspect that the animal might have rabies.

Giving First Aid Care for Animal Bites

If the wound is deep or extensive, bleeding heavily or uncontrollably, or carries a high risk for infection (e.g., a puncture wound), medical care will be needed. The person may need stitches, a tetanus booster shot or both. If the wound is bleeding heavily, take steps to control bleeding.

If the bleeding is minimal, stop any minor bleeding using direct pressure. Then, wash the wound with soap and water and then rinse with clean, running water. Apply a small amount of antibiotic wound ointment, cream or gel

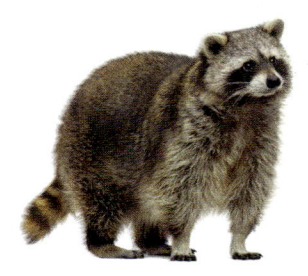

> **Box 7-8 Rabies**
>
> Rabies is a serious infection that attacks the brain and spinal cord and causes death if it is not treated. The virus that causes rabies is spread when an animal that has the disease bites another animal or a person. Wild animals (such as foxes, skunks, bats and raccoons) can carry rabies. Pets and livestock can also carry rabies if they are not vaccinated against it.
>
> Animals with rabies may act strangely. For example, those that are usually active at night may be active in the daytime. A wild animal that usually tries to avoid people might not run away when people are in the area. Rabid animals may drool, appear to be partially paralyzed or act aggressively or strangely quiet.
>
> Call 9-1-1 or tell someone to do so if a person is bitten by an animal that could have rabies. If possible, try to remember details about the animal's behavior and appearance, and where you last saw it. When you call 9-1-1 or the designated emergency number, the dispatcher will direct the proper authorities, such as animal control, to the scene.
>
> A person who is bitten by an animal that might have rabies must get medical attention immediately. Treatment for rabies includes a series of injections to build up immunity that will help fight the disease.

to the wound if the person has no known allergies or sensitivities to the ingredients, and then cover the wound with a dressing and bandage. The person should monitor the wound over the next several days to make sure that it is healing well with no signs of infection.

Venomous Snake Bites

Venomous snakes found in the United States include rattlesnakes, copperheads, cottonmouths (water moccasins) and coral snakes (Table 7-1). Prompt medical care significantly reduces the likelihood of dying from a venomous snake bite. Most deaths from venomous snake bites occur because the person had an allergic reaction to the venom or is in poor health, or because too much time passed before they received medical care.

Recognizing Venomous Snake Bites

Signs and symptoms of a possibly venomous snakebite include a pair of puncture wounds and localized redness, pain and swelling in the area of the bite.

Call 9-1-1 and get equipment immediately, or tell someone to do so, for any snakebite. If you are not sure whether the snake bite was caused by a venomous snake, call 9-1-1 anyway. Do not waste time trying or take the risk to find and capture the snake for identification, and do not wait for life-threatening signs and symptoms of poisoning to appear.

Giving First Aid Care for Venomous Snake Bites

After calling 9-1-1, keep the injured area still and lower than the heart. The person should walk only if absolutely necessary. Wash the wound with soap and water and cover the bite with a clean, dry dressing.

Pressure immobilization bandaging, with the use of an elastic bandage, may be considered by those trained in proper application following the suspected bite of a coral snake in the United States if the transport time to the hospital may be prolonged. However, pressure immobilization bandaging *should not be used* following the bite of a pit viper in the United States and Canada. Pit vipers include rattlesnakes, cottonmouths (water moccasins) and copperheads.

Applying an elastic (pressure immobilization) bandage after a coral snake bite will help to slow the spread of the venom through the lymphatic system, control swelling and provide support. To apply an elastic bandage:

- Check the skin on the side of the bite farthest away from the heart for feeling, warmth and color.
- Place the end of the bandage against the skin, beginning at the point farthest from the heart.
- To cover a long body section, such as an arm or calf, use overlapping turns and gently stretch the bandage

TABLE 7-1 Venomous Snakes

SNAKE	USUALLY FOUND
Rattlesnake	- Across the United States - Mountains, prairies, deserts and beaches - Sunning themselves near logs, boulders or in open areas
Copperhead	- Eastern United States, extending as far west as Texas - Forests, rocky areas and near sources of water like swamps and rivers
Cottonmouth (water moccasin)	- Southeastern United States - Frequently found in and around water (wetland areas, rivers and lakes)
Coral snake **Note:** *To differentiate coral snakes from nonvenomous king snakes, which have similar coloration but in a different pattern, think "Red on yellow, dangerous fellow."*	- Southern United States - Wooded, sandy or marshy areas - Tend to hide in leaf piles and burrow into the ground

as you wrap. To cover a joint, such as the knee or ankle, use overlapping figure-eight turns to support the joint (Figure 7-4, A–B).
- Check the snugness of the bandage—it should be snug, but you should be able to slide a finger easily underneath it.
- Check again for feeling, warmth and color, especially in the fingers and toes, after you have applied the elastic bandage. By checking before and after bandaging, you may be able to tell if any changes (e.g., tingling or numbness, cool or pale skin) are from the elastic bandage or the injury.

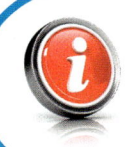

Myth-Information. *Actions such as applying a tourniquet, cutting the wound, applying suction, applying ice or applying electricity can help to slow the spread of venom throughout the body. None of these measures are effective for slowing the spread of venom. In fact, they are likely to cause pain and injury. Your time is better spent seeking medical attention as quickly as possible.*

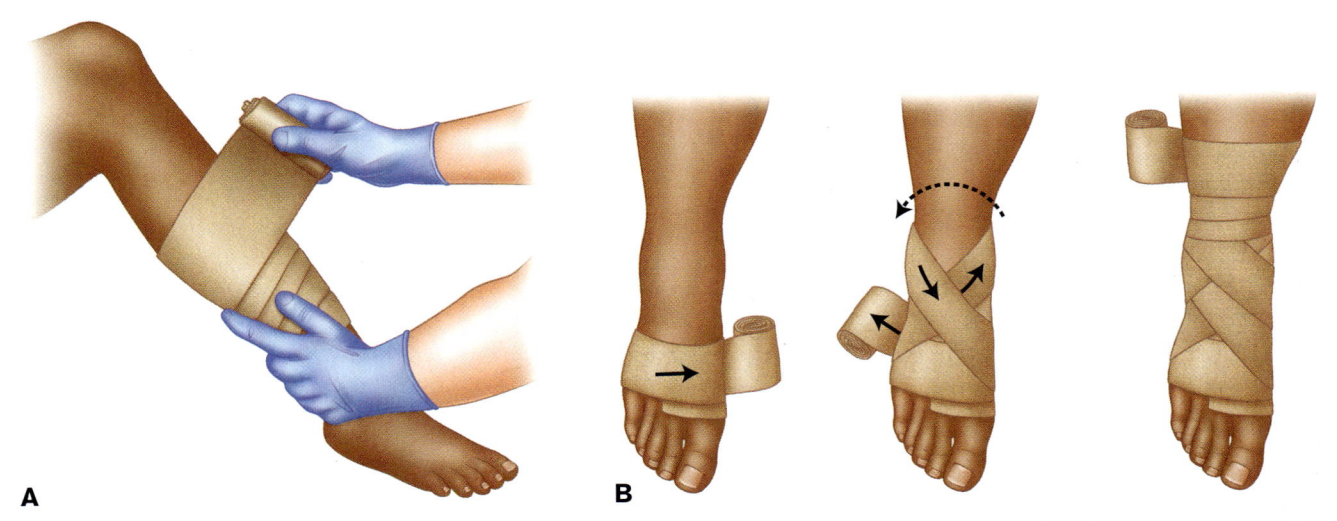

Figure 7-4. To apply a pressure immobilization bandage over a long body section, use overlapping turns and gently stretch the bandage as you wrap (A). To cover a joint, use overlapping figure-eight turns (B).

Spider Bites

Few spiders in the United States can cause serious illness or death. The bites of harmless spiders cause reactions similar to that of a bee sting (e.g., swelling, redness, and stinging or pain at the site).

Dangerous spiders that live in the United States include the brown recluse spider (also known as the violin or fiddleback spider) and the black widow spider (Table 7-2). The bites of the black widow and brown recluse spiders can, in rare cases, kill a person.

Recognizing Spider Bites

Signs and symptoms of spider bites depend on the amount of venom injected and the person's sensitivity to the venom. Most spider bites heal with no adverse effects or scarring. Signs and symptoms of venomous spider bites can seem identical to those of other conditions and therefore can be difficult to recognize. The only way to be certain that a spider has bitten a person is to have witnessed it.

If you suspect that someone has been bitten by a black widow spider or brown recluse spider, call 9-1-1 and get equipment or tell someone to do so.

TABLE 7-2 Venomous Spiders	
SPIDER	**USUALLY FOUND**
Black widow spider	■ Across the United States, but most common in the southern states ■ Outdoors: woodpiles, rock piles, brush piles, hollow stumps, rodent burrows, sheds and garages ■ Indoors: cluttered, undisturbed areas in attics, basements and crawlspaces
Brown recluse spider	■ Midwestern and southeastern United States ■ Under porches and in woodpiles

Widow Spiders

Widow spiders can be black, red or brown. The black widow spider is black with a reddish hourglass shape on the underside of its body and is the most venomous of the widow spiders. The bite of the black widow spider is the most painful and deadly of the widow spiders, especially in very young children and older adults. The bite usually causes an immediate sharp pinprick pain, followed by dull pain in the area of the bite. However, the person often does not know that they have been bitten until the person starts to feel ill or notices a bite mark or swelling. Other signs and symptoms of a black widow spider bite include:

- Rigid muscles in the shoulders, chest, back and abdomen.
- Restlessness.
- Anxiety.
- Dizziness.
- Headache.
- Excessive sweating.
- Weakness.
- Drooping or swelling of the eyelids.

Brown Recluse Spiders

The brown recluse spider has a distinctive violin-shaped pattern on the back of its front body section. The bite of the brown recluse spider may produce little or no pain initially. Pain in the area of the bite develops an hour or more later. A blood-filled blister forms under the surface of the skin, sometimes in a target or bull's-eye pattern. Over time, the blister increases in size and eventually ruptures, leading to tissue destruction and a black scab.

Giving First Aid Care for Spider Bites

If you suspect that someone has been bitten by a black widow spider or brown recluse spider, after calling 9-1-1 wash the area with soap and water. Apply a cold pack wrapped in a thin, dry towel. Keep the bitten area elevated and as still as possible.

To care for a spider bite from a harmless spider, wash the area with soap and water; apply an antibiotic wound ointment, cream or gel to the wound if the person has no known allergies or sensitivities to the ingredients. Applying a cold pack wrapped in a thin, dry towel can help to reduce pain and swelling.

Tick Bites

Ticks attach themselves to any warm-blooded animal with which they come into direct contact, including people. When ticks attach themselves to the skin, they can spread pathogens from their mouths into the person's body. These pathogens can cause serious illnesses, such as Lyme disease and Rocky Mountain spotted fever. Box 7-9 describes strategies for limiting exposure to ticks.

Box 7-9 Limiting Exposure to Ticks

Ticks are found in wooded, brushy areas; in tall grass; and in leaf litter on the ground. When engaging in activities in environments where ticks are likely to be, lower your risk for picking up a tick by using the following strategies.

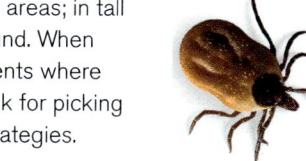

- Limit the amount of exposed skin. Wear long-sleeved shirts and long pants. Tuck your shirt into your pants and your pant legs into your socks or boots.
- Wear light-colored clothing to make it easier to see ticks on your clothing.
- Stay in the midcle of trails. Avoid underbrush and tall grass.
- Conduct a full-body check for ticks after being outdoors.
- Check the scalp, under the arms, in and around the ears, inside the navel, around the waist, behind the knees and between the legs. If you are outdoors for an extended period of time, check several times throughout the day.
- Consider using an insect repellent if you will be in a grassy or wooded area for a long period of time or if you know that the tick population in the area is high. Use repellents sparingly. One application will last 4 to 8 hours. Heavier or more frequent applications do not increase effectiveness.

○ DEET is the active ingredient in many insect repellents. The amount of DEET contained in the product can range from less than 10 percent to over 30 percent. The more DEET that a product contains, the longer it will provide protection. Products with 30 percent DEET are as safe as products with 10 percent DEET when used properly.

- Apply products that contain DEET only once a day, or according to the manufacturer's instructions.
- Do not use DEET on infants younger than 2 months.
- Do not use a product that combines a DEET-containing insect repellent with sunscreen. Sunscreens wash off and need to be reapplied often. DEET does not wash off with water. Repeating applications may increase absorption of DEET through the skin, possibly leading to toxicity.

○ To apply repellent to your face, first spray it on your hands and then apply it from your hands to your face. Avoid sensitive areas such as the lips and eyes.
○ Never put repellents on children's hands. They may put them in their eyes or mouth.
○ Never use repellents on an open wound or irritated skin.

To lower the risk for tick-borne illnesses, always check for ticks immediately after outdoor activities. Most experts believe that the longer the tick stays attached to the skin, the greater the chances are of infection, so it is a good practice to check for ticks at least once daily after having been outdoors. Get equipment and promptly remove any ticks that you find before they become swollen with blood.

To remove a tick, put on gloves. Using fine-tipped, pointed tweezers with a smooth inside surface, grasp the tick at the head as close to the skin as possible. Pull upward slowly and steadily without twisting until the tick releases its hold (Figure 7-5). Seal the tick in a container to help the healthcare provider with identifying the type of tick later. Wash the area with soap and warm water and then apply an antibiotic wound ointment, cream or gel if the person has no known allergies or sensitivities to the ingredients. If you are unable to remove the tick, or if you think that the tick's mouth parts are still embedded in the skin, the person should see a healthcare provider.

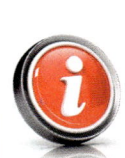

> **Myth-Information.** *To remove a tick, burn it off with a match or smother it with petroleum jelly or nail polish.* These folk remedies are not the best way to go about removing a tick. They rely on the tick detaching itself, which could take hours. As long as the tick's mouth parts are in contact with the skin, the tick is potentially transmitting disease. The goal is to remove the tick in one piece as quickly as possible. The best tool for doing this is a pair of fine-tipped tweezers or a special tick removal tool, such as a tick key.

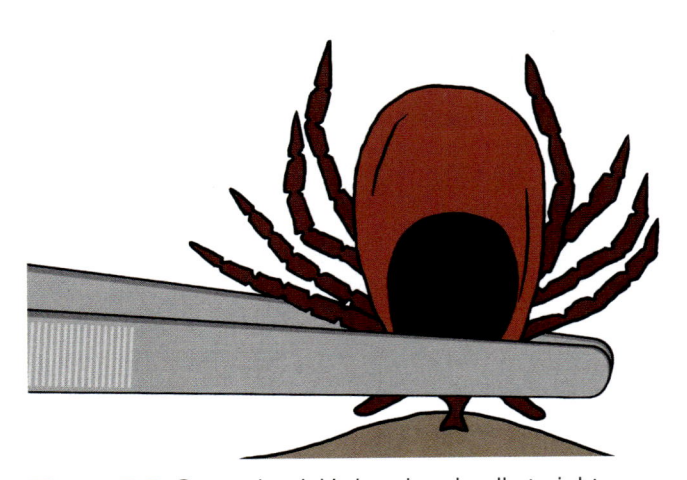

Figure 7-5. Grasp the tick's head and pull straight up.

The person should be monitored for several days for signs and symptoms of infection as a result of the tick exposure. Common signs and symptoms of tick-borne illnesses include rashes, fever, muscle and joint aches and pains, and fatigue.

Insect Stings

Most of the time, insect stings are merely uncomfortable. However, allergic reactions and anaphylaxis are always a concern.

Recognizing Insect Stings

Signs and symptoms of an insect sting include a quick, sharp pain at the site of the sting, often accompanied by pain, itching, swelling and redness. You may see the stinger still embedded in the skin. If the person is allergic to insect stings, the person will show signs and symptoms of an allergic reaction or anaphylaxis (see Chapter 5).

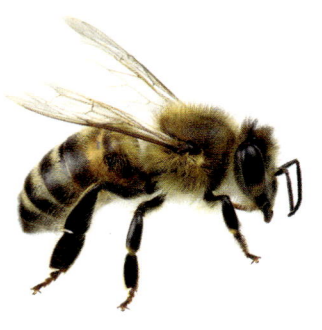

If the person is showing signs and symptoms of anaphylaxis, call 9-1-1 immediately and get equipment or tell someone to do so. If you do not need to call 9-1-1, get equipment or tell someone to do so.

Giving First Aid Care for Insect Stings

In the case of anaphylaxis, after calling 9-1-1 give appropriate first aid care (see Chapter 5: Sudden Illness).

For an uncomplicated insect sting it is important to remove the stinger as quickly as possible. It is best to use clean fingernails or tweezers to grasp and pull the stinger out of the skin. Wash the area with soap and warm water and then apply an antibiotic wound ointment, cream or gel if the person has no known allergies or sensitivities to the ingredients. To reduce swelling and pain, apply a cold pack wrapped in a thin, dry towel to the site.

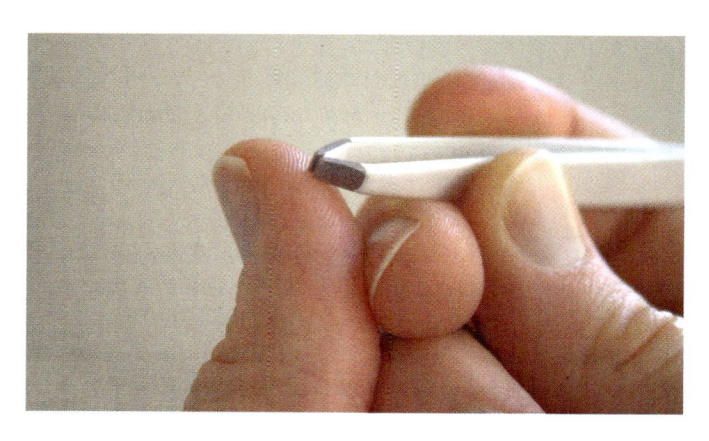

Scorpion Stings
Scorpions live in dry regions, such as the southwestern United States and Mexico. They live under rocks, logs and the bark of certain trees. They are most active at night. Like spiders, only a few species of scorpions have a sting that can cause death.

Recognizing Scorpion Stings
A scorpion sting causes pain, tingling, burning and numbness at the site. Life-threatening signs and symptoms that affect the whole body (such as numbness, difficulty breathing and seizures) may develop.

Giving First Aid Care for Scorpion Stings
It is difficult to distinguish highly poisonous scorpions from nonpoisonous scorpions, so treat every scorpion sting as a medical emergency and seek immediate medical care.

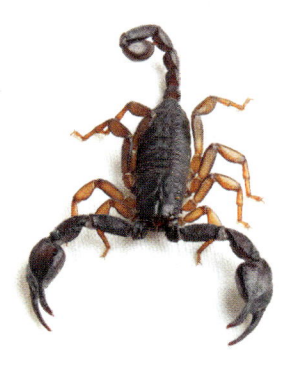

Marine Life Stings
Many forms of marine life (such as jellyfish, stingrays, sea urchins, stinging coral and spiny fish) cause stinging wounds (Table 7-3). Stings from marine life can have effects that range from merely painful to very serious (such as allergic reactions that can cause breathing and heart problems, paralysis or even death).

Recognizing Marine Life Stings
Signs and symptoms of marine life stings include pain and swelling at the site. You may also see a puncture wound or laceration. If the person is allergic to marine life stings, the person will show signs and symptoms of an allergic reaction or anaphylaxis (see Chapter 5).

Call 9-1-1 and get equipment, or tell someone to do so, if the person has been stung by a lethal jellyfish, does not know what stung them, has a history of allergic reactions to marine life stings, is stung on the face or neck, or you note signs and symptoms of shock or anaphylaxis, including trouble breathing. If you do not need to call 9-1-1, get equipment or tell someone to do so.

Giving First Aid Care for Marine Life Stings
Jellyfish Stings
Get the person out of the water as soon as possible, then take steps to remove any remaining tentacles and then neutralize the toxin and reduce pain.

Carefully remove any tentacles with a gloved hand, a hand wrapped in a plastic bag or a towel, or by using a blunt object such as a stick or plastic utensil. Lifting or pulling the tentacles off of the skin is preferable to scraping them off. If you do not have these items to remove any remaining tentacles, you can use seawater to flush the area.

After removing any remaining tentacles, immerse the affected area in water as hot as the person can tolerate without scalding them (no more than about 113° F [45° C] if the temperature can be measured) for at least 20 minutes or until the pain is relieved. If hot water immersion or a shower is not available, use a chemical heat pack or another hot item, such as a hot rock or hot sand. You should wrap a heat pack or hot items in a thin, dry towel to protect the skin from a burn.

If heat sources are not available, or after you have applied heat, you can apply lidocaine gel to relieve pain, if available. Do not rub the area or apply an elastic (pressure immobilization) bandage.

Stingray, Sea Urchin or Spiny Fish Stings
If you know the sting is from a stingray, sea urchin or spiny fish, flush the wound with tap water. Ocean water also may be used. Keep the injured part still and soak the affected area in water as hot as the person can tolerate for at least 20 minutes or until the pain is relieved. Check with a healthcare provider to determine if a tetanus

TABLE 7-3 Venomous Marine Life	
MARINE LIFE	**USUALLY FOUND**
Jellyfish	■ East and west coasts of the continental United States
Portuguese man-of-war (bluebottle jellyfish)	■ Tropical and subtropical waters
Stingray	■ Tropical and subtropical waters
Sea urchin	■ Oceans all over the world (warm and cold water) ■ In rock pools and mud, on wave-exposed rocks, on coral reefs, in kelp forests and in sea grass beds

shot is needed and monitor the wound for signs and symptoms of infection.

Exposure to Rash-Causing Plants

Plants such as poison ivy, poison sumac and poison oak (Table 7-4) are covered with an oil called **urushiol** that causes an allergic skin reaction in many people. In people who are sensitive to urushiol, touching or brushing against the plant or other items contaminated with urushiol causes an itchy, red rash with bumps or blisters. The rash can range from irritating to incapacitating, depending on the person's sensitivity, the amount of exposure and the rash's location. If urushiol is inhaled via smoke caused by burning the plants, severe reactions can result, including irritation of the lungs and swelling of the throat.

Prevention is the best strategy. Although "leaves of three, let it be" is a good guideline for identifying poison ivy and poison oak, rash-causing plants vary in appearance depending on the species and time of year. It is a good idea to familiarize yourself with the appearance of the rash-causing plants in your area. If you will be engaging in activities where you could potentially be exposed to a

TABLE 7-4 Rash-Causing Plants

PLANT	USUALLY FOUND
Poison ivy	■ Throughout the United States, except for California, Alaska and Hawaii
Poison oak	■ Southeastern United States and along the West Coast
Poison sumac	■ Eastern and southeastern United States (especially prevalent along the Mississippi River and in boggy areas of the southeast) ■ Texas

rash-causing plant, wear a long-sleeved shirt, long pants and boots. Applying a pre-contact barrier cream or lotion before you go outside can help prevent urushiol from contacting your skin and causing a rash. Similarly, washing with a specialized skin cleanser designed to remove urushiol or a degreasing soap (such as dishwashing liquid) and plenty of water as soon as you come in from outside can remove the urushiol from your skin and may prevent a rash from developing, or it may minimize the severity of the rash if one does develop. Wash tools, work gloves and clothing too because urushiol can remain on these surfaces and transfer to your skin the next time you use the item.

If exposure does result in a rash, apply calamine lotion or hydrocortisone cream to the area to reduce itching and blistering. An oral antihistamine may also help to relieve itching. If the rash is severe or on a sensitive part of the body (such as the face or groin), the person should see a healthcare provider. Call 9-1-1 and get equipment, or tell someone to do so, if the person experiences a severe allergic reaction or is having trouble breathing. If you do not need to call 9-1-1, get equipment or tell someone to do so.

Lightning-Strike Injuries

Lightning travels at speeds of up to 300 miles per second. Anything tall—a tower, tree or person—can become a path for the electrical current (Box 7-10). Lightning can "flash" over a person's body or it can travel through blood vessels and nerves to reach the ground. The electrical energy can cause burn injuries and cardiac arrest. When the force of the lightning strike is sufficient to throw the person through the air, traumatic injuries such as fractures or dislocations can result.

Box 7-10 Avoiding Lightning-Strike Injuries

Taking cover is the best strategy for preventing lightning-strike injuries. If you are outdoors, seek cover in a substantial building or a fully enclosed vehicle at the first sound of thunder or sight of lightning, even if it is not raining. Remember the 30/30 rule: take cover when the time between a flash of lightning and a roll of thunder is 30 seconds or less and remain under cover until 30 minutes after the last flash of lightning was seen or the last roll of thunder was heard. If you are outside and cannot reach safety inside of a building, look for a low area. Avoid high ground, tall trees that stand alone, wide-open spaces (such as meadows) and structures such as sheds, dugouts, bleachers and picnic pavilions. These areas are not safe in a thunderstorm. If no safe shelter is available, squat with your feet together and your arms wrapped around your legs. Stay low but do not lie flat. The less of your body that is in contact with the ground, the better.

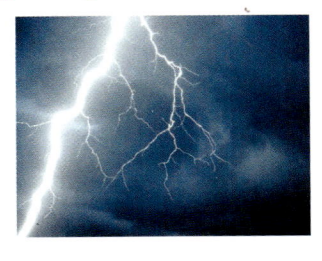

Recognizing Lightning-Strike Injuries

A person who has been struck by lightning may seem dazed and confused, or they may be unresponsive. The person may be having difficulty breathing, or they may not be breathing at all. The person may have burn injuries; open wounds; or muscle, bone or joint injuries. It may be possible to see an entry and exit wound for the lightning but due to the extremely high energy, it may not be easy to identify.

Call 9-1-1 and get equipment immediately, or tell someone to do so, if a person is struck by lightning.

Giving First Aid Care for Lightning-Strike Injuries

After calling 9-1-1, if the person is unresponsive and not breathing or only gasping, give CPR and use an AED if you are trained in these skills. Give care for any other conditions that you find, such as burns; muscle, bone or joint injuries; or shock. Even if the person does not seem to have serious injuries and quickly recovers after the incident, they should still see a healthcare provider for follow-up evaluation and care.

Appendices

Appendix A: Emergency Moves

Appendix B: Injury Prevention

Appendix C: Skill Practice Sheets for Core Course

Appendix D: Skill Practice Sheets for Skill Boosts

APPENDIX A
Emergency Moves

Generally speaking, you should avoid moving an injured or ill person to give care. Unnecessary movement can cause additional injury and pain and may complicate the person's recovery. However, under the following conditions, it would be appropriate to move an injured or ill person.

- You must move the person to protect them from immediate danger (such as fire, flood or poisonous gas). However, you should only attempt this if you can reach the person and remove them from the area without endangering yourself.
- You must move the person to reach another person who may have a more serious injury or illness.
- You must move the person to give proper care. For example, it may be necessary to move a person who needs CPR onto a hard, flat surface.
- You have to move the person to call 9-1-1 or obtain emergency care, such as when you are in the wilderness away from communication.

If you must move a person in an emergency situation, the goal is to do so without injuring yourself or causing additional injury to the person. General principles include:

- Keep the person's head, neck and back in a straight line without bending or twisting as you move them.
- Support the head and neck while minimizing movement.
- Use good body dynamics to avoid injury to yourself.

The following common emergency moves can be done by one or two people and with minimal or no equipment. The situation will dictate which move you should use.

MOVE	WHEN TO USE IT	HOW TO DO IT
Walking Assist*	To move a person who can walk but needs help	1. Place the person's arm around your shoulder or waist (depending on how tall the person is) and hold it in place with one hand. 2. Support the person with your other hand around their waist. (Another responder can also support the person in the same way on the other side.)
Two-Person Seat Carry*	To move a responsive person who is not seriously injured	1. Put one arm under the person's thighs and the other across their back, under their arms. Have a second responder do the same. 2. Interlock your arms with the other responder's arms under the person's legs and across the person's back. 3. Lift the person in the "seat" formed by your interlocked arms.
Clothes Drag	To move a responsive or unresponsive person who may have a head, neck or back injury	1. Grasp the person's shirt behind the neck, gathering enough material so that you have a firm grip. 2. Cradle the person's head with the shirt and your hands and, keeping their head midline without lifting it, pull them to safety.

* Do not use this emergency move if you suspect that the person has a head, neck or spinal injury.

MOVE	WHEN TO USE IT	HOW TO DO IT
Blanket Drag	To move a responsive or unresponsive person	1. Fold the blanket in half lengthwise, and place it so that the fold is alongside the person's body. 2. Take the top layer of the folded blanket, and roll it toward the person's body. 3. Position yourself so that the person is between you and the blanket. 4. Put one hand on the person's shoulder and the other on their hip and roll the person onto their side, toward you, and then pull the blanket toward you so that it is against the person's body. 5. Roll the person onto their back, onto the blanket. 6. Pull the side of the blanket that was rolled up toward yourself, so that the person is in the middle of the blanket. 7. Gather the blanket at the person's head, supporting their head and keeping it midline, and pull them to safety.
Ankle Drag	To move a person who is too large to move another way	1. Cross the person's arms over their chest. 2. Firmly grasp the person's ankles. 3. Move backward, pulling the person in a straight line and being careful not to bump their head.

APPENDIX B
Injury Prevention

General Strategies for Reducing the Risk for Injury

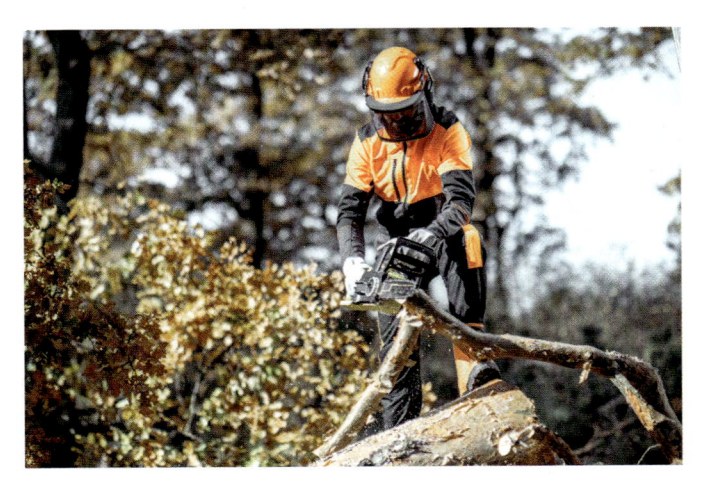

- Think and act with safety in mind.
- Be aware of your environment and surroundings.
- Dress appropriately for the weather and your planned activity.
- Read and follow instructions and safety guidelines.
- Use safety equipment that is available to you (e.g., seat belts, helmets, protective eyewear and footwear), including personal protective equipment.
- Get trained in first aid, CPR and AED use, and keep your knowledge and skills current. To enroll in a Red Cross First Aid/CPR/AED class, visit redcross.org.
- Have an emergency action plan (Box B-1).

Vehicle Safety

- Do not use alcohol or drugs while operating a motor vehicle.
- Do not drive distracted. Texting, emailing or talking on a mobile phone; eating or drinking; talking to passengers; reading; using navigation systems; operating audiovisual equipment; daydreaming; and putting on makeup are hazardous activities when you are behind the wheel.
- Do not drive drowsy. Lack of sleep affects your ability to operate a vehicle safely, even if you do not actually fall asleep at the wheel. When you are not well rested, your reaction time is slowed, and your judgment is impaired. Know the warning signs that you are too tired

Box B-1 Developing an Emergency Action Plan

Emergencies happen quickly. There may not be time to consider what to do, only time to react. Having an emergency action plan in place and being familiar with the procedures it contains can save precious minutes when every minute counts. To create an emergency action plan:

1. Identify the types of emergencies that could occur. Think about potential injuries, illnesses, weather events and other situations (such as power failures) that are likely to occur in your specific setting.
2. Develop and write down the procedure that is to be followed in the event of each emergency. Include:
   - How the plan is activated (call to internal number, over the radio, etc.).
   - The signal or communication that will be used to indicate that the emergency action plan should be activated (such as a whistle blast).
   - The steps for responding to the emergency and who is responsible for each step.
   - The procedure for calling 9-1-1 or the designated emergency number and directing emergency medical services (EMS) personnel to the scene.
   - What follow-up actions should be taken, if any.
3. Identify equipment that is needed to respond to the potential emergencies you have identified and stock it in an easily accessible place.

Review the emergency action plan with family members and practice it regularly so that the procedures it contains become second nature. Periodically review the emergency action plan and update it as necessary.

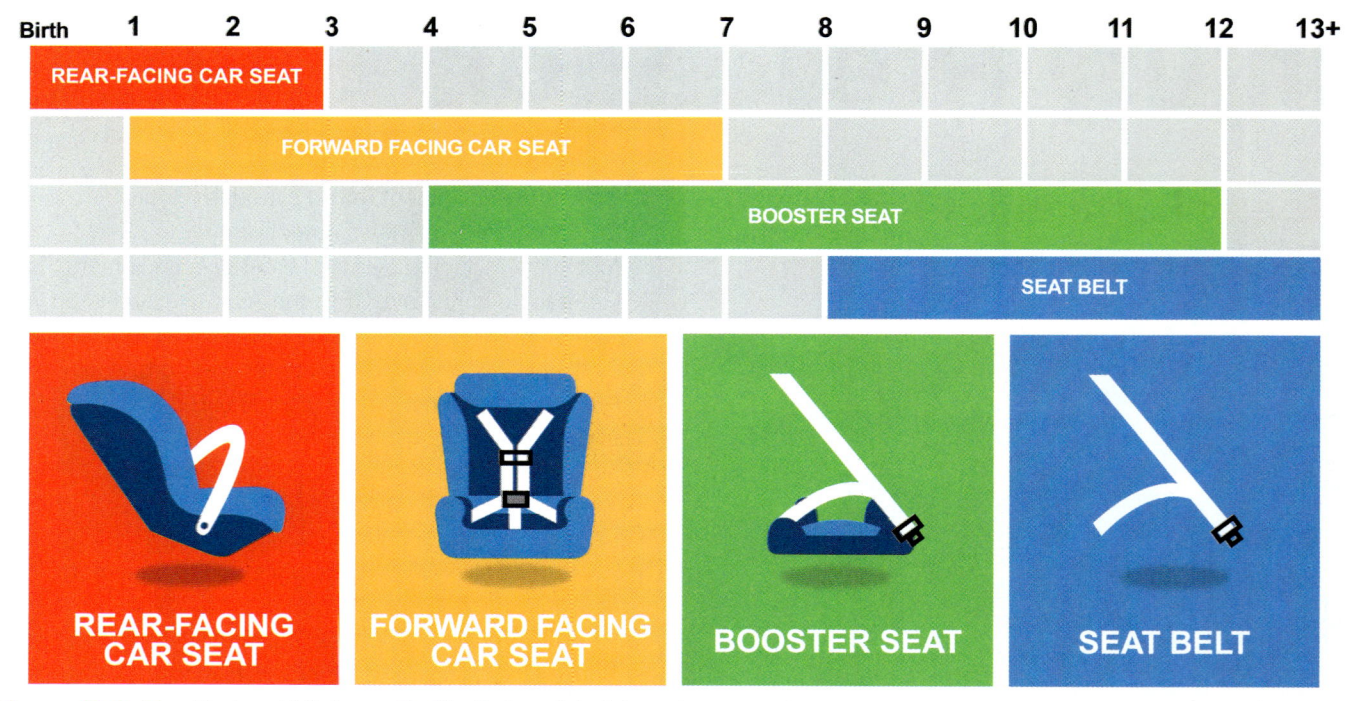

Figure B-1. The National Highway Traffic Safety Administration provides car seat recommendations for children from birth through 12 years.

to drive: yawning or blinking frequently, drifting from your lane, missing an exit or not being able to recall driving for the last several miles. Pull over to rest or change drivers. Opening the window for fresh air or drinking a caffeinated beverage will not keep you alert enough to continue driving.
- Always wear your seat belt.
- Always have infants and children younger than 12 years ride in the back seat in safety seats that are approved for the child's age and size (Figure B-1). The amount of force created by a deploying airbag can kill or severely injure an infant or child occupying the front seat, even if the infant or child is in a rear-facing safety seat. Make sure that the safety seat is installed correctly in your vehicle. Visit the National Highway Traffic Safety Administration website (nhtsa.gov) for information about choosing an appropriate child safety seat and using it correctly. If you need help installing the safety seat or want to be sure that you have installed the seat correctly, visit safecar.gov to find a nearby child safety seat inspection station.
- Never leave a child alone in a car, even for a few minutes, and always check the back seat of the vehicle before you lock it and walk away. Temperatures inside the car can reach deadly levels quickly, even when the temperature outside is moderate.

Fire Safety

- Install a smoke alarm and carbon monoxide detector on every floor of your home. Check the batteries once a month and change the batteries at least every 6 months or per the manufacturer's recommendations.
- Make sure that your home has at least one working, easily accessible fire extinguisher, and make sure everyone in your home knows how to use it.
- Have fireplaces and chimneys inspected annually and perform cleaning and repairs as necessary.
- If you have more than one floor, have approved escape devices that allow exit from above the first floor if internal stairs are inaccessible.
- Develop and practice a fire escape plan with your family. Gather everyone together at a convenient time. For each floor of your home, sketch a floor plan, noting rooms, doors, windows and hallways. Use arrows to

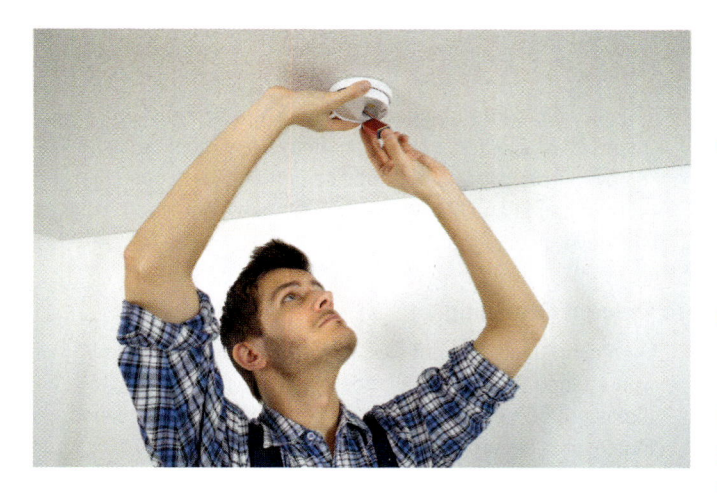

indicate two ways (if possible) to get out of each room. Teach family members to leave the building first, then call 9-1-1 or the designated emergency number. No one should re-enter the burning building for any reason. To escape through a door, feel the door first. Do not open it if it is hot.
- If smoke is present, crawl low.
- If escape is not possible, stay in the room and call 9-1-1 or the designated emergency number, even if rescuers are already outside.

Safety at Home

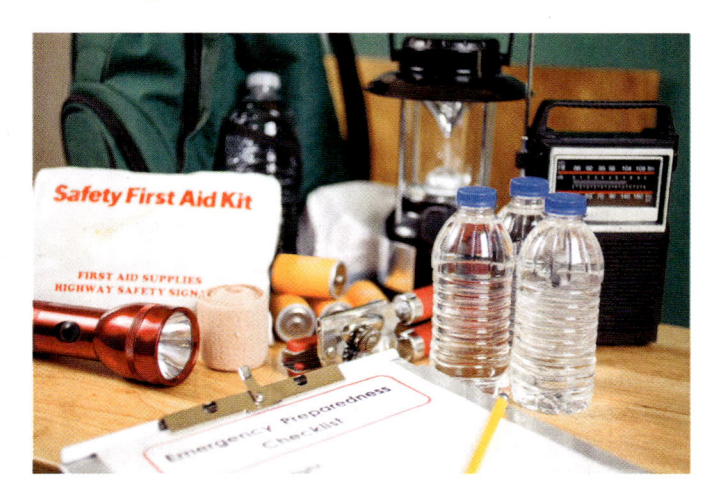

- Enter emergency numbers in your mobile phone's contact list and post them near every phone in your home. Include 9-1-1 or the designated emergency number, the national Poison Help hotline (1-800-222-1222), and the phone numbers of your family's healthcare providers, as well as any other important numbers.
- Make an emergency preparedness kit and have an emergency preparedness plan in place. Visit redcross.org to obtain an emergency preparedness kit or for more information about how to prepare for disasters and other emergencies.
- Box B-2 contains a checklist of special safety considerations for households with young children.

Preventing Slips, Trips and Falls
- Make sure that stairways and hallways are well lit.
- Make sure that stairways and hallways are free of clutter.
- Equip stairways with handrails and use nonslip treads or securely fastened rugs.
- Secure rugs to the floor with double-sided tape.
- Ensure that cords for lamps and other items are not placed where someone can trip over them.
- Clean up spills promptly.
- Place a mat with a suction base on the bottom of the tub if the tub does not have built-in nonslip strips.
- If a member of your household has impaired mobility, install handrails in the bathtub or shower and beside the toilet.

Preventing Burns and Fires
- Set the water heater at a temperature of 120° F or less to prevent scalding. If your household contains children or older adults, the water temperature should be lower, between 100° F and 115° F.
- Keep flammable items, such as curtains, away from heat sources, such as space heaters.
- Do not wear loose clothing when cooking.
- When you are using the stove, use the back burners and turn pot and pan handles toward the back of the stove so that they are out of the reach of children.
- Do not use extension cords or overload outlets.

Preventing Firearm Accidents
- Keep firearms in the home unloaded in a locked place, out of the reach of children. Store ammunition separately in a locked location.
- Obtain the knowledge and skills you need to handle firearms safely.

Box B-2 Safety Checklist for Households with Young Children

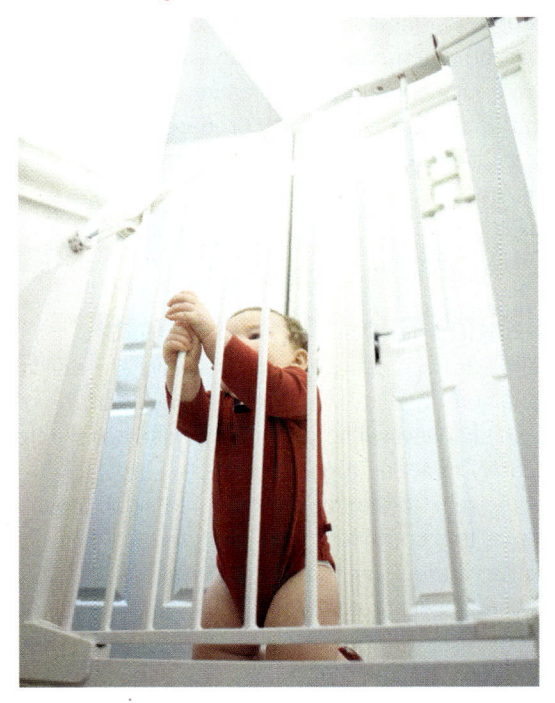

To Prevent Fire and Burns
- Matches and lighters are stored out of the reach of children.
- Space heaters, if used, are placed out of the reach of children and away from curtains.
- Pot and pan handles are turned toward the back of the stove and out of the reach of children.

To Prevent Electrical Shock
- Safety covers are placed on all unused electrical outlets.
- Loose cords are secured and out of the way.
- Electrical appliances are away from sinks, tubs, toilets and other sources of water.

To Prevent Choking, Suffocation and Strangulation
- Small objects are kept out of children's reach.
- Toys are age appropriate and pose no choking hazard. Items such as coolers and plastic storage containers that a child could get trapped in are stored in a safe place that is not accessible to the child.
- Lidded toy boxes have lightweight, removable lids with supports to keep the lids open and air vents to allow air flow when the lid is closed.
- The crib mattress fits into the crib snugly, and all soft objects and loose bedding (such as toys, blankets, bumper pads and pillows) are removed from the crib. The only thing in the crib is a mattress with a tightly fitted sheet.
- Drape and blind cords are wound up and not dangling. Make sure they are out of reach of children.
- Objects with cords, strings and ribbons are kept out of the reach of children. Hanging crib toys, like mobiles, are removed from cribs when the baby first begins to push up on their hands and knees or when the baby is 5 months old, whichever occurs first.

To Prevent Drowning
- Swimming pools and hot tubs are completely surrounded with a fence that has a self-closing and self-latching gate that is out of the reach of a child. Hot tubs are covered, and the cover is secured.
- Kiddie pools, bathtubs and sinks are immediately emptied after each use.
- Toilet lids are kept down when not in use.
- Bathroom and laundry room doors are closed at all times.
- Buckets or other containers with standing water are securely covered or emptied of water and stored upside-down and out of children's reach.

To Prevent Poisoning
- Cleaning supplies, laundry supplies, car maintenance supplies, pesticides and other household chemicals are stored in locked cabinets and are out of the reach of children.
- Houseplants are kept out of reach.
- Medicine is kept in a locked storage place that children cannot reach.
- Packages containing potential poisons are closed securely after each use, and the container is promptly returned to a locked cabinet. (**Note:** There is no such thing as "childproof" packaging.)

To Prevent Falls and Tipping Injuries
- Safety gates are installed at all open stairways in homes with toddlers and babies. (**Note:** Pressure gates, which attach to the walls with pressure rather than with screws, should not be installed at the top of stairs. This type of gate can give way if a child leans on it.)
- Windows and balcony doors have childproof latches or window guards.
- Balconies have barriers to prevent children from slipping through the bars.
- Large, heavy items (such as television sets, microwaves, fish tanks, dressers, bookcases and heavy appliances) are properly secured to the wall to prevent them from tipping over onto a child if the child climbs or hangs on them.

To Prevent Wounds
- Knives, hand tools, power tools, razor blades, scissors, guns, ammunition and other objects that can cause injury are stored in locked cabinets or locked storage areas.
- Corner guards are installed on all sharp furniture edges.

Safety at Work

At work, participate in any workplace safety programs your employer offers. Make sure you know:

- Your place of employment's emergency action plan and fire evacuation procedures.
- How to activate your emergency response team and how to call 9-1-1 or the designated emergency number.
- The location of the nearest fire extinguisher, automated external defibrillator (AED) and first aid kit.
- How to use recommended safety equipment and how to follow safety procedures if you work in an environment where hazards exist.

Safety at Play

Enjoy sports and other recreational activities safely by making sure equipment is in good working order and following accepted guidelines for the activity. Wear all recommended safety equipment while playing. Before undertaking an activity that is unfamiliar to you, such as boating, skiing or riding a motorcycle, take lessons to learn how to perform the activity safely.

Water Safety

- Learn to swim and obtain the knowledge and skills you need to prevent, recognize and respond to aquatic emergencies. Knowing how to swim is a basic life skill that everyone should possess. The American Red Cross Swimming and Water Safety program teaches people to be safe in, on and around the water through water safety courses, water orientation classes for infants and toddlers, and comprehensive Learn-to-Swim courses for people of all ages and abilities.
- Use a U.S. Coast Guard–approved life jacket. Young children, weak or inexperienced swimmers and nonswimmers should always wear a U.S. Coast Guard–approved life jacket whenever they are in, on or around the water. Even strong swimmers should wear a U.S. Coast Guard–approved life jacket when engaging in certain aquatic activities, such as boating.
- Do not use alcohol or drugs while engaging in aquatic activities.
- Never swim alone. Swim only in designated areas and areas supervised by a lifeguard.
- Closely supervise children in, on or near water, even when a lifeguard is present. Stay within arm's reach of the child.
- Read and obey all rules and posted signs. Pay special attention to water-depth markings and "no diving" signs.
- Enter the water feetfirst, unless you are in an area that is clearly marked for diving.
- Watch out for the dangerous "too's": too tired, too cold, too far away from safety, too much sun and too much strenuous activity.

Bicycle Safety

- Always wear an approved helmet. Children should wear a helmet even if they are still riding along the sidewalk on training wheels. Look for a helmet that has been approved by the American National Standards Institute (ANSI) or Consumer Products Safety Commission (CPSC) and make sure that the helmet is the correct size and that it fits comfortably and securely. For more information about helmet laws in your area, conduct an Internet search or contact state or local officials.
- Avoid riding on roads that are busy or have no shoulder.
- Wear reflective clothing at night.
- Use a headlight, taillight and high-visibility strobe lights on your bicycle wheels.
- Keep bicycles properly maintained.

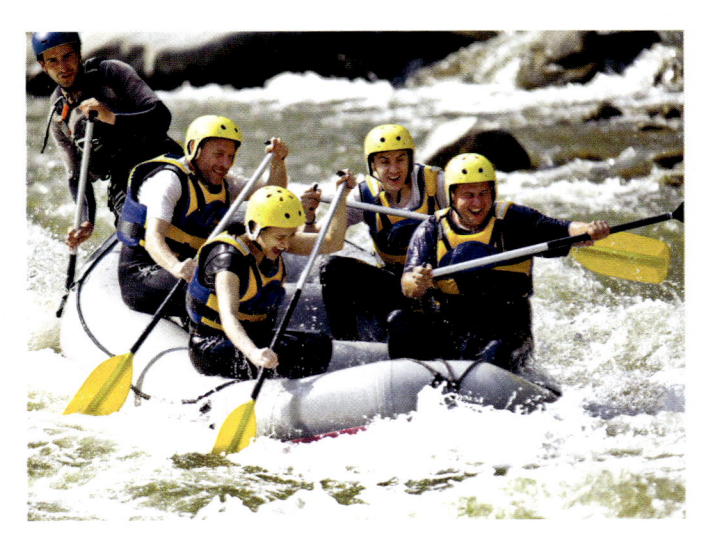

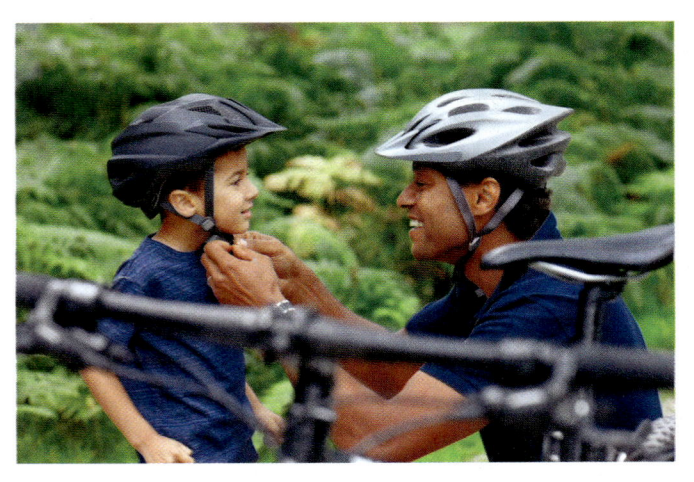

Safety for Runners, Joggers and Walkers

- Plan your route carefully and exercise in well-lit, well-populated areas.
- Consider exercising with another person.
- Pay attention to your environment and surroundings. Consider doing without music so you can hear sounds and warnings.
- Avoid roads that do not easily accommodate pedestrian traffic.
- If you must exercise outdoors after dark, wear reflective clothing and run, jog or walk facing traffic.
- Be alert for cars pulling out at intersections and driveways.

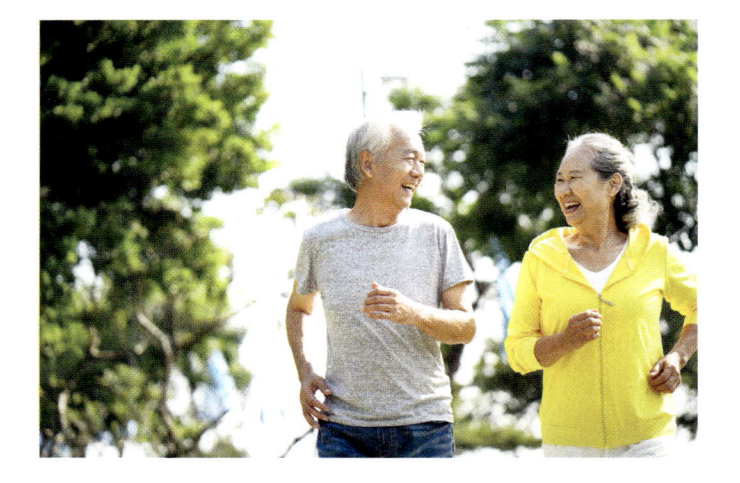

APPENDIX C
Skill Practice Sheets for Core Course

Skill Practice Sheet: Checking a Person Who Appears Unresponsive. **166**

Skill Practice Sheet: Giving Chest Compressions to Adults **168**

Skill Practice Sheet: Giving Breaths to Adults with a Face Shield. **169**

Skill Practice Sheet: Giving Breaths to Adults with a Pocket Mask. **170**

Skill Practice Sheet: Giving CPR Cycles to Adults. **171**

Skill Practice Sheet: Using an AED for Adults **172**

Skill Practice Sheet: Giving Chest Compressions to Children. **174**

Skill Practice Sheet: Giving Breaths to Children with a Face Shield **176**

Skill Practice Sheet: Giving Breaths to Children with a Pocket Mask **177**

Skill Practice Sheet: Giving CPR Cycles to Children **178**

Skill Practice Sheet: Giving CPR Cycles to Infants **179**

Skill Practice Sheet: Using an AED for Children and Infants **180**

Skill Practice Sheet: Giving Back Blows and Abdominal Thrusts to Adults and Children **182**

Skill Practice Sheet: Giving Back Blows and Chest Thrusts to Infants **184**

Skill Practice Sheet: Using Direct Pressure to Control Life-Threatening Bleeding. **186**

Note: *Skill Practice Sheets are used for hands-on skill practice during instructor-led skills sessions.*

SKILL PRACTICE SHEET

Checking a Person Who Appears Unresponsive

EACH PARTICIPANT WILL CHECK A PERSON WHO APPEARS UNRESPONSIVE FROM CHECKING THE SCENE THROUGH VERBALIZING THE NEED FOR CARE.	
1. Check the scene before entering to ensure safety. - Verbalize that the scene is safe.	
2. Check the person: Form an initial impression and obtain consent. - Form an initial impression about what's going on with the person as you approach them. - Identify any life-threatening conditions, such as appearing unresponsive, appearing not to be breathing, life-threatening bleeding or another life-threatening condition. - Verbalize that the person appears unresponsive and consent is implied.	
3. Put on gloves.	
4. Check for responsiveness, breathing, life-threatening bleeding and other life-threatening conditions. - Shout to get person's attention, using person's name if known. - If person does not respond, tap shoulder (adult/child) or foot (infant). - Shout again while checking for breathing, life-threatening bleeding and other life-threatening conditions. - Verbalize that the person does not respond, is not breathing, and does not appear to have life-threatening bleeding or other life-threatening conditions.	

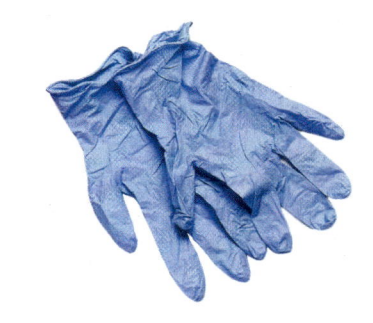

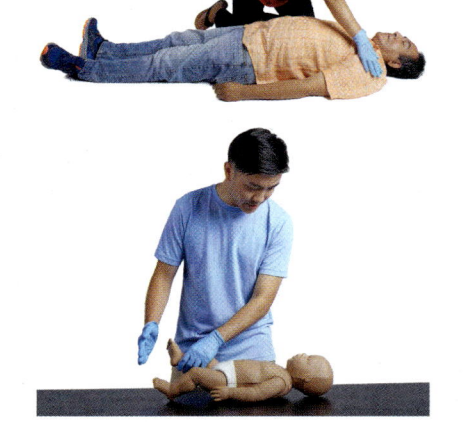

166 Appendix C | Skill Practice Sheets for Core Course

SKILL PRACTICE SHEET

5. Call 9-1-1 and get equipment.
- Tell Bystander, "You. Call 9-1-1 and get an AED and first aid kit."
- Bystander repeats, "I'll call 9-1-1 and get an AED and first aid kit."

6. Give care according to the conditions that you find and your level of knowledge and training.
- Verbalize the need for care.

American Red Cross | Appendices

SKILL PRACTICE SHEET

Giving Chest Compressions to Adults

EACH PARTICIPANT SHOULD GIVE FIVE SETS OF 30 COMPRESSIONS.	
1. Ensure the person is on their back on a firm, flat surface.	
2. Kneel beside the person. ■ Your knees should be near the person's body and spread about shoulder width apart.	
3. Use correct hand placement. ■ Place the heel of one hand in the center of their chest, with your other hand on top. ■ Interlace your fingers and make sure they are up off the chest.	
4. Use correct body position. ■ Position your body so that your shoulders are directly over your hands. ■ Lock your elbows to keep your arms straight.	
5. Give 30 compressions. ■ Push hard and fast (at least 2 inches; 100 to 120 compressions per minute).	**x 30**
6. Allow chest to return to its normal position after each compression.	
7. Give four more sets of compressions.* ■ Take a brief break between each set of compressions. *Practice only; in an emergency give sets of 30 compressions followed by 2 breaths.	**+ 4 more sets**

168   Appendix C | Skill Practice Sheets for Core Course

SKILL PRACTICE SHEET

Giving Breaths to Adults with a Face Shield

EACH PARTICIPANT SHOULD GIVE **FIVE SETS** OF **2 BREATHS**.	
1. **Place face shield** over person's face, ensuring the one-way valve is over their mouth.	
2. **Open the airway** to a past-neutral position using the head-tilt/chin-lift technique.	
3. Pinch nose shut, take a normal breath and **make a complete seal** over person's mouth with your own mouth.	
4. Give **1st breath**. ■ Blow into the person's mouth for about 1 second, enough to make the chest begin to rise. ■ Look to see that the chest rises. **Note:** *If you do not see chest rise, retilt head and ensure a proper seal before giving 2nd breath.*	
5. Pause between the breaths to **allow for the chest to fall and the air to exit**.	**Pause**
6. Give **2nd breath**. ■ Take another breath, make a seal, then give 2nd breath.	
7. Give **four more sets of breaths**.* ■ Take a brief break between each set of breaths. ** Practice only; in an emergency give sets of 30 compressions followed by 2 breaths.*	**+ 4 more sets**

American Red Cross | Appendices 169

SKILL PRACTICE SHEET

Giving Breaths to Adults with a Pocket Mask

EACH PARTICIPANT SHOULD GIVE FIVE SETS OF 2 BREATHS.	
1. Place the mask at the bridge of the nose and lower it over the person's nose and mouth.	
2. Seal the mask and **open the airway**. ■ Place the space of your hand between your thumb and index finger at the top of the mask above the valve. ■ Place your remaining fingers on the side of the person's face. ■ Place the thumb of your other hand along the base of the mask and place your bent index finger under the person's chin. ■ Lift the person's face into the mask and open the airway to a past-neutral position by tilting the head back.	
3. Give 1st breath. ■ Take a normal breath, make a complete seal over the mask valve with your mouth and blow into the person's mouth for about 1 second, enough to make the chest begin to rise. ■ Look to see that the chest rises. **Note:** *If you do not see chest rise, retilt head and ensure a proper seal before giving 2nd breath.*	
4. Pause between the breaths to allow for the chest to fall and the air to exit.	**Pause**
5. Give 2nd breath. ■ Take another breath, make a seal, then give 2nd breath.	
6. Give four more sets of breaths.* ■ Take a brief break between each set of breaths. * *Practice only; in an emergency give sets of 30 compressions followed by 2 breaths.*	**+ 4 more sets**

SKILL PRACTICE SHEET

Giving CPR Cycles to Adults

EACH PARTICIPANT SHOULD PERFORM THREE CPR CYCLES OF 30 CHEST COMPRESSIONS AND 2 BREATHS.

1. **Give 30 chest compressions.**
   - Push hard and fast (at least 2 inches; 100 to 120 compressions per minute).
   - Use correct hand placement.
   - Allow chest to return to its normal position.

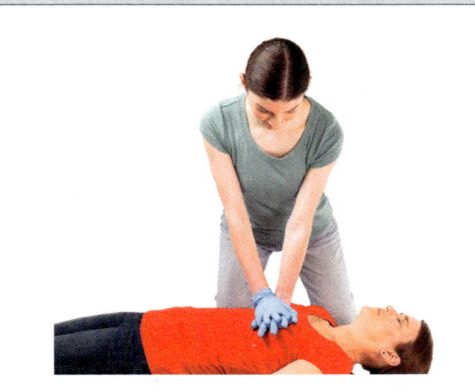

2. **Give 2 breaths.**
   - Each breath should last about 1 second and make the chest begin to rise.
   - Minimize interruptions to chest compressions to give breaths to **less than 10 seconds**.

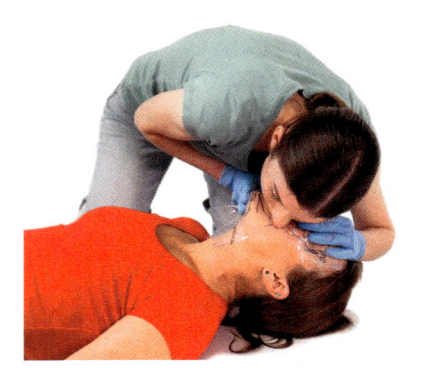

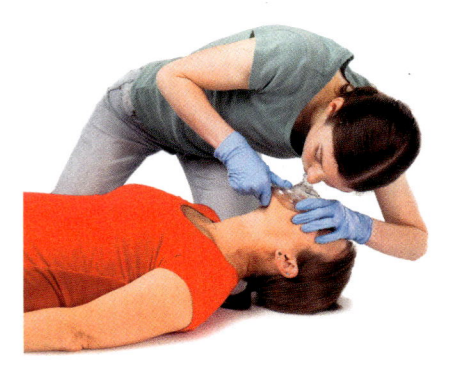

3. **Give two more sets** of 30 compressions and 2 breaths.

+ 2 more sets

American Red Cross | Appendices 171

SKILL PRACTICE SHEET

Using an AED for Adults

EACH PARTICIPANT SHOULD OPERATE THE AED AND START CPR AFTER PUSHING THE SHOCK BUTTON.

1. Turn on AED and follow the voice prompts.	
2. Remove all clothing covering the chest, if necessary.	
3. Attach pads correctly. ■ Place one pad on upper right side of chest. ■ Place one pad on lower left side of chest, a few inches below the left armpit. ■ Pads should not touch.	
4. Plug the pad connector cable into the AED, if necessary.	
5. Clear for analysis.	

172 Appendix C | Skill Practice Sheets for Core Course

SKILL PRACTICE SHEET

6. **Clear** for shock.	**Clear**
7. **Push shock button** to deliver shock.	
8. Immediately get into position to start **CPR**. **Note:** *Skill practice ends here.*	

American Red Cross | Appendices

SKILL PRACTICE SHEET

Giving Chest Compressions to Children

EACH PARTICIPANT SHOULD GIVE FIVE SETS OF 30 COMPRESSIONS.	
1. Ensure that the child is on their back on a firm, flat surface.	
2. Kneel beside the child. ■ Your knees should be near the child's body and spread about shoulder width apart.	
3. Use correct hand placement. ■ Place the heel of one hand in the center of their chest, with your other hand on top. ■ Interlace your fingers and make sure they are up off the chest. ■ **For a smaller child, you may use one hand to give compressions.**	
4. Use correct body position. ■ Position yourself so your shoulders are directly over your hands. Lock your elbows to keep your arms straight.	

SKILL PRACTICE SHEET

5. Give 30 compressions. ■ Push hard and fast (about 2 inches; 100 to 120 compressions per minute).	**x 30**
6. Allow chest to return to its normal position after each compression.	
7. Give four more sets of compressions.* Take a brief break between each set of compressions. *Practice only; in an emergency give sets of 30 compressions followed by 2 breaths.*	**+ 4 more sets**

SKILL PRACTICE SHEET

Giving Breaths to Children with a Face Shield

EACH PARTICIPANT SHOULD GIVE **FIVE SETS** OF **2** BREATHS.	
1. **Place face shield** over child's face, ensuring the one-way valve is over their mouth.	
2. **Open the airway** to a slightly past-neutral position using the head-tilt/chin-lift technique.	
3. Pinch nose shut, take a normal breath and **make a complete seal** over person's mouth with your own mouth.	
4. Give **1st breath**. ■ Blow into the child's mouth for about 1 second, enough to make the chest begin to rise. ■ Look to see that the chest rises. **Note:** *If you do not see chest rise, retilt head and ensure a proper seal before giving 2nd breath.*	
5. Pause between the breaths to **allow for the chest to fall and the air to exit**.	**Pause**
6. Give **2nd breath**. ■ Take another breath, make a seal, then give 2nd breath.	
7. Give **four more sets of breaths**.* ■ Take a brief break between each set of breaths. ** Practice only; in an emergency give sets of 30 compressions followed by 2 breaths.*	**+ 4 more sets**

176 Appendix C | Skill Practice Sheets for Core Course

SKILL PRACTICE SHEET

Giving Breaths to Children with a Pocket Mask

EACH PARTICIPANT SHOULD GIVE FIVE SETS OF 2 BREATHS.	
1. Place the mask at the bridge of the nose and lower it over the child's nose and mouth.	
2. Seal the mask and open the airway. • Place the space of your hand between your thumb and index finger at the top of the mask above the valve. • Place your remaining fingers on the side of the child's face. • Place the thumb of your other hand along the base of the mask and place your bent index finger under the child's chin. • Lift the child's face into the mask and open the airway to a slightly past-neutral position by tilting the head back.	
3. Give 1st breath. • Take a normal breath, make a complete seal over the mask valve with your mouth and blow into the child's mouth for about 1 second, enough to make the chest begin to rise. • Look to see that the chest rises. **Note:** *If you do not see chest rise, retilt head and ensure a proper seal before giving 2nd breath.*	
4. Pause between the breaths to **allow for the chest to fall and the air to exit**.	**Pause**
5. Give 2nd breath. • Take another breath, make a seal, then give 2nd breath.	
6. Give four more sets of breaths.* • Take a brief break between each set of breaths. ** Practice only; in an emergency give sets of 30 compressions followed by 2 breaths.*	**+ 4 more sets**

American Red Cross | Appendices 177

SKILL PRACTICE SHEET

Giving CPR Cycles to Children

EACH PARTICIPANT SHOULD PERFORM THREE CPR CYCLES OF 30 CHEST COMPRESSIONS AND 2 BREATHS.

1. **Give 30 chest compressions.**
   - Push hard and fast (about 2 inches; 100 to 120 compressions per minute).
   - Use correct hand placement.
     - Place the heel of one hand in the center of their chest with your other hand on top.
     - Interlace your fingers and make sure they are up off the chest.
   - For a smaller child, you may use one hand to give compressions.
   - Allow chest to return to its normal position.

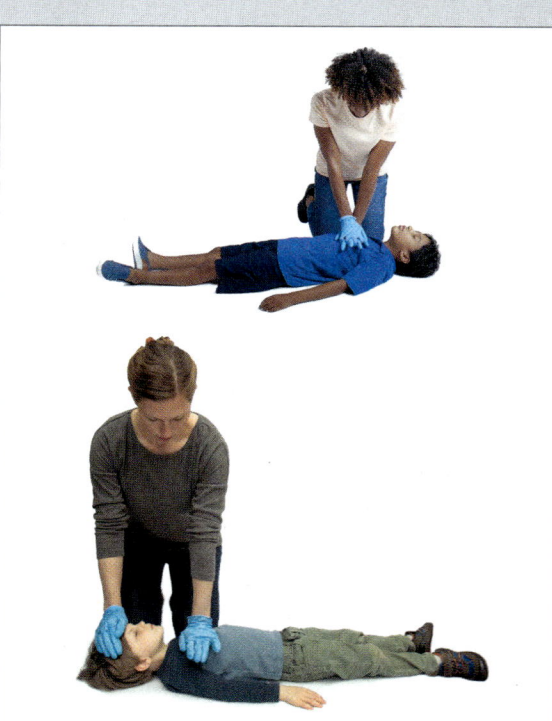

2. **Give 2 breaths.**
   - Each breath should last about 1 second and make the chest begin to rise.
   - Minimize interruptions to chest compressions to give breaths to **less than 10 seconds**.

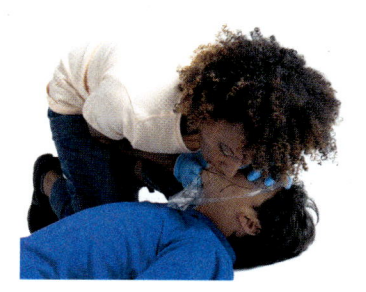

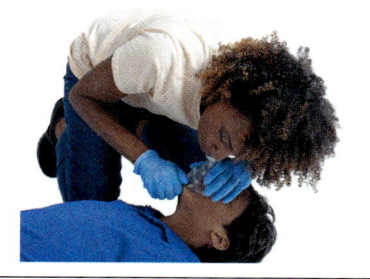

3. **Give two more sets of 30 compressions and 2 breaths.**

+ 2 more sets

178 Appendix C | Skill Practice Sheets for Core Course

SKILL PRACTICE SHEET

Giving CPR Cycles to Infants

EACH PARTICIPANT SHOULD PERFORM THREE CPR CYCLES OF 30 CHEST COMPRESSIONS AND 2 BREATHS.	
1. Ensure the infant is on their back on a firm, flat surface.	
2. Use correct body position. ■ Stand or kneel to the side of the infant, with your hips at a slight angle.	

3. Give 30 chest compressions.
■ Push hard and fast (about 1½ inches; 100 to 120 per minute).
■ Use correct hand technique (encircling thumbs technique).
  • Place both thumbs (side-by-side) on the center of the infant's chest just below the nipple line.
  • Use other fingers to encircle the infant's chest toward the back, providing support.
■ Use both thumbs at the same time to press down on the infant's chest.
■ Allow chest to return to its normal position.
	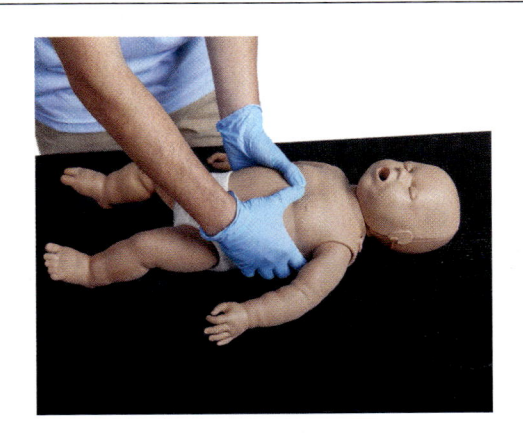

4. Give 2 breaths. ■ Maintain an open airway in the neutral position. ■ Each breath should last about 1 second and make the chest begin to rise. ■ Pause between the breaths to allow the infant's chest to fall and the air to exit. ■ Minimize interruptions to chest compressions to give breaths to **less than 10 seconds**.	
5. Give two more sets of 30 compressions and 2 breaths.	**+ 2 more sets**

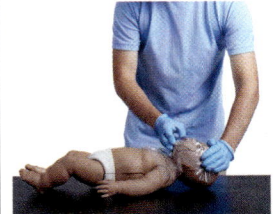

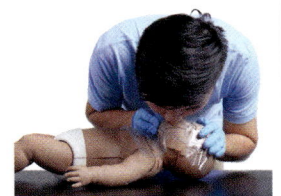

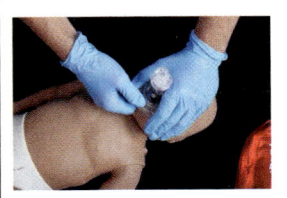

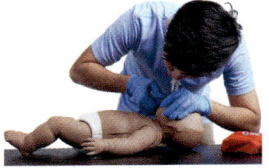

American Red Cross | Appendices

SKILL PRACTICE SHEET

Using an AED for Children and Infants

EACH PARTICIPANT SHOULD OPERATE THE AED AND START CPR AFTER PUSHING THE SHOCK BUTTON.	
1. Turn on AED.	
2. Remove all clothing covering the chest, if necessary.	
3. Choose appropriate pads. ■ Use pediatric pads or pediatric settings for children and infants up to 8 years of age and/or weighing less than 55 pounds (25 kg). ■ Use adult pads for children older than 8 years of age and/or weighing more than 55 pounds (25 kg).	
4. Attach pads correctly. ■ **Children**: Place one pad on upper right side of chest and one pad on lower left side of chest, a few inches below the left armpit. Pads should not touch. If pads touch, use front/back pad placement. ■ **Infants**: Always use the front/back pad placement. Place one pad in the middle of the chest and one pad on the back between the shoulder blades.	

Appendix C | Skill Practice Sheets for Core Course

SKILL PRACTICE SHEET

5. Plug the pad connector cable into the AED, if necessary.	
6. Clear for analysis.	
7. Clear for shock.	**Clear**
8. Push the shock button to deliver shock.	
9. Immediately start CPR, beginning with compressions.	

American Red Cross | Appendices

SKILL PRACTICE SHEET

Giving Back Blows and Abdominal Thrusts to Adults and Children

EACH PARTICIPANT SHOULD PERFORM FIVE CYCLES OF 5 BACK BLOWS AND 5 ABDOMINAL THRUSTS.	
BACK BLOWS. (ONLY SIMULATE STRIKING THE PERSON WHILE PRACTICING THIS SKILL.)	
1. Position self to the side and slightly behind choking person. ■ For a small child, you may need to kneel behind them rather than stand.	
2. Place one arm diagonally across person's chest and **bend them forward** at the waist. ■ The person's upper body should be as parallel to the ground as possible.	
3. Give 5 back blows. ■ Simulate* firmly striking the person to give 5 back blows between the shoulder blades with the heel of one hand. ■ Each of the back blows should be separate from the others. *Practice only; in an emergency strike the person's back firmly.*	
ABDOMINAL THRUSTS. (ONLY SIMULATE GIVING ABDOMINAL THRUSTS WHILE PRACTICING THIS SKILL.)	
4. Find the person's navel with two fingers.	
5. Move behind the person and **place your front foot in between the person's feet** with your knees slightly bent to provide balance and stability. ■ For a young child, you may need to **kneel behind them** rather than stand.	

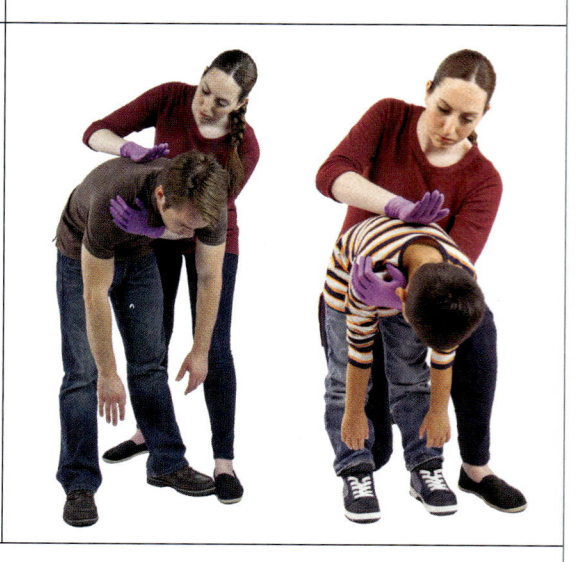

SKILL PRACTICE SHEET

6. Make a fist with your other hand and **place the thumb side against the person's stomach,** right above your fingers.

7. Take your first hand and **cover your fist** with that hand.

8. Give 5 abdominal thrusts.

- Simulate* pulling inward and upward to give 5 abdominal thrusts.
- Each of the abdominal thrusts should be separate from the others.

Practice only; in an emergency pull inward and upward to give an abdominal thrust.

American Red Cross | Appendices

SKILL PRACTICE SHEET

Giving Back Blows and Chest Thrusts to Infants

EACH PARTICIPANT SHOULD PERFORM FIVE CYCLES OF 5 BACK BLOWS AND 5 CHEST THRUSTS.

BACK BLOWS

1. Place the infant's back along your forearm.
- Cradle the back of the infant's head with your hand.

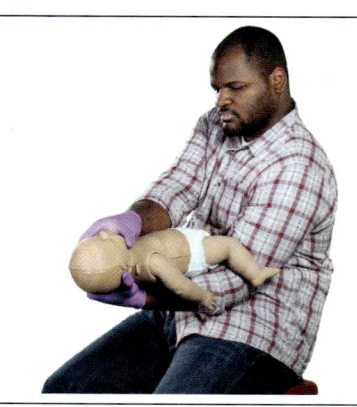

2. Place your other forearm on the infant's front.
- Support the infant's jaw with the thumb and fingers; do not cover the infant's face.

3. Turn the infant to a face-down position and hold them along your forearm using your thigh for support.
- Keep the infant's head lower than their body.

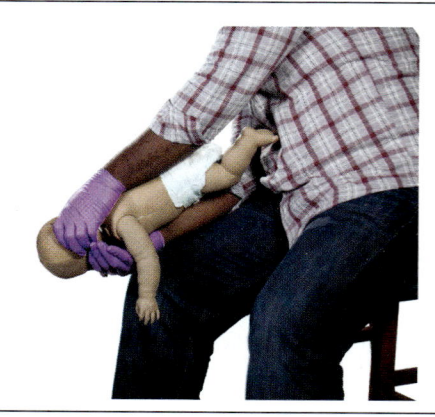

4. Give 5 firm back blows.
- Use the heel of your hand to give back blows between the infant's shoulder blades.
- Keep your fingers up to avoid hitting the infant's head or neck.
- Each of the back blows should be separate from the others.

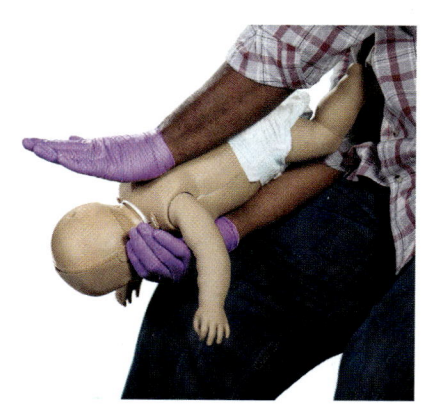

184 Appendix C | Skill Practice Sheets for Core Course

SKILL PRACTICE SHEET

CHEST THRUSTS

5. Position the infant between your forearms.
- Support the head and neck.
- Turn the infant face-up.
- Lower the infant onto your thigh with their head lower than their chest.

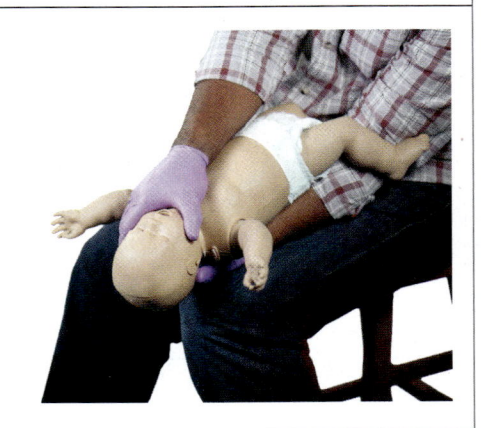

6. Place two fingers in the center of the infant's chest, just below the nipple line.

7. Give 5 quick chest thrusts about 1½ inches deep.
- Let the chest return to its normal position in between each chest thrust, keeping your fingers in contact with the chest.
- Each chest thrust should be separate from the others.
- Support the infant's head, neck and back while giving chest thrusts.

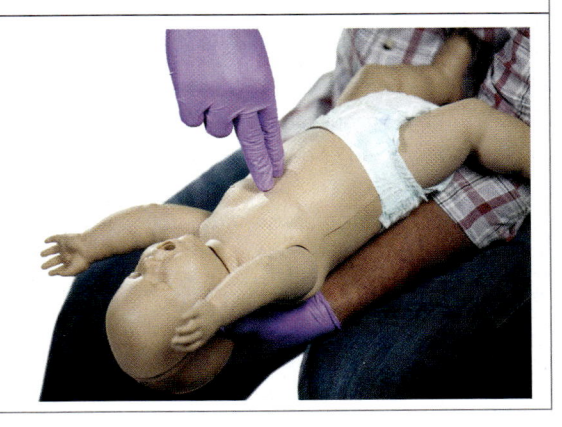

SKILL PRACTICE SHEET

Using Direct Pressure to Control Life-Threatening Bleeding

1. Place the dressing on the wound.*

- Ensure good contact with the bleeding surfaces of the wound.

Use a hemostatic dressing if available.

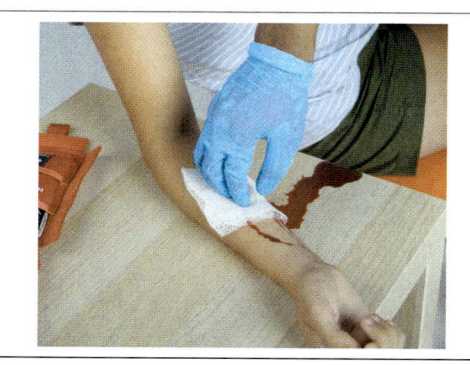

2. Apply steady, firm pressure directly over the wound until the bleeding stops.

- Put one hand on top of the dressing and put your other hand on top.
- Position your shoulders over your hands and lock your elbows.
- Push down as hard as you can.
- If blood soaks through the original gauze pad, you do not need to do anything, but you can put another gauze pad on top. Replace the new gauze pad as necessary if blood soaks through the pads.

Note: Do not remove the original gauze pad and **do not** stack multiple gauze pads.

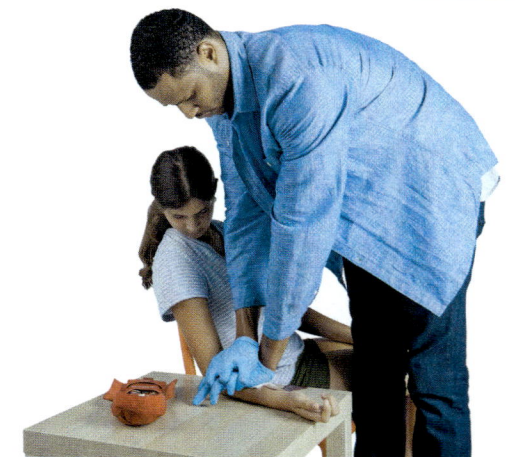

3. Hold direct pressure until:

- The bleeding stops.
- A tourniquet is applied (for life-threatening bleeding from an arm or leg) and the bleeding has stopped.
- Another person relieves you.
- You are too exhausted to continue.
- The situation becomes unsafe.

186 Appendix C | Skill Practice Sheets for Core Course

SKILL PRACTICE SHEET

If bleeding stops before EMS arrives:

4. Apply a roller bandage.

- Check for circulation beyond the injury.
- Apply the bandage over the dressing and secure it firmly to keep pressure on the wound.
  - Place the end of a bandage on the dressing at a 45-degree angle.
  - Continue wrapping the bandage over the dressing.
  - Tape to secure the dressing.
- Check again for circulation beyond the injury. If there is any change, the bandage may be too tight; carefully loosen the bandage.

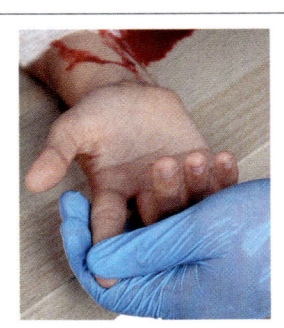

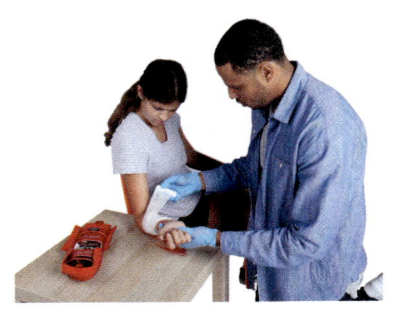

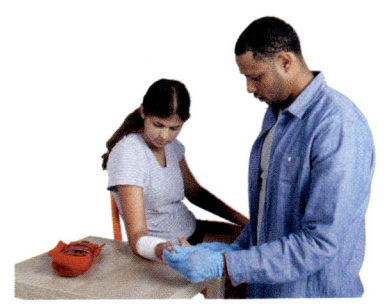

APPENDIX D
Skill Practice Sheets for Skill Boosts

Skill Practice Sheet: Administering Quick-Relief Medication Using an Inhaler **190**

Skill Practice Sheet: Administering Quick-Relief Medication Using a Nebulizer **191**

Skill Practice Sheet: Administering Epinephrine Using an Auto-Injector **193**

Skill Practice Sheet: Administering Naloxone Using a Nasal Spray **195**

Skill Practice Sheet: Administering Naloxone Using a Nasal Atomizer **196**

Skill Practice Sheet: Using Direct Pressure to Control Life-Threatening Bleeding **197**

Skill Practice Sheet: Using Direct Pressure and a Windlass Rod Tourniquet to Control Life-Threatening Bleeding **199**

Skill Practice Sheet: Using Direct Pressure and a Ratcheting Tourniquet to Control Life-Threatening Bleeding **201**

Skill Practice Sheet: Using Direct Pressure and an Elastic Tourniquet to Control Life-Threatening Bleeding **203**

Skill Practice Sheet: Wound Packing **205**

Skill Practice Sheet: Applying a Rigid Splint to a Leg **206**

Skill Practice Sheet: Applying a Sling and Binder **208**

Skill Practice Sheet: Applying a Vacuum Splint to a Leg **210**

Note: *Skill Practice Sheets are used for hands-on skill practice during instructor-led skills sessions.*

SKILL PRACTICE SHEET

Administering Quick-Relief Medication Using an Inhaler

1. **Verify the medication** with the person.
   - Check the label for the medication name and expiration date.

2. **Shake the inhaler** and **remove the mouthpiece cover**.

3. **Attach a spacing device** (and a **face mask** for a young child or infant) to the inhaler.

4. **Tell the person to breathe out** as much as possible through the mouth.

5. Have the person **place their lips tightly around the mouthpiece** (or **place the face mask over the child's or infant's nose and mouth**).

6. **Firmly press the inhaler canister** to release the medicine into the spacer.

7. Tell the person to take a **slow deep breath** and then to **hold their breath for 5 to 10 seconds**.
   - If they can't take a slow, deep breath OR they are using a spacer with a face mask, tell them to take **several normal breaths** from the spacer.

8. **Note the time of administration and any change in their condition**.

190 Appendix D | Skill Practice Sheets for Skill Boosts

SKILL PRACTICE SHEET

Administering Quick-Relief Medication Using a Nebulizer

1. Verify the medication with the person. ■ Check the label for the medication name and expiration date.	
2. Connect the tubing to the bottom of the medicine cup.	
3. Remove the cap of the medicine cup and **fill it with the prescribed amount of liquid medication**. **Note:** *Make sure the medicine cup remains upright.*	
4. Put the cap back onto the medicine cup and **connect the tubing to the air compressor**.	
5. Attach a mouthpiece OR a face mask to the medicine cup.	
6. Turn the nebulizer on and make sure it is misting.	

(Continued on next page)

American Red Cross | Appendices 191

SKILL PRACTICE SHEET

Administering Quick-Relief Medication Using a Nebulizer continued

7. Place the mouthpiece and have the person bite down to seal it in the person's mouth **OR place the face mask** over the person's nose and mouth.	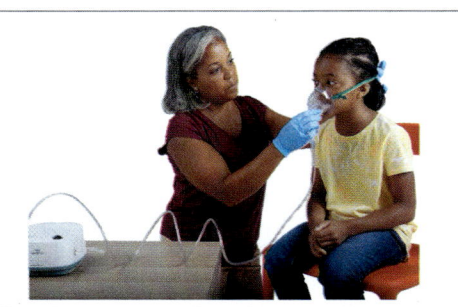
8. Tell the person to take slow and deep breaths through the mouth (mouthpiece) or mouth and nose (face mask) until all the medicine is used. ■ Occasionally tap the sides of the nebulizer to help the medicine drop to where it can be misted.	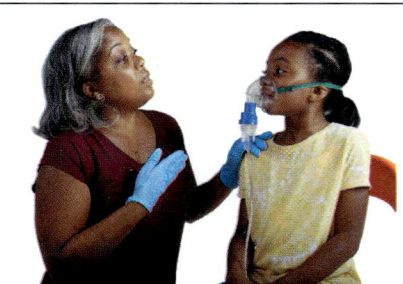
9. After all the medication has been given, **remove the mouthpiece** from the person's mouth **OR take the mask off** the person. Then, turn off the nebulizer.	
10. Note the time of administration and any **change in their condition**.	

192 Appendix D | Skill Practice Sheets for Skill Boosts

SKILL PRACTICE SHEET

Administering Epinephrine Using an Auto-Injector

1. **Verify the medication** with the person.
   - Check the label for the medication name and expiration date.

2. **Remove the cap and any safety device** on the auto-injector.

3. **Locate the outside middle of one thigh** to use as the injection site.

4. **Hold the person's leg firmly.**
   - With one hand, hold the person's leg firmly to limit movement while you administer the medication.

5. **Administer the medication.**
   - With your other hand, administer the medication.
   - Quickly and firmly push the auto-injector tip into the person's thigh at a 90-degree angle.
   - Hold it in place for 3 seconds after a click is heard.

   Note: It's OK to do this through clothing, if necessary.

(Continued on next page)

American Red Cross | Appendices

SKILL PRACTICE SHEET

Administering Epinephrine Using an Auto-Injector continued

6. Massage the injection area for 10 seconds.	
7. Note the time of administration and any change in their condition.	

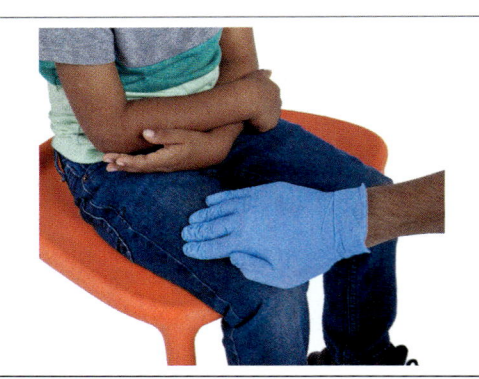

SKILL PRACTICE SHEET

Administering Naloxone Using a Nasal Spray

1. Verify the medication. ■ Check the label for the medication name and expiration date.	
2. Hold the naloxone device with your thumb on the bottom of the plunger and two fingers on either side of the nozzle.	
3. Place and hold the tip of the nozzle in either nostril until your fingers touch the bottom of the person's nose.	
4. Press the plunger firmly to release the dose into the person's nose.	

American Red Cross | Appendices 195

SKILL PRACTICE SHEET

Administering Naloxone Using a Nasal Atomizer

1. **Verify the medication.**
   - Check the label for the medication name and expiration date.

2. **Uncap the naloxone medication vial** and the **syringe OR uncap the prefilled syringe.**

3. **Attach the medication vial onto the syringe, if necessary.**

4. **Screw the nasal atomizer spray device onto the top of the syringe.**

5. **Spray half of the medication into each nostril.**

SKILL PRACTICE SHEET

Using Direct Pressure to Control Life-Threatening Bleeding

1. Place the dressing on the wound.*

- Ensure good contact with the bleeding surfaces of the wound.

Use a hemostatic dressing if available.

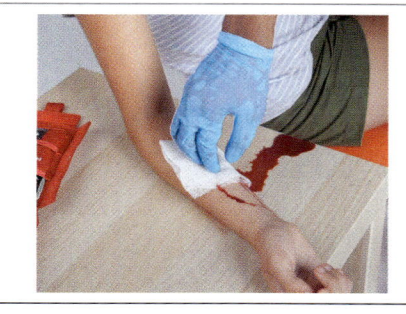

2. Apply steady, firm pressure directly over the wound until the bleeding stops.

- Put one hand on top of the dressing and put your other hand on top.
- Position your shoulders over your hands and lock your elbows.
- Push down as hard as you can.
- If blood soaks through the original gauze pad, you do not need to do anything, but you can put another gauze pad on top. Replace the new gauze pad as necessary if blood soaks through the pads.

Note: Do not remove the original gauze pad and **do not** stack multiple gauze pads.

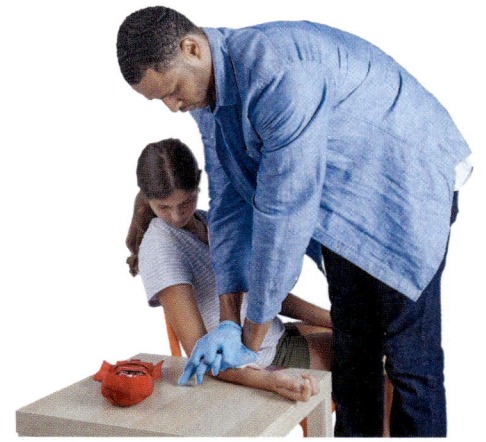

3. Hold direct pressure until:

- The bleeding stops.
- A tourniquet is applied (for life-threatening bleeding from an arm or leg) and the bleeding has stopped.
- Another person relieves you.
- You are too exhausted to continue.
- The situation becomes unsafe.

(Continued on next page)

SKILL PRACTICE SHEET

Using Direct Pressure to Control Life-Threatening Bleeding continued

If bleeding stops before EMS arrives:

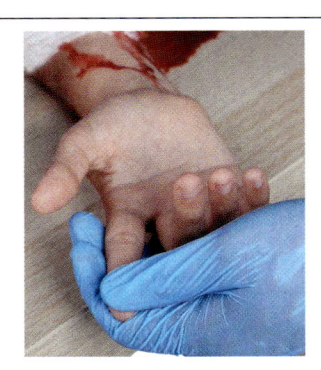

4. Apply a roller bandage.

- Check for circulation beyond the injury.
- Apply the bandage over the dressing and secure it firmly to keep pressure on the wound.
  - Place the end of a bandage on the dressing at a 45-degree angle.
  - Continue wrapping the bandage over the dressing.
  - Tape to secure the dressing.
- Check again for circulation beyond the injury. If there is any change, the bandage may be too tight; carefully loosen the bandage.

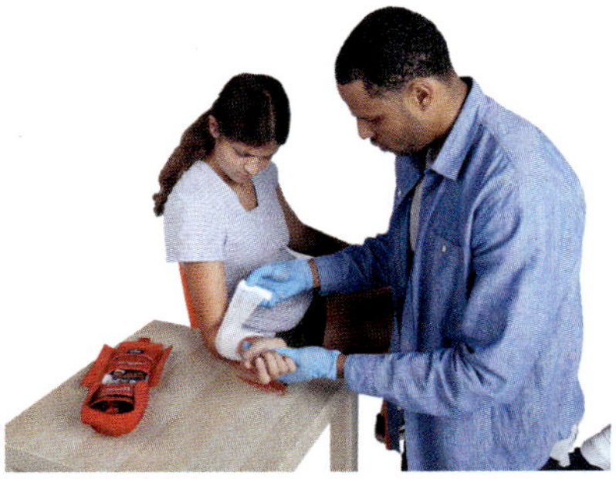

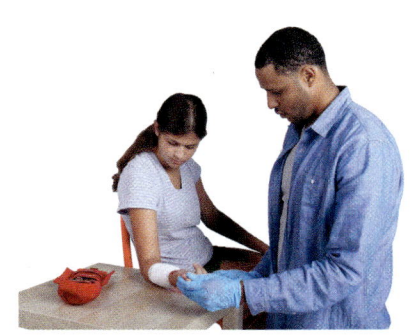

SKILL PRACTICE SHEET

Using Direct Pressure and a Windlass Rod Tourniquet to Control Life-Threatening Bleeding

The steps in this skill practice sheet are a guide to using a Windlass Rod Tourniquet. Always follow the instructions of the particular tourniquet to which you have access.

1. **Place the dressing on the wound.***

   * Use a hemostatic dressing if available.

2. **Apply steady, firm pressure directly over the wound until the tourniquet is available.**

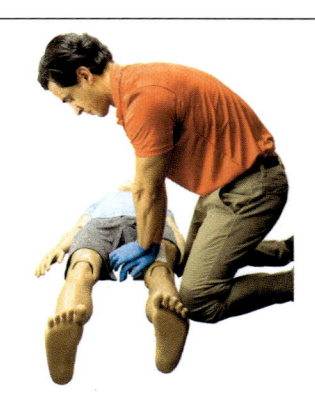

3. **Continue to apply direct pressure until a tourniquet is available.**
   - Once a tourniquet is available, have a member of your group continue applying direct pressure while you apply the tourniquet.
   - If you are practicing alone, use your knee to apply pressure while you apply the tourniquet.

4. **Position the tourniquet.**
   - Place the tourniquet around the limb, 2 to 3 inches above the wound between the wound and the heart.
   - Do not place the tourniquet on top of the wound or a joint.
   - If the wound is over a joint, apply the tourniquet 2 to 3 inches above the joint.

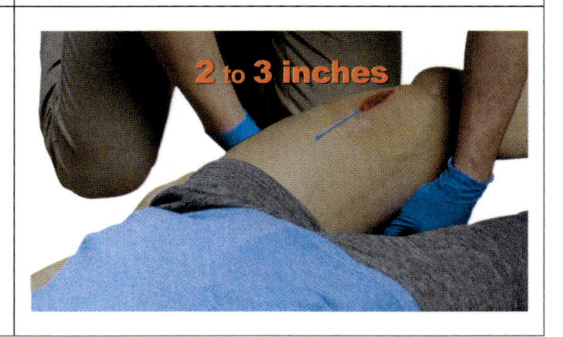

(Continued on next page)

American Red Cross | Appendices 199

SKILL PRACTICE SHEET

Using Direct Pressure and a Windlass Rod Tourniquet to Control Life-Threatening Bleeding continued

5. Buckle the tourniquet.
- Attach the buckle or pass the end of the strap through the buckle.

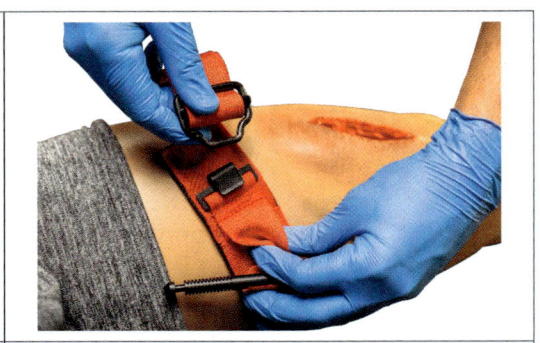

6. PULL.
- Pull the free end of the strap until the tourniquet is as tight as possible around the arm or leg.
- Make sure there is no room between the tourniquet and the limb before activating the tightening mechanism.
- If the strap has a hook-and-loop fastener, securely fasten the strap back onto itself after you have pulled the tourniquet as tight as possible around the arm or leg.
- If the tourniquet is not tight enough around the leg, it may be beneficial to move the tourniquet closer on the limb to the core of the body where the extremity is thicker.

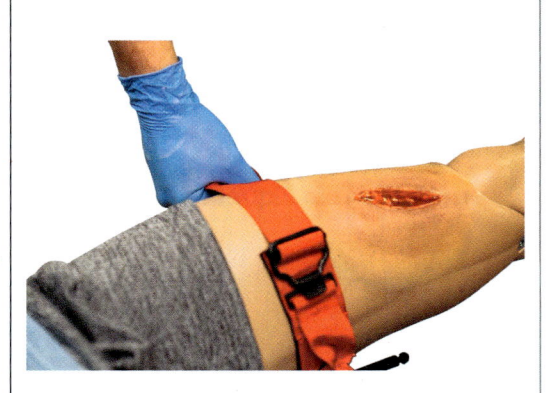

7. TWIST.
- Twist the rod until the bleeding stops or until you cannot twist it anymore.

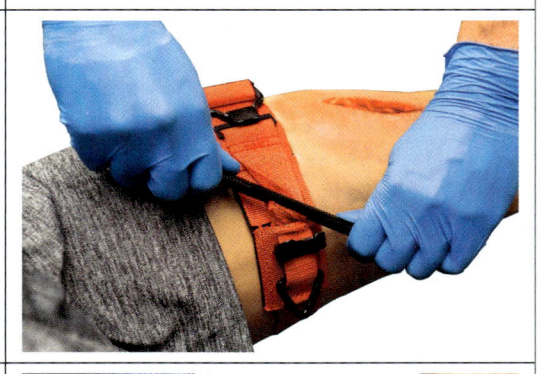

8. CLIP.
- Clip the rod in place to prevent the rod from untwisting and to keep the tourniquet tight.

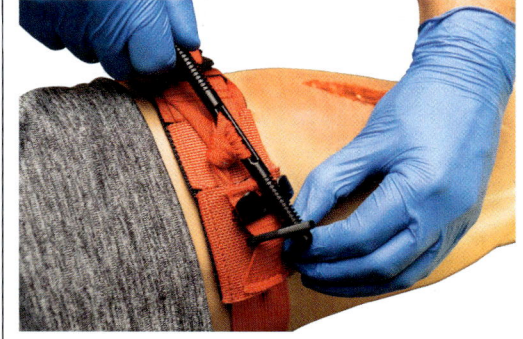

SKILL PRACTICE SHEET

Using Direct Pressure and a Ratcheting Tourniquet to Control Life-Threatening Bleeding

The steps in this skill practice sheet are a guide to using a Ratcheting Tourniquet. Always follow the instructions of the particular tourniquet to which you have access.

Note: *There are adult and child sizes: TX-3/TX-1. Both adult and child work exactly the same way.*

1. **Place the dressing on the wound.***

   * *Use a hemostatic dressing if available.*

2. **Apply steady, firm pressure directly over the wound until the tourniquet is available.**

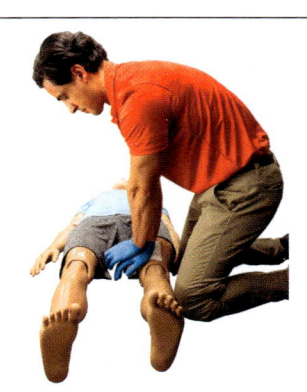

3. **Continue to apply direct pressure until a tourniquet is available.**
   - Once a tourniquet is available, have a member of your group continue applying direct pressure while you apply the tourniquet.
   - If you are practicing alone, use your knee to apply pressure while you apply the tourniquet.

4. **Position the tourniquet.**
   - Place the tourniquet around the limb, 2 to 3 inches above the wound.
   - Avoid placing the tourniquet on top of the wound or a joint.
   - If the wound is over a joint, apply the tourniquet 2 to 3 inches above the joint.

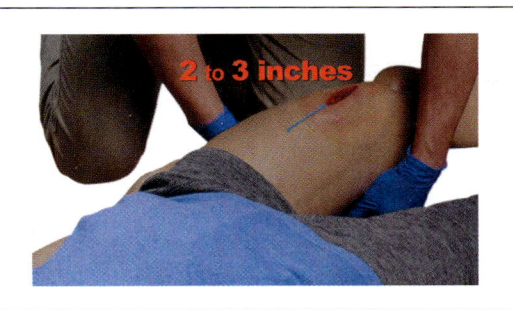

(Continued on next page)

American Red Cross | Appendices 201

SKILL PRACTICE SHEET

Using Direct Pressure and a Ratcheting Tourniquet to Control Life-Threatening Bleeding continued

5. PULL Tight.

- Pull tight on the loop to tighten the strap as tight as possible around the arm or leg.
- Make sure there is no room between the tourniquet and the limb before activating the tightening mechanism.
- If the tourniquet is not tight enough around the leg, it may be beneficial to move the tourniquet closer on the limb to the core of the body where the extremity is thicker.

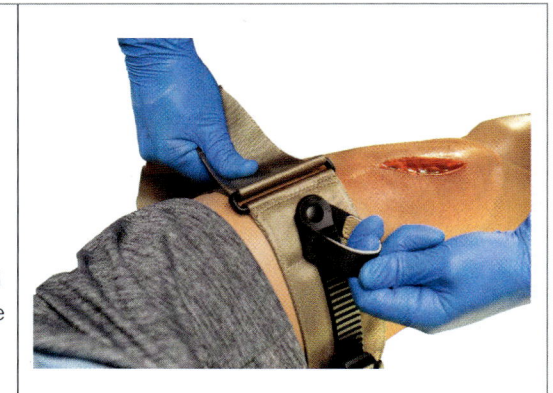

6. LIFT.

- Lift the buckle to tighten the tourniquet.
- Keep lifting up on the buckle until the bleeding stops or you cannot lift it up anymore.
- Ratcheting tourniquets are self-securing.

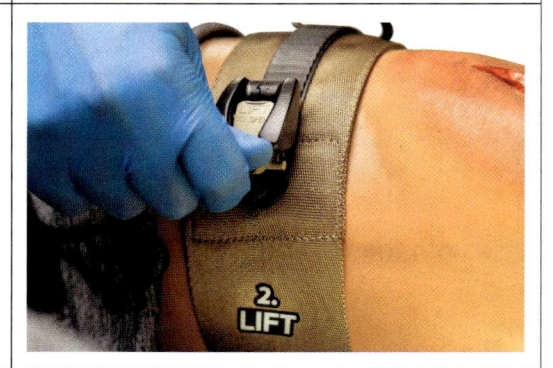

SKILL PRACTICE SHEET

Using Direct Pressure and an Elastic Tourniquet to Control Life-Threatening Bleeding

The steps in this skill practice sheet are a guide to using an Elastic Tourniquet. Always follow the instructions of the particular tourniquet to which you have access.

1. Place the dressing on the wound.*

* Use a hemostatic dressing if available.

2. Apply steady, firm pressure directly over the wound until the tourniquet is available.

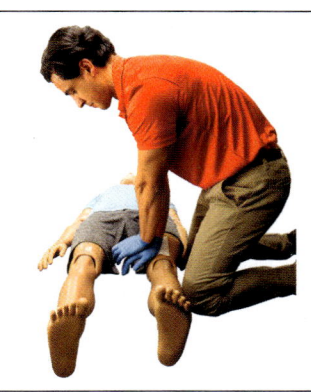

3. Continue to apply direct pressure until a tourniquet is available.

- Once a tourniquet is available, have a member of your group continue applying direct pressure while you apply the tourniquet.
- If you are practicing alone, use your knee to apply pressure while you apply the tourniquet.

4. WRAP.

- Wrap the tourniquet around the limb, 2 to 3 inches above the wound.
- Avoid placing the tourniquet on top of the wound or a joint.
- If the wound is over a joint, apply the tourniquet 2 to 3 inches above the joint.

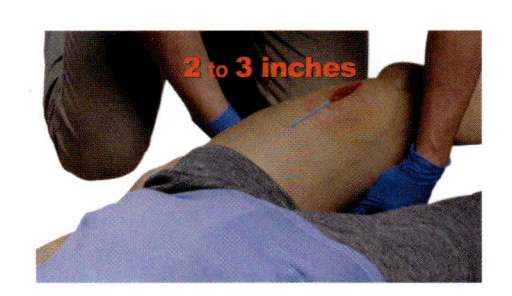

(Continued on next page)

American Red Cross | Appendices 203

SKILL PRACTICE SHEET

Using Direct Pressure and an Elastic Tourniquet to Control Life-Threatening Bleeding continued

5. PULL.

- Continue wrapping the tourniquet around the limb, stretching and pulling it as tight as possible with each wrap.
- You will know you are stretching and pulling it tight enough when you see a change in the shapes on the tourniquet from ovals to circles and diamonds to squares.

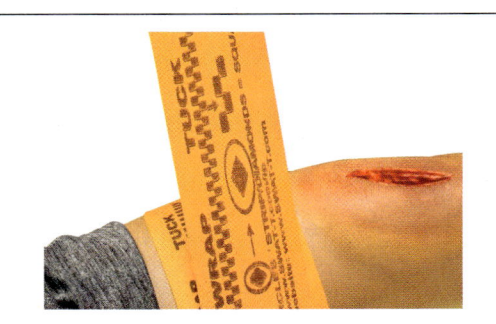

6. TUCK.

- As you near the end of the tourniquet, pull and wrap tightly, lifting up the last wrap to create a loop.
- Tuck the free end of the tourniquet underneath the loop to secure the tourniquet.

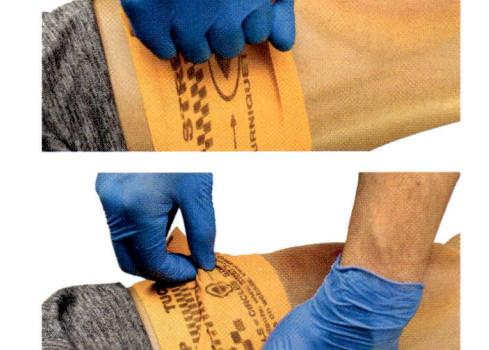

SKILL PRACTICE SHEET

Wound Packing

1. Locate the source of the bleeding within the wound.	
2. Place the dressing into the wound cavity directly onto the bleeding source.* ** Use a hemostatic dressing if available.*	
3. Continue packing the entire wound cavity. ■ While holding pressure on the bleeding source, continue packing the entire wound cavity until it is tightly packed.	
4. Apply direct pressure.	

American Red Cross | Appendices

SKILL PRACTICE SHEET

Applying a Rigid Splint to a Leg

1. Support the injured body part. ■ Support the injured body part above and below the site of the injury. **Note:** *The ground provides support for a leg injury.*	
2. Check for circulation and sensation beyond the injured area.	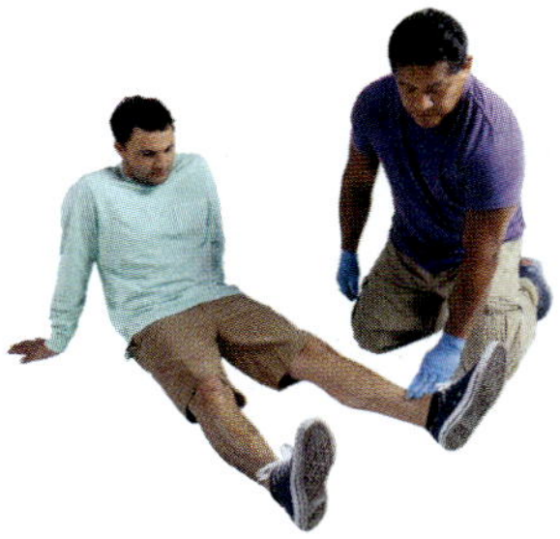
3. Place bandages. ■ Slide several folded triangular bandages under the leg, where there is a gap between the leg and the ground. ■ Slide them above and below the injured body part.	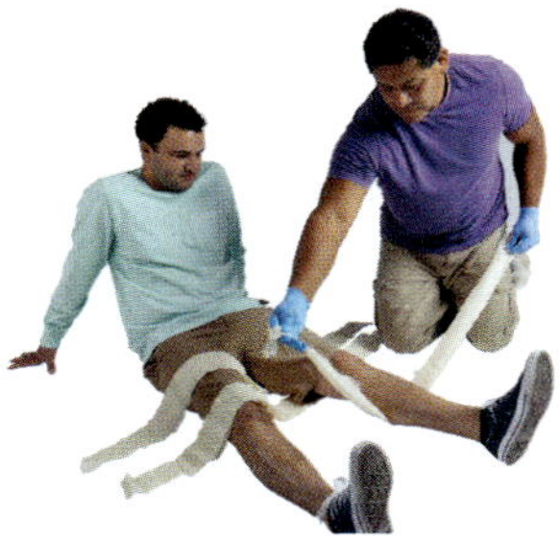
4. Place rigid splints. ■ Place two appropriately sized rigid splints *along* the two sides of the injured leg, ensuring that they extend to either the bone or joint above and below the injured area.	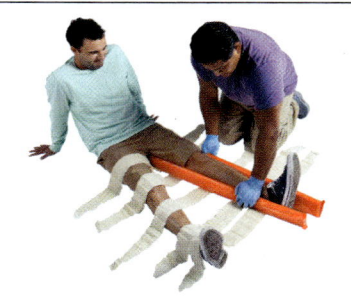
5. Secure the splints. ■ Secure the splints by tying the triangular bandages above and below the injured body part. ■ Tie the triangular bandages from bottom to top, but tie the bandage around the foot last.	

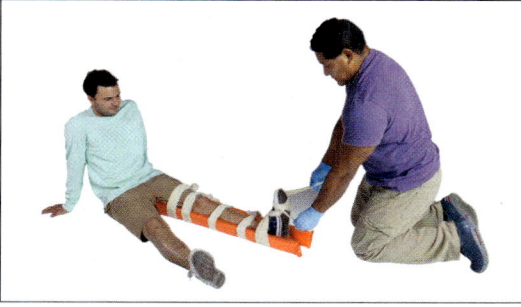

SKILL PRACTICE SHEET

6. Recheck for circulation and sensation.

- Recheck for circulation and sensation beyond the injured area.

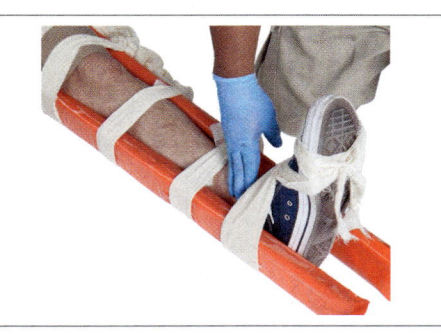

SKILL PRACTICE SHEET

Applying a Sling and Binder

1. **Support the injured body part.**
   - Support the injured body part above and below the site of the injury.

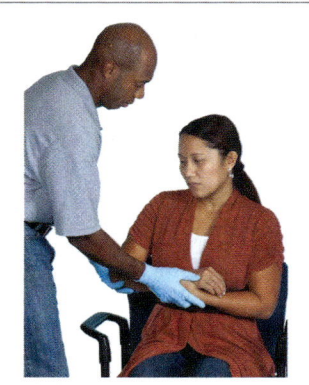

2. **Check for circulation and sensation** **beyond the injured area.**

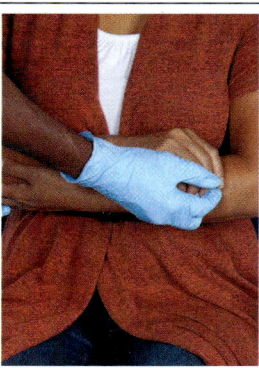

3. **Place the bandage.**
   - Place a triangular bandage under the injured arm and over the uninjured shoulder to form a sling.

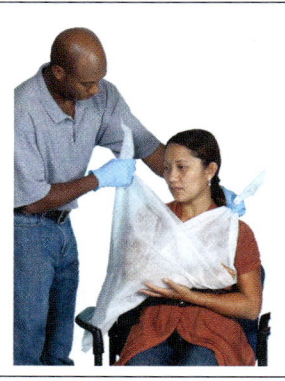

4. **Tie the sling.**
   - Tie the ends of the sling at the side of the neck.
   - Use gauze to pad between the knot and the skin to lessen discomfort.

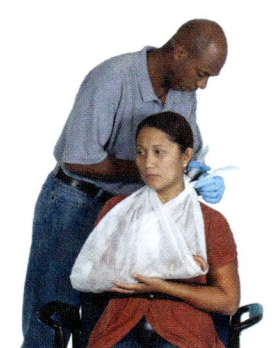

SKILL PRACTICE SHEET

5. Bind the injured body part to the chest with a folded triangular bandage.

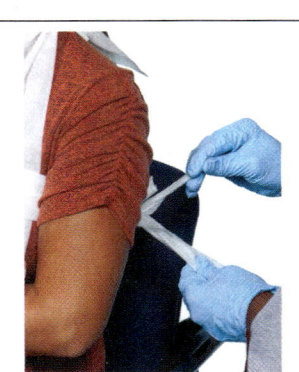

6. Recheck for circulation and sensation beyond the injured area.

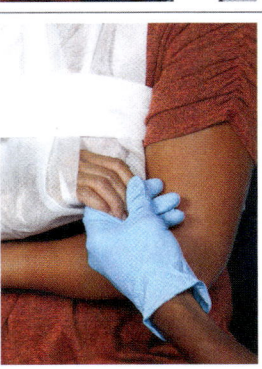

American Red Cross | Appendices

SKILL PRACTICE SHEET

Applying a Vacuum Splint to a Leg

1. Support the injured body part. ■ Support the injured body part above and below the site of the injury. **Note:** *The ground provides support for a leg injury.*	
2. Check for circulation and sensation **beyond the injured area.**	
3. Place the splint flat on the ground **with the valve side down.**	
4. Push the valve to equalize air pressure. ■ Remove the red cap from the valve and push in on the red end of the valve to equalize the air pressure in the splint.	
5. Distribute the beads throughout the splint evenly.	
6. Place the splint under the injured limb. ■ Ensure that the splint extends to either the bone or joint above and below the injured area. ■ Make sure that at least one strap is above the suspected fracture site and at least one strap is below the suspected fracture site. **Note:** *Do not attach the splint straps to secure the splint at this time.*	

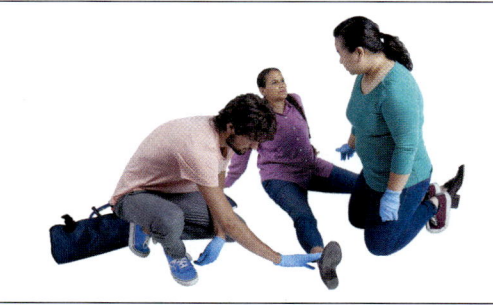

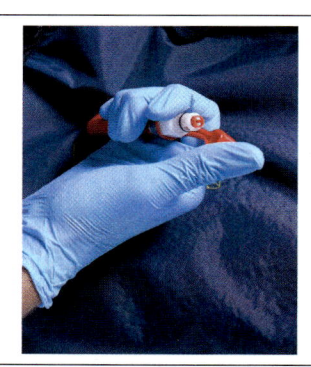

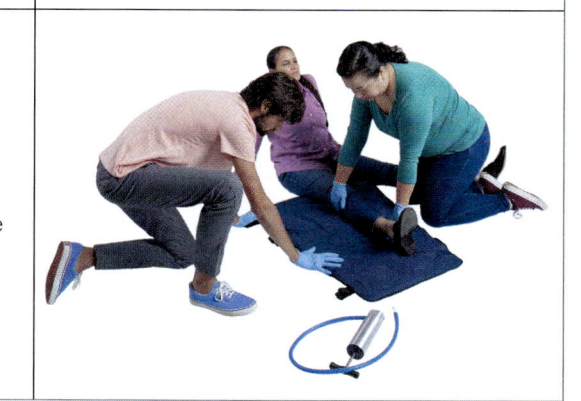

SKILL PRACTICE SHEET

7. Conform the splint around the injured limb.

- Do not overlap the splint edges.

Note: If the splint does not conform easily, you can adjust it by allowing air to enter the splint.

- Leave a 1-inch open space along the length of the splint to allow for visualization of the injured limb.

Note: If the splint is too wide, you can fold the edge without the straps back on itself to form a narrower splint.

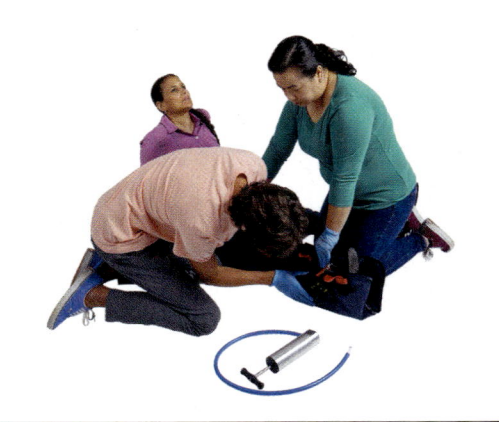

8. Hold the splint in place.

- Ask the coach to assist you by holding the splint in place by grasping both edges of the splint above and below the fracture site while you operate the pump.

9. Connect the pump hose to the valve.

- You should hear a "click" when the connection has been made.

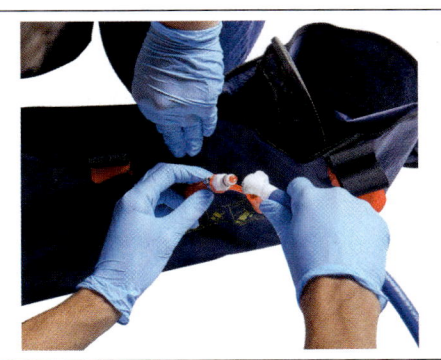

10. Operate the pump to remove the air from the splint.

- Keep pumping until the splint is rigid around the injured limb.
- You will feel resistance when enough air has been removed from the splint.

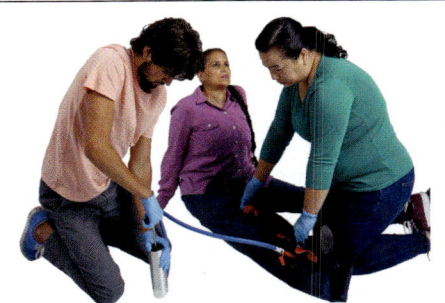

11. Remove the pump hose from the valve by pressing the metal tab on the pump hose coupling and replace red cap.

(Continued on next page)

American Red Cross | Appendices

SKILL PRACTICE SHEET

Applying a Vacuum Splint to a Leg continued

12. Attach the splint straps around the splint to secure it in place.

- Attach the straps from bottom to top, but attach the strap around the foot last.

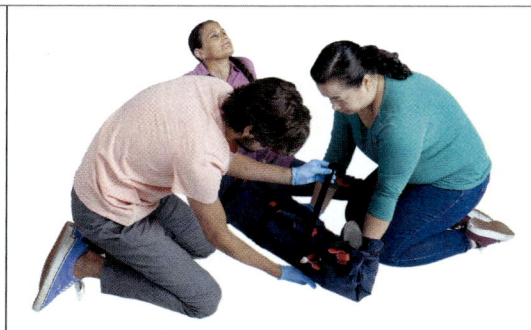

13. Recheck for circulation and sensation beyond the injured area.

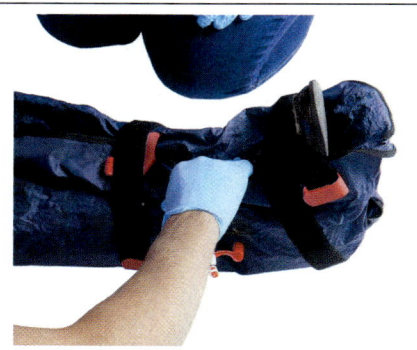

Glossary

A

Abdominal thrusts: inward and upward thrusts just above the navel, used in combination with back blows to force the object out of the airway when a person is choking

Abrasion: an open wound that occurs when something rubs roughly against the skin, causing damage to the skin's surface

Abuse: the willful infliction of injury or harm on another

Acute illness: an illness that strikes suddenly and usually only lasts for a short period of time

Adolescent: someone from the onset of puberty through adulthood

Agonal breaths: isolated or infrequent gasping in the absence of normal breathing. Agonal breaths *do not* represent the presence of breathing when checking the person.

Airborne pathogens: disease-causing microorganisms that are expelled into the air when an infected person breathes, coughs or sneezes

Airborne transmission: infection spread through exposure to infectious agent-containing respiratory droplets comprised of smaller droplets (usually less than 5 micrometers) that can remain suspended in the air for longer periods of time and can travel greater distances (usually greater than 6 feet) and time (typically hours)

Anaphylaxis: a severe, life-threatening allergic reaction

Antihistamine: a medication that counteracts the effects of histamine, a chemical released by the body during an allergic reaction

Asthma: a chronic illness in which certain substances or conditions (triggers) cause inflammation and narrowing of the airways, making breathing difficult

Asthma action plan: a written plan that the person develops with his or her healthcare provider that details daily management of the condition as well as how to handle an asthma attack

Asthma triggers: substances or conditions that initiate an asthma attack when the person is exposed to them

Aura: an unusual sensation or feeling that may signal the onset of a seizure in some people

Avulsion: an open wound that occurs when a portion of the skin, and sometimes the underlying tissue, is partially or completely torn away

B

Back blows: blows between the shoulder blades, used in combination with abdominal thrusts to force the object out of the airway when a person is choking

Bandage: a strip of material used to hold a dressing in place and to control bleeding

Bloodborne pathogens: disease-causing microorganisms that are spread when blood from an infected person enters the bloodstream of a person who is not infected

Blunt trauma: injury caused by impact with a flat object or surface

Brain contusion: bruising of the brain tissue

Brain hematoma: bleeding into the space between the brain and the skull

Breathing barriers: devices used to protect the responder from contact with exhaled air, saliva and other body fluids, such as blood, when giving breaths

Bronchiolitis: an infection of the lower airway that can cause difficulty breathing

Bruise (contusion): a type of closed wound that occurs when the small blood vessels under the surface of the skin are damaged and blood leaks into the surrounding tissues

Burn: a traumatic injury to the skin (and sometimes the underlying tissues as well) caused by contact with extreme heat, chemicals, radiation or electricity

C

Cardiac arrest: a condition that occurs when the heart stops beating or beats too ineffectively to circulate blood to the brain and other vital organs

Cardiac Chain of Survival: six actions that, when performed in rapid succession, increase a person's likelihood of surviving cardiac arrest

Chest thrusts: quick thrusts into the center of a person's chest used to help remove an obstruction when someone is choking

Child: someone from the age of 1 year to the onset of puberty. One can use the evidence of breast development in girls and underarm hair development in boys (usually around the age of 12 years) to help determine onset of puberty.

Chronic illness: an illness that a person lives with on an ongoing basis and that often requires continuous treatment to manage

Closed wound: a wound where the surface of the skin is intact but the underlying tissues are injured

Compression-only CPR: a CPR technique that involves giving continuous chest compressions, with no breaths

Concussion: a traumatic brain injury that alters the way the brain functions

Consent: permission to give care

Convulsions: uncontrolled body movements caused by contraction of the muscles due to electric activity in the brain

CPR: cardiopulmonary resuscitation; a skill involving compressing the chest and giving breaths that is used when a person is in cardiac arrest to keep oxygenated blood moving to the brain and other vital organs until advanced medical help arrives

Croup (laryngotracheobronchitis): an infection of the upper airway that causes difficulty breathing and a harsh, repetitive, bark-like cough; common in children younger than 5 years

D

Dehydration: too little fluid in the body

Depth of compressions: the depth to which one pushes down on the chest to give compressions during CPR. It differs by age group: Adults: at least 2 inches; Children: about 2 inches; Infants: about 1½ inches.

Diabetes: a chronic condition characterized by the body's inability to process glucose (sugar) in the bloodstream

Diffuse axonal injury: tearing of nerves due to traumatic injury

Dislocation: an injury that occurs when the bones that meet at a joint move out of their normal position

Dressing: a pad that is placed directly on a wound to absorb blood and other fluids and promote clotting

Droplet transmission: infection spread through exposure to infectious agent-containing respiratory droplets (i.e., larger particles) that are propelled through the air for short distances due to coughing, sneezing, talking or being in close contact with an infected person

E

Emergency medical services (EMS) system: a network of professionals linked together to provide the best care for people in all types of emergencies

Epiglottitis: swelling of the epiglottis (the piece of cartilage that covers the trachea), usually caused by a bacterial infection

Epilepsy: a chronic seizure disorder that can often be controlled with medication

Epinephrine: a drug that stimulates certain parts of the body and can be used to slow or stop the effects of anaphylaxis

Epinephrine auto-injector: a syringe system, available by prescription only, that contains a single dose of epinephrine, which allows administration by those who may not be trained in giving injections

External bleeding: bleeding that is visible on the outside of the body

F

Face shield: a breathing barrier used to protect the responder from contact with exhaled breath, saliva and other body fluids, such as blood, as they give breaths; consists of a flat piece of thin plastic and a one-way valve. This term is also often used to describe a plastic shield worn in front of the face to protect the eyes and face from exposure.

Febrile seizure: a convulsion brought on by a fever in an infant or small child

Flow of blood: the movement of blood

Fracture: a complete break, a chip or a crack in a bone

Frostbite: an injury caused by freezing of the skin and underlying tissues as a result of prolonged exposure to freezing or subfreezing temperatures

G

Good Samaritan laws: laws that protect people against claims of negligence when they give emergency care in good faith without accepting anything in return

H

Head-tilt/chin-lift maneuver: a technique used to open the airway

Heart attack: a condition that occurs when blood flow to part of the heart muscle is blocked, causing cells in the affected area of the heart muscle to die

Heat cramps: painful muscle spasms, usually in the legs and abdomen, caused by loss of fluids and electrolytes as a result of sweating

Heat exhaustion: a condition that occurs when fluids lost through sweating are not replaced

Heat stroke: a life-threatening condition that occurs when the body's cooling system is completely overwhelmed and stops working

Hemostatic dressing: a dressing treated with a substance that promotes clot formation

Hepatitis: inflammation of the liver, an organ that performs many vital functions for the body

High-quality CPR: CPR that includes correct hand placement and body position; compressing the chest at a rate of 100 to 120 compressions per minute; compressing the chest to a depth of at least 2 inches; allowing the chest to return to its normal position between each compression; minimizing necessary interruptions to chest compressions, and if there is an interruption keep it to less than 10 seconds; and avoiding excessive breaths. Each breath should last about 1 second and cause the chest to begin to rise.

HIV: a virus that invades and destroys the cells that help us to fight off infections

Hyperglycemia: excessively high blood glucose levels

Hyperventilation: breathing that is faster and often deeper than normal

Hypoglycemia: excessively low blood glucose levels

Hypothermia: a condition that occurs when the body loses heat faster than it can produce heat, causing the core body temperature to fall below 95° F (35° C)

I

Implied consent: permission to give care that is not expressly granted by the person but is assumed because circumstances exist that would lead a reasonable person to believe that the person would give consent if they were able to

Infant: someone under the age of 1 year

Influenza: a viral illness that is spread when virus-containing droplets are released into the air when an infected person coughs or sneezes

Insulin: a hormone secreted by the pancreas that causes glucose to be moved from the bloodstream into the cells, where it is used for energy

Internal bleeding: bleeding that occurs inside the body, into a body cavity or space

L

Laceration: a cut, commonly caused by a sharp object such as broken glass or a knife

Lay responder: a nonprofessional responder who gives care in an emergency situation

Long-term control medications: medications taken regularly to help prevent asthma attacks by reducing inflammation and swelling and making the airways less sensitive to triggers

Lung contusion: bruising of the lung tissue

O

Open wound: a wound where the skin's surface is broken

Opioids: drugs that are prescribed to reduce pain and can be used for events such as after surgeries or serious injuries, or for cancer pain. There are also illegal derivates of opioids, such as heroin.

Opioid overdose: exposure to an amount of opioid higher than is prescribed. Symptoms of an opioid overdose include evidence of opioid use and decreased breathing effort, for example, breathing slowly and perhaps only a few times a minute, and gasping or gurgling, unresponsiveness, bluish or grayish colored skin and cardiac arrest.

P

Paradoxical breathing: abnormal movement of the chest wall when a person breathes. (When the person inhales, the injured area draws in while the rest of the chest expands and when the person exhales, the injured area expands while the rest of the chest draws in.)

Paralysis: the loss of movement

Paraplegia: paralysis that affects both legs and the lower trunk

Pathogens: harmful microorganisms that can cause disease

Penetrating trauma: trauma that occurs when the body is pierced by or impaled on an object

Personal protective equipment (PPE): devices used to prevent pathogens from contaminating the skin, mucous membranes or clothing

Pneumothorax: collapse of a lung caused by an abnormal collection of air in the space between the lung and the chest wall

Pocket mask: a transparent, flexible device that creates a seal over the person's nose and mouth with a one-way valve to allow the responder to give rescue breaths without making mouth-to-mouth contact or inhaling exhaled air; a type of breathing barrier

Poison exposure: exposure to any substance that causes injury, illness or death if it enters the body or touches the surface of the body

Puncture wound: an open wound that occurs when an object, such as a nail or an animal's tooth, pierces the skin

Q

Quadriplegia: paralysis that affects both arms, the trunk and both legs

Quick-relief (rescue) medications: medications taken when a person is experiencing an acute asthma attack to open the airways right away

R

Rate of compressions: the rate at which one pushes down on the chest to give compressions during CPR. The compression rate during CPR is between 100 and 120 per minute for all age groups (adult, child and infant).

Respiratory arrest: absence of breathing

Respiratory distress: difficulty breathing

S

Scene size-up: a brief survey done prior to entering the scene of an emergency to ensure safety, form an initial impression about what happened and the nature of the person's illness or injury, identify any life-threatening conditions, and determine necessary resources

Seizure: a temporary and involuntary change in body movement, function, sensation, awareness or behavior that results from abnormal electrical activity in the brain

Shock: a progressive, life-threatening condition in which the circulatory system fails to deliver enough oxygen-rich blood to the body's tissues and organs, causing organs and body systems to begin to fail

Shout-tap-shout sequence: sequence used to check for responsiveness. Shout, using the person's name if you know it. If there is no response, tap the person's shoulder (if the person is an adult or child) or the bottom of the foot (for an infant) and shout again.

Splint: immobilization of a body part to limit motion, or the device used to limit the motion of a body part

Sprain: an injury that occurs when a ligament is stretched, torn or damaged. (Ligaments connect bones to bones at the joints.)

Strain: an injury that occurs when a tendon or muscle is stretched, torn or damaged. (Tendons connect muscles to bones.)

Stroke: a condition that occurs when blood flow to part of the brain is interrupted, causing cells in the affected area of the brain to die

Sudden cardiac arrest: cardiac arrest that happens suddenly and without any warning signs

T

Tetanus: a severe bacterial infection that can result from a puncture wound or a deep laceration

Thermoregulation: the body's ability to maintain an internal temperature within an acceptable range despite external conditions

Tourniquet: a device placed around an arm or leg to apply pressure and compress blood vessels and stop blood flow to a wound to treat life-threatening bleeding

Tracheostomy: a surgically created opening in the front of the neck that opens into the trachea (windpipe) to form an alternate route for breathing when the upper airway is blocked or damaged

Transient ischemic attack (TIA): a condition that occurs when blood flow to part of the brain is temporarily interrupted, causing stroke-like signs and symptoms that then go away

Traumatic amputation: the loss of a body part as a result of an injury

Triggers: a substance or condition that normally causes no reaction in one person but creates an overreaction in the body of another person on exposure, leading to inflammation

Tuberculosis: a bacterial infection of the lungs that is spread through airborne transmission from one person to another

U

Urushiol: an oil on plants such as poison ivy, poison sumac and poison oak that causes an allergic skin reaction in many people

V

Ventricular fibrillation (V-fib): an abnormal heart rhythm in which the heart muscle simply quivers (fibrillates) weakly instead of contracting strongly so that there is no circulation

Ventricular tachycardia (V-tach): an abnormal heart rhythm in which the heart muscle contracts too fast for effective blood circulation, which can lead to cardiac arrest

Volume of blood: the amount of blood present

W

Wheezing: a high-pitched, noisy breathing and/or whistling sound during exhalation

Wound: an injury that results when the skin or other tissues of the body are damaged

Sources

American Academy of Allergy, Asthma and Immunology. *Food Allergy.* https://www.aaaai.org/Conditions-Treatments/Allergies/Food-Allergy. Accessed January 2021.

American College of Surgeons. *Stop the Bleed, Save a Life: What Everyone Should Know to Stop Bleeding After an Injury.* https://www.bleedingcontrol.org/-/media/bleedingcontrol/files/stop-the-bleed-booklet.ashx. Accessed January 2021.

American Diabetes Association. *Hyperglycemia (High Blood Glucose).* https://www.diabetes.org/healthy-living/medication-treatments/blood-glucose-testing-and-control/hyperglycemia. Accessed January 2021.

American Diabetes Association. *Hypoglycemia (Low Blood Sugar).* https://www.diabetes.org/healthy-living/medication-treatments/blood-glucose-testing-and-control/hypoglycemia. Accessed January 2021.

American Family Physician. *Practical Tips for Preventing a Sickle Cell Crisis.* https://www.aafp.org/afp/2000/0301/p1363.html. Accessed January 2021.

American Heart Association. *CPR Facts and Stats.* https://cpr.heart.org/en/resources/cpr-facts-and-stats. Accessed January 2021.

American Heart Association. *Telecommunicator CPR (T-CPR).* https://cpr.heart.org/en/resuscitation-science/telecommunicator-cpr. Accessed January 2021.

American Lung Association. *Asthma.* https://www.lung.org/lung-health-diseases/lung-disease-lookup/asthma. Accessed January 2021.

The American National Red Cross. 2019. *Basic Life Support Participant's Manual.*

The American National Red Cross. 2021. *First Aid for Severe Trauma Handbook.*

The American National Red Cross. 2020. *Focused Updates and Guidelines 2020.*

American National Standards Institute. *Workplace First Aid Kits—ANSI/ISEA Z308-2015—Classes, Types, and the Standard.* https://blog.ansi.org/2018/06/workplace-first-aid-kits-ansi-isea-z308-2015/#gref. Accessed January 2021.

American National Standards Institute and International Safety Equipment Association. *Minimum Requirements for Workplace First Aid Kits and Supplies.* https://dir.nv.gov/uploadedFiles/dirnvgov/content/News/Useful%20Guidance%20for%20First%20Aid%20Kits.pdf. Accessed January 2021.

Asthma and Allergy Foundation of America: *Asthma Overview.* https://www.aafa.org/asthma.aspx. Accessed January 2021.

Celox Medical. *The Best of the 3-Minute Compression Gauzes.* https://www.celoxmedical.com/cx-product/celox-gauze/. Accessed January 2021.

Centers for Disease Control and Prevention. https://www.cdc.gov/. Accessed January 2021.

Centers for Disease Control and Prevention. *Prevent Lyme Disease.* https://www.cdc.gov/ncezid/dvbd/media/lymedisease.html. Accessed January 2021.

Congress.gov. *Patient Self-Determination Act of 1994.* https://www.congress.gov/bill/101st-congress/house-bill/4449. Accessed January 2021.

Home Safety Council. *Poison Prevention Tips.* https://www.homesafetycouncil.org/SafetyGuide/sg_poison_w001.asp. Accessed January 2021.

International Liaison Committee on Resuscitation (ILCOR). https://www.ilcor.org/. Accessed January 2021.

Journal of Emergency Medical Services. *Use of Hemostatic Dressings in Civilian EMS.* https://www.jems.com/2008/02/29/use-hemostatic-dressings-civil/. Accessed January 2021.

MayoClinic.com. *Hypothermia: Symptoms and Causes.* https://www.mayoclinic.org/diseases-conditions/hypothermia/symptoms-causes/syc-20352682. Accessed January 2021.

MedlinePlus. *Epiglottitis.* https://www.nlm.nih.gov/medlineplus/ency/article/000605.htm. Accessed January 2021.

MedlinePlus. *Hypothermia.* http://www.nlm.nih.gov/medlineplus/hypothermia.html. Accessed January 2021.

MedlinePlus. *Transient Ischemic Attack.* https://medlineplus.gov/transientischemicattack.html. Accessed January 2021.

National Center for Biotechnology Information, U.S. National Library of Medicine. Sickle Cell Crisis. https://www.ncbi.nlm.nih.gov/books/NBK526064/. Accessed January 2021.

National Highway Traffic Safety Administration. *Car Seats and Booster Seats.* https://www.nhtsa.gov/equipment/car-seats-and-booster-seats. Accessed January 2021.

Nursing 2021. *Wrapping an Ankle with an Elastic Compression Bandage.* https://journals.lww.com/nursing/Citation/2009/12000/Wrapping_an_ankle_with_an_elastic_compression.5.aspx. Accessed January 2021.

Real First Aid. *A Brief Guide to Haemostatic Agents.* https://www.realfirstaid.co.uk/haemostatics. Accessed January 2021.

Recreational Equipment, Inc. (REI). *Layering Basics.* https://www.rei.com/learn/expert-advice/layering-basics.html. Accessed January 2021.

Sickle Cell Disease News. *Here's What Triggers a Sickle Cell Crisis for Me.* https://sicklecellanemianews.com/2020/10/09/what-causes-sickle-cell-crisis/. Accessed January 2021.

Sickle Cell Disease News. *How I Manage a Sickle Cell Crisis at Home.* https://sicklecellanemianews.com/2020/10/23/how-manage-sickle-cell-crisis-home-tips/. Accessed January 2021.

TeensHealth. *Sickle Cell Crisis (Pain).* https://kidshealth.org/en/teens/sickle-crisis.html. Accessed January 2021.

United States Code, Title 42, Section 1395 cc (a)(1)(Q)(A). https://www.govinfo.gov/app/details/USCODE-2010-title42/USCODE-2010-title42-chap7-subchapXVIII-partE-sec1395cc. Accessed January 2021.

United States Department of Health and Human Services. *The Poison Help Line.* https://poisonhelp.hrsa.gov/. Accessed January 2021.

United States Department of Justice. *Burn Injuries in Child Abuse.* https://www.ncjrs.gov/pdffiles/91190-6.pdf. Accessed January 2021.

United States Department of Labor. *OSHA's Heat Illness Prevention Campaign.* https://www.osha.gov/heat. Accessed January 2021.

United States Federal Communications Commission. *Wireless 911 Service.* https://www.fcc.gov/consumers/guides/911-wireless-services. Accessed January 2021.

WebMD. *What Is a Sickle Cell Crisis?* https://www.webmd.com/a-to-z-guides/sickle-cell-crisis#1. Accessed January 2021.

Photography Credits

Chapter 1

Page 5   iStock.com/lostinbids
Page 10 iStock.com/GrabillCreative
Page 10 TheWikiContributor (derivative author)/DoerNoc (original author)
Page 10 iStock.com/NickyBlade
Page 13 iStock.com/photovs
Page 13 MegaPixel/Shutterstock.com
Page 17 iStock.com/Nastco
Page 21 iStock.com/releon8211
Page 22 iStock.com/GrapeImages

Chapter 2

Page 39 iStock.com/coffeekai

Chapter 3

Page 50 Gelpi/Shutterstock.com
Page 50 TY Lim/Shutterstock.com
Page 50 Syda Productions/Shutterstock.com
Page 57 Michelle Lala Clark Photography

Chapter 4

Page 66 iStock.com/Tim UR
Page 66 iStock.com/FineArtCraig
Page 67 iStock.com/Pixel_away
Page 70 cyperc stock/Shutterstock.com
Page 70 cyperc stock/Shutterstock.com

Chapter 5

Page 80 iStock.com/GrabillCreative
Page 83 iStock.com/koya79
Page 85 iStock.com/kwanchaichaiudom
Page 85 iStock.com/urtoicurto
Page 88 Allison Herreid/Shutterstock.com
Page 88 Peter Waters/Shutterstock.com
Page 88 Mrs.Rungnapa akthaisong/Shutterstock.com
Page 89 kaleo

Page 90 Steve Heap/Shutterstock.com
Page 90 iStock.com/spukkato
Page 92 Bob LoCicero/Shutterstock.com
Page 92 iStock.com/digitalskillet
Page 98 CGN089/Shutterstock.com
Page 99 iStock.com/evrim ertik
Page 100 iStock.com/parinyabinsuk

Chapter 6

Page 106 iStock.com/Andrii Zorii
Page 106 iStock.com/helovi
Page 106 iStock.com/RapidEye
Page 113 iStock.com/digitalskillet

Chapter 7

Page 123 iStock.com/Nes
Page 125 iStock.com/cveiv
Page 126 iStock.com/industryview
Page 127 iStock.com/Evgen_Prozhyrko
Page 127 iStock.com/robeo
Page 128 iStock.com/Daisy-Daisy
Page 129 danielo/Shutterstock.com
Page 133 ALPA PROD/Shutterstock.com
Page 138 iStock.com/Cineberg
Page 138 iStock.com/skibreck
Page 141 iStock.com/red_pepper82
Page 141 iStock.com/Devonyu
Page 141 Scott Rothstein/Shutterstock.com
Page 142 iStock.com/Mod Quaint
Page 143 iStock.com/Gannet77
Page 143 AppleZoomZoom/Shutterstock.com
Page 143 iStock.com/Ivan-balvan
Page 143 iStock.com/Kameleon007
Page 144 Penn State Pesticide Education Program and Pennsylvania Poison Centers
Page 146 Eric Isselee/Shutterstock.com
Page 146 iStock.com/stevelenzphoto
Page 146 iStock.com/amwu
Page 146 iStock.com/negaprion
Page 146 iStock.com/texcroc
Page 147 iStock.com/stephanie phillips
Page 147 iStock.com/Schiz-Art
Page 148 iStock.com/andriano_cz
Page 149 Centers for Disease Control and Prevention, National Center for Emerging and Zoonotic Infectious Diseases, Division of Vector-Borne Diseases
Page 150 Dan Alto/Shutterstock.com
Page 150 iStock.com/rainmax
Page 151 iStock.com/Mshake
Page 151 Yann hubert/Shutterstock.com

Page 151 iStock.com/naturediver
Page 151 iStock.com/naturediver
Page 152 Dwight Smith/Shutterstock.com
Page 152 Dwight Smith/Shutterstock.com
Page 152 Courtesy of www.poison-ivy.org
Page 153 iStock.com/Molnár ákos

Appendix B

Page 159 iStock.com/RossHelen
Page 161 iStock.com/AndreyPopov
Page 161 iStock.com/fstop123
Page 162 iStock.com/MartinPrescott
Page 163 iStock.com/VlLevi
Page 163 iStock.com/Dean Mitchell
Page 164 iStock.com/imtmphoto

Appendix C

Page 178 Michelle Lala Clark Photography

Index

abdominal injuries, 135
abdominal thrusts, 67–68, 69, 72–73
   Skill Practice Sheet for giving, 182–183
abrasions, 106–107
absorbed poisons, 141
abused or neglected person, 20
acquired immunodeficiency syndrome (AIDS), 4
ACS. *See* acute chest syndrome (ACS)
acute chest syndrome (ACS), 98
acute illness, 80
adolescent, definition of, 50. *See also* children
advanced life support, in Cardiac Chain of Survival
   for adults, 31
   for children, 50–51
AED. *See* automated external defibrillator (AED)
agonal breaths, 30
AIDS. *See* acquired immunodeficiency syndrome (AIDS)
airborne pathogens, 4
airborne transmission, 4
alcoholic drink, for hypothermia, 140
alcohol poisoning, 142, 143
allergic reactions, 89–90. *See also* anaphylaxis
allergies, in mnemonic SAM, 17
amputations, traumatic, 112
anaphylaxis
   allergic reactions and, 88–90
   calling 9-1-1 for, 23, 81
   in children, 89
   definition of, 88
   first aid care for, 89–90
   recognition of, 88
   respiratory distress in, 84, 85
anatomic splint, 132
ankle drag, 158
antihistamines, for anaphylaxis, 90
appearances, unusual, 11, 12
arrhythmia (irregular heartbeat), 40
aspirin
   for fever, in children and infants, 99
   for heart attack, 84
asthma, definition of, 86
asthma attack
   asthma action plan for, 86
   first aid care for, 86–88, 100–101
   recognition of, 86, 87
   triggers for, 86
aura, 95

automated external defibrillator (AED)
   for adults, 38–43, 45–47, 172–173
   for children, 54–64, 189–181
   environmental considerations when using, 40
   facts/fiction about, 40–41
   for infants, 54–56, 61–64, 180–181
   maintenance of, 39
   with one first responder, 39, 42
   pads for
      with feedback device, 42
      placement of, 55–56, 59, 180
   person-specific considerations when using, 40
   Skill Practice Sheets for using, 172–173, 180–181
   with two or more first responders, 42–43
   using, 38–43
avulsions, 106, 107

BAC. *See* blood alcohol concentration (BAC)
back blows
   for adult or child who is choking, 67, 68, 182–183
   for infant who is choking, 70, 72–73, 184–185
   Skill Practice Sheets for giving, 182–185
bandages, 109–110
   application of, 109–110
   pressure immobilization with, 145, 147, 150
   roller, 9, 108, 109, 112, 117, 132, 187, 198
   triangular, 9, 132, 206
"bandage splitting" technique, 109
behaviors, unusual, 11, 17
bicycle safety, 163
bites, 144–149
   animal, 113, 144–145
   human, 113
   rabies and, 145
   spider, 147–148
   tick, 148–149
   venomous snake, 145–147
black widow spider, 147, 148
blanket drag, 158
bleeding
   control kit, 5
   non-life-threatening, 112–114
   re-bleeding, monitoring for, 110, 118
   See also life-threatening bleeding
blood, volume and flow of, 107
blood alcohol concentration (BAC), 143
bloodborne illnesses, 4

bloodborne pathogens, 4
blunt trauma
    to chest, 133
    internal bleeding and, 114
body piercings, AED pads and, 40
bone injuries. *See* muscle, bone, and joint injuries
BPD. *See* bronchopulmonary dysplasia (BPD)
brain contusion, 128
brain damage, 30, 31, 38, 50
brain hematoma, 128
brain injuries, 128
breathing barriers, 6–7
    face shields, 6–7
    pocket masks, 7, 32, 34, 36–37, 45, 52–54, 58, 62, 170, 177
breaths
    for adults, 34–37, 44–45, 169–170
    for children, 51, 53, 58, 176–177
    Skill Practice Sheets for giving, 169–170, 176–177
bronchiolitis, 86
bronchopulmonary dysplasia (BPD), 84
brown recluse spider, 147, 148
bruise (contusion), 114
burns, 124–127
    causes of, 124–125, 127
    chemical, 126–127
    classification of, 126
    definition of, 124
    electrical, 127
    first aid care for, 125–127
    household safety and, 162
    signs, symptoms, and severity of, 125

call 9-1-1, 20–22. *See also* 9-1-1
carbohydrates, for heat-related illnesses, 136, 137
carbon monoxide poisoning, 142, 143
cardboard splints, 131
cardiac arrest
    agonal breaths and, 30
    Cardiac Chain of Survival and, 30–31
    in children, 50–51
    definition of, 29
    diagnosing and treating cause of, 31, 51
    first aid care for, 30–31
    integrated post–cardiac arrest care and, 51
    recognition of, 30
    recovery from, 51
    sudden, 30
Cardiac Chain of Survival
    for adults, 30–31
    pediatric, 50–51

cardiopulmonary resuscitation (CPR), 31
    for adults, 29–47
        AED and, 38–43, 45–47, 172–173
        breaths in, 34–37, 44–45, 169–170
        cardiac arrest and, 30–31
        chest compressions in, 32–34, 44, 168
        compression-only, 38
        cycles in, 32, 37, 45, 171
        giving, 32–38, 44–45
        high-quality, components of, 31
        instructions given over the phone for, by EMS dispatchers, 10, 22
        moving the person needing, 23, 157–158
        positioning for, 32, 33, 34, 44, 168
        telephone, 38
    for children, 49–64
        AED and, 54–64, 180–181
        breaths in, 51, 53, 58, 176–177
        cardiac arrest and, 50–51
        chest compressions in, 51, 52, 53, 57, 174–175
        cycles in, 53, 58, 178–179
        differences among adults and, 51–56
        high-quality, components of, 51
        positioning for, 51, 52
caring for an ill or injured person, 22–24
    caring before calling 9-1-1, 23
    in CHECK-CALL-CARE emergency actions steps, 12–13
    emotional aspects of, 24
    general guidelines for, 22
    moving or transporting, 23, 24
    positioning for, 23, 24
car seats, 160
cell phones. *See* mobile phones
cellulitis, 113
CHECK-CALL-CARE emergency actions steps. *See* emergency action steps (CHECK/CALL/CARE)
checking an ill or injured person, 15–20, 25–26
    for abuse and neglect, 20
    in CHECK-CALL-CARE emergency actions steps, 12–13
    consent in, obtaining, 15–16
    focused check in, 19–20
    gathering information in, strategies for, 18–19
    initial impression in, forming, 15
    interviewing person in, 16–20, 25–26
    mnemonic SAM for, 16–20
    unresponsive person and, 16, 25, 166–167
checking the scene, 13

chest compressions
    for adults, 32–34, 44, 168
    for children, 51, 52, 53, 57, 174–175
    Skill Practice Sheets for giving, 168, 174–175
chest hair, AED pads and, 40
chest injuries, 133–134
chest thrusts
    for adult or child who is choking, 68, 69
    for infant who is choking, 70–71, 184–185
    Skill Practice Sheet for giving, 184–185
childproof packaging, 142, 162
children
    abused or neglected, recognition of, 20
    anaphylaxis in, 89
    asthma in, 86–88, 100–101
    bicycle safety for, 163
    breathing barriers for, 7, 52–54, 58, 176–177
    burns in, 125, 161, 162
    cardiac arrest in, 50–51
    car seats for, 160
    cold-related illness in, 138
    concussions in, 129
    CPR for, 49–64
    definition of, 50
    dehydration in, 100
    diabetic emergencies in, 93–94
    diarrhea in, 100
    fever in, 99
    firearm accidents and, 161
    gathering information from, 17, 18
    heat-related illness in, 136
    interviewing parents or guardians of, 17
    life-threatening external bleeding in, 21
    Pediatric Cardiac Chain of Survival for, 50–51
    poison exposure in, 141–142, 162
    respiratory distress in, 85–86
    rib fractures in, 133–134
    safety checklist for home of, 162
    spinal cord injuries in, 127
    sudden illness in, 81
    tourniquets for, 111
    vehicle safety for, 160
    vomiting in, 100
    water safety for, 163
choking
    first aid care for, 67–71, 182–185
    household safety and, 162
    in infants, 70–71, 184–185
    recognition of, 66–67
    special situations in, 69
    unresponsive person and, 68, 70, 71

chronic illness, 80
chronic obstructive pulmonary disease (COPD), 84
closed wounds, minor, 114–115
clothes drag, 157
cold-related illnesses, 138–140
combustible materials, AEDs and, 40
compression-only CPR, 34, 38
compression wrap, 131
concussions, 128–129
consciousness, level of, 20, 21, 96, 114, 134, 135, 137
consent, 15–16
contusion (bruise), 114, 128
convulsions, 95
COPD. *See* chronic obstructive pulmonary disease (COPD)
copperheads, 145, 146
coral snakes, 145, 146
cottonmouths (water moccasins), 145, 146
CPR. *See* cardiopulmonary resuscitation (CPR)
cravat fold, 132
croup (laryngotracheobronchitis), 86
C-splint, 131
cycles, CPR
    for adults, 32, 37, 45, 171
    for children, 53, 58, 178–179
    for infants, 53, 179
    Skill Practice Sheets for giving, 171, 178–179

DEET, 148
defibrillation, 31, 40, 41. *See also* automated external defibrillator (AED)
dehydration, 100
dental injuries, 133
depth of compressions, 54
diabetes, definition of, 92
diabetic emergencies, 92–94
    in children, 93–94
    first aid care for, 93–94
    recognition of, 93
    sugar for, acceptable forms of, 93–94
diarrhea, 100
diffuse axonal injury, 128
digital medical identification tag, 9
direct pressure, 107–109, 116–121
disabilities, gathering information from people with, 18–19
dislocation, 130
distracted driving, 159
DPI. *See* dry powder inhaler (DPI)
dressings, 108
driving under the influence, 159
droplet transmission of pathogens, 4–5

drowning
   cardiac arrest and, 30, 32, 37, 50, 51
   in-water rescues and, 13, 14
   "Reach or throw, don't go!," 14
   water safety, 162–163
drug overdose, 91–92, 143
dry powder inhaler (DPI), 87

elastic wrap tourniquet, 111
electrical shock, delivered by an AED, 31, 38
electrical shock, preventing, 162
electrolytes, for heat-related illnesses, 136, 137
embedded objects, open wounds with, 112
emergency
   action plan, developing, 159
   activating EMS system for, 21
   conditions, 21
   definition of, 8
   first aid kits and supplies for, 9
   preparing for, 8–10
   signs of, 11–12
   situations, 21
emergency action steps (CHECK/CALL/CARE), 12–24
   call 9-1-1, 20–22
   caring for an ill or injured person, 22–24
   checking an ill or injured person, 15–20, 25–26
   checking the scene, 13
   confidence in taking, tips for, 12
emergency medical services (EMS) system
   when to activate, 21
   your role in, 10–11
emergency moves, 157–158
encircling thumbs technique, 53–54, 61, 71, 75, 179
environmental emergencies, 136–153
   bites and stings, 144–151
   cold-related, 138–140
   general approach to, 124
   heat-related, 136–138
   lightning-strike injuries, 153
   poison exposure, 141–144
   rash-causing plants, 151–152
epilepsy, 94
epinephrine, 81, 89–90, 103–104
epinephrine auto-injector, 89–90, 103–104
   Skill Practice Sheet for using, 193–194
equipment, cleaning and disinfecting, 8
exposure incident, handling, 8

face shields, 6–7
   for adults, 32, 34, 36, 44, 52, 169
   for children, 52, 54, 58, 176

   for infants, 52, 54, 62
   Skill Practice Sheets for using, 169, 176
fainting, 97–98
falls, 114, 161, 162
FAST check for recognizing stroke, 96, 97
fatigue, extreme, 80, 82, 83
fever, 94, 99
fire safety, 160–161, 162
first aid kits, 5, 9
flail chest, 134
flammable materials, AEDs and, 40
flow of blood, 107
focused check, 19–20
fracture, 130
frostbite, 140
full-thickness burns, 126

gauze dressings, 108
glucose (sugar), 92
Good Samaritan laws, 12

hand sanitizers, alcohol-based, 5
handwashing, 5
Hank's Balanced Salt Solution, 133
head, neck, and spinal injuries, 127–129
head-tilt/chin-lift maneuver
   for adults, 32, 34, 35, 36, 44, 52, 169
   for children, 51, 52, 54, 58, 62, 176
heart attack, 82–84
heat, for muscle, bone or joint injury, 131
heat cramps, 136
heat exhaustion, 137
heat-related illnesses, 136–138
heat stroke, 138
hemostatic dressings, 108
hepatitis B and C, 4
high-quality CPR, 31, 51
HIV. *See* human immunodeficiency virus (HIV)
household safety, 161–162
   burns, 161, 162
   choking, suffocation, and strangulation, 162
   drowning, 162
   electrical shock, 162
   firearm accidents, 161
   fires, 161, 162
   poisoning, 162
   slips, trips, and falls, 161, 162
   tipping injuries, 162
   wound prevention, 162
human immunodeficiency virus (HIV), 4, 6
hydrogen peroxide to clean a wound, 114
hyperglycemia, 92, 93

hypoglycemia, 92, 93
hypothermia, 138–140
    burns and, 126
    definition of, 138
    dressing for cold weather to avoid, 139
    first aid care for, 139–140
    recognition of, 139

ICDs. *See* implantable cardioverter defibrillators (ICDs)
implantable cardioverter defibrillators (ICDs), 40
inclement weather, AEDs and, 40
infants
    AED for, 54–56, 61–64
    breathing barriers for, 7, 52, 54, 62
    cardiac arrest in, 50–51
    choking in, 70–71, 184–185
    CPR for, 51–56, 61–64, 179
    definition of, 50
    dehydration in, 100
    diarrhea in, 100
    fever in, 99
    infection in, 99–100
    interviewing parents or guardians of, 17
    life-threatening external bleeding in, 21
    Pediatric Cardiac Chain of Survival for, 50–51
    respiratory distress in, 85–86
    sudden illness in, 81
    vomiting in, 100
infection
    in children and infants, 99–100
    exposure incident and, 8
    lowering risk for, 4–8, 12
    open wounds and, 113
    pathogens and, 4–7
    risk of, when giving first aid care, 4
influenza, 4
information, strategies for gathering, 18–19
inhalers, 87, 101–102, 190
injuries, 124–135
    abdominal, 135
    burns, 124–127
    chest, 133–134
    general approach to, 124
    head, neck, and spinal, 127–129
    mouth, 133
    muscle, bone, and joint, 130–132
    nose, 133
    pelvic, 135
    recognition of, 124
injury prevention, 159–164
    emergency action plan for, developing, 159
    fire safety and, 160–161, 162
    general strategies for, 159
    at home, 161–162
    at play, 163–164
    vehicle safety and, 159, 160
    at work, 163
insulin, 92
integrated post–cardiac arrest care, 51
interviewing injured or ill persons, 16–20, 25–26
in-water rescues, 13, 14

jellyfish stings, 150, 151
jewelry, AED pads and, 40
joggers, safety measures for, 164
joint injuries. *See* muscle, bone, and joint injuries

lacerations, 106, 107
language barriers, 16, 19
laryngotracheobronchitis (croup), 86
latex allergy, 6
latex-free disposable gloves, 5–6, 7
lay responder, 10, 29, 33
legal protections, 12
lethal poisons, 142, 143
life-threatening bleeding
    bandages for, 109–110
    direct pressure for, 107–109, 116–121, 186–187, 197–205
    external, 107–111, 116–121
    first aid care for, 107
    internal, 114
    recognition of, 107
    Skill Practice Sheets for controlling, 186–187, 197–205
    tourniquets for, 110–111, 119–121
    traumatic amputations and, 112
    wound packing for, 108, 110, 205
light-headedness, 80, 83
lightning-strike injuries, 153
lip injuries, 133
long-term control medications for asthma, 87
lung contusion, 134

MDI. *See* metered dose inhaler (MDI)
medical identification tags, 9, 10, 19, 26, 80
medications, administering and assisting with, 81–82
medications and medical conditions, in SAM, 17
metal surfaces, AED pads and, 40
metered dose inhaler (MDI), 87
mini-strokes, 96
mobile phones
    calling 9-1-1 from, 22, 38, 69
    emergency telephone numbers in, 9, 161

mobile phones *(Continued)*
   medical information in, 9
   vehicle safety and, 159
mouth injuries, 133
mouth-to-nose breathing, 35
mouth-to-stoma breathing, 36
moving an injured or ill person, 23, 24
muscle, bone, and joint injuries, 130–132
   cause of, 130
   first aid care for, 131–132
   recognition of, 130–131
   splints for, 131–132, 206–212

naloxone, 91–92
   Skill Practice Sheets for administering, 195, 196
nasal atomizer, 91, 92, 196
nasal spray, 91, 92, 195
nebulizers, 87, 191–192
neck injuries, 127–129
neutral position, 52, 53, 54, 62, 179
9-1-1
   calling from mobile phone, 22, 38, 69
   in CHECK-CALL-CARE emergency actions steps, 12–13
   decide whether to call first or give care first, 22, 23
   information for dispatcher when calling, 22
   when to call, 12, 20, 21
noises, unusual, 11
nosebleed, 133
nose injuries, 133

odors, unusual, 11
older people
   abuse in, 20
   burns in, 125, 161
   cold-related illnesses in, 138
   gathering information from, 18
   heat-related illnesses in, 136
   pelvic injuries in, 135
   poison exposure in, 141–142
   stroke in, 96
one-hand technique, 52, 54, 57, 61
open wounds, 106–114
   from bites, 113
   bleeding from, 107–111, 112, 114, 116–121
   with embedded objects, 112
   infection and, 113
   stitches for, 113
   tetanus infection and, 113
   traumatic amputations and, 112
   types of, 106–107

opioid overdose, 91–92, 143
opioids, 90
osteomyelitis, 113

pacemakers, AED pads and, 40
padded board, 131, 132
paradoxical breathing, 134
paralysis, 127–128
paraplegia, 127–128
partial-thickness burns, 126
past-neutral position
   for adults, 32, 34, 36, 37, 44, 45, 52, 53, 169, 170
   for children, 52, 53, 58, 176
pathogens, 4–7
   airborne transmission of, 4
   bloodborne, 4
   definition of, 4
   droplet transmission of, 4–5
   exposure to, limiting, 5–7
PCMs. *See* physical counterpressure maneuvers (PCMs)
pelvic injuries, 135
penetrating trauma, 114
personal protective equipment (PPE), 5–7
physical counterpressure maneuvers (PCMs), 98
pit vipers, 145
play, safety at, 163–164
   for bicycles, 163
   for runners, joggers and walkers, 164
   for water, 163
pneumothorax, 134
pocket masks, 7
   for adults, 32, 34, 36–37, 45, 52, 170
   for children, 7, 52, 53, 54, 58, 177
   for infants, 7, 54, 62
   Skill Practice Sheets for using, 170, 177
poison control centers, 144
poison exposure, 141–144
   first aid care for, 143, 144
   inducing vomiting for, 144
   lethal, 142, 143
   prevention of, 162
   recognition of, 142–143
   unintentional, 141–142
poison ivy, 151–152
poison oak, 151–152
Poison sumac, 151–152
Portuguese man-of-war (bluebottle jellyfish), 151
positioning
   for adult CPR, 32, 33, 34, 44, 168
   incorrect, 33

neutral, 52, 53, 54, 62, 179
past-neutral, 32, 34, 36, 37, 44, 45, 52, 53, 58, 169, 170, 176
for pediatric CPR, 51, 52
recovery, 23, 24
for sudden illness, 81
PPE. *See* personal protective equipment (PPE)
pregnancy, AEDs and, 40
pressure gates, 162
pressure immobilization bandages, 145, 147, 150
puncture wounds, 106, 107

quadriplegia, 128
quick-relief medications for asthma, 87–88
    Skill Practice Sheets for administering, 190–192

rabies, 145
rash-causing plants, 151–152
rate of compressions, 54
rattlesnakes, 145, 146
reaching assist, 14
recovery position, 23, 24
respiratory arrest, 84
respiratory distress, 84–86
rib fractures, 134
rigid splints, 131–132, 206–207, 210–212
roller bandage, 9, 108, 109, 112, 117, 132, 187, 198
rubbing alcohol for fever, 99
runners, safety measures for, 164

safety gates, 162
salt tablets, for heat cramps, 137
SAM mnemonic, 16–17
SAM splint, 131
scene, checking (scene size-up), 13
seat belts, 160
sea urchin stings, 150–151
seizures, 94–95, 99
shock, 95–96
shout-tap-shout sequence, 16, 44
sickle cell crisis, 98
sights, unpleasant, 11, 12
skin color, changes in, 80
sleepy drivers, 159, 160
sling and binder, 131–132, 208–209
slips, preventing, 161
small-volume nebulizer, 87
smells, unpleasant, 11, 12
soft splints, 131–132
sounds, unpleasant, 11, 12
spinal injuries, 127–129

spiny fish stings, 150–151
splints
    Skill Practice Sheets for applying, 206–207, 210–212
    types of, 131–132
sprain, 130
stingray stings, 150–151
stings, 149–151
    insect, 149
    marine life, 150–151
    scorpion, 150
stitches, 113
strain, 130
strangulation, preventing, 162
stroke, 96–97
sucking chest wounds, 134
sudden cardiac arrest, 30
sudden illness
    cause of, 80
    first aid care for, 81–82
    medications for, 81–82
    positioning for, 81
    recognition of, 80–81
suffocation, preventing, 162
superficial burns, 126
surfaces, cleaning and disinfecting, 8

telephone CPR, 38
tetanus infection, 113, 150, 151
throwing assist, 14
TIAs. *See* transient ischemic attacks (TIAs)
tipping injuries, preventing, 162
tongue injuries, 133
tooth, missing, 133
tourniquets, 110–111, 119–121
    pediatric considerations for using, 111
    Skill Practice Sheets for using, 199–204
tracheostomy, 36
transdermal medication patches, AED pads and, 40
transient ischemic attacks (TIAs), 96
transporting an injured or ill person, 23, 24
traumatic amputations, 112
triangular bandages, 9, 132, 206
trips, preventing, 161
tuberculosis, 4
two-finger technique, 52, 54, 61, 71
two-person seat carry, 157
two-thumb/encircling hands technique. *See* encircling thumbs technique
TX-1 pediatric ratcheting tourniquet, 111
TX-3 ratcheting medical tourniquet, 111

unresponsive person
    checking, 16, 25, 44, 166–167
    in choking, 68, 70, 71
    first aid care for, 16, 44
urushiol, 151–152

vacuum splint, 132, 210–212
vehicle safety, 159, 160
ventricular fibrillation (V-fib), 38
ventricular tachycardia (V-tach), 38
volume of blood, 107
vomiting
    aspiration and, 23
    of blood, 21
    first aid care for, 100
    in giving breaths, 34, 35
    in poison exposure, 142, 143, 144

wading assist, 14
walking, safety measures for, 164
walking assist, 157
water, AEDs and, 40
water moccasins (cottonmouths), 145, 146
water safety, 163
wheezing, 86
windlass rod tourniquet, 111, 119–121
work, safety at, 163
wound packing, 108, 110, 205
wounds, 105–121
    household safety and, 162
    minor closed, 114–115
    open, 106–114